TRANSFORMATIONAL LEADERSHIP IN NURSING

Elaine Sorensen Marshall, PhD, RN, FAAN, is a former Berneice Castella Distinguished Professor and Chair, Department of Health Restoration and Care Systems Management, University of Texas Health Science Center School of Nursing, San Antonio. Formerly, she was Professor and Endowed Chair, School of Nursing, Georgia Southern University, Statesboro, Georgia, and Dean of the College of Nursing, Brigham Young University, Provo, Utah, while she also served as a member of the board of trustees of Intermountain Healthcare in Utah. She has authored four books and has published more than 50 peer-reviewed journal articles, as well as 11 book chapters. She has served in national elected and appointed leadership positions for the American Association of Colleges of Nursing, the American Association for the History of Nursing, and the Western Institute of Nursing. Her work has been awarded the New Professional Book Award from the National Council on Family Relations, the Lavinia Dock Award from the AAHN, and the Jo Eleanor Elliott Leadership Award from the Western Institute of Nursing.

Marion E. Broome, PhD, RN, FAAN, is the Ruby Wilson Professor of Nursing, Dean, and Vice Chancellor for Nursing Affairs at Duke University, Durham, North Carolina, and Associate Vice President for Academic Affairs for Nursing at Duke University Health System. Prior to joining Duke, she was dean of the Indiana University School of Nursing, Indianapolis, Indiana, where she was awarded the rank of Distinguished Professor. Her research has been published in more than 110 papers in 50 refereed nursing, medical, and interdisciplinary journals. She also has published five books and 15 book chapters and consumer publications. She has served in a variety of leadership positions, including as a member of the National Advisory Council for the National Institute of Nursing Research, as president of the Society for Pediatric Nurses, and as a member of the governing boards for the Association for the Care of Children's Health and the Midwest Nursing Research Society. Currently, she is editor-in-chief of *Nursing Outlook*, the official journal of the American Academy of Nursing and the Council for the Advancement of Nursing Science. Selected honors include Outstanding Alumnus for Georgia Health Sciences University and the University of South Carolina. In 2012, she was selected to receive the National League for Nursing Award for Outstanding Leadership in Nursing Education. In 2014, she was awarded the President's Medal for Excellence at Indiana University.

TRANSFORMATIONAL LEADERSHIP IN NURSING

From Expert Clinician to Influential Leader

Second Edition

Elaine Sorensen Marshall, PhD, RN, FAAN
Marion E. Broome, PhD, RN, FAAN

Editors

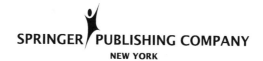

SPRINGER PUBLISHING COMPANY
NEW YORK

Springer Publishing Company, LLC
11 West 42nd Street
New York, NY 10036
www.springerpub.com

Acquisitions Editor: Margaret Zuccarini
Senior Production Editor: Kris Parrish
Composition: diacriTech

ISBN: 978-0-8261-9398-8
e-book ISBN: 978-0-8261-9399-5
Instructor's PowerPoints: 978-0-8261-9401-5

Instructor's materials are available to qualified adopters by e-mailing textbook@springerpub.com.

16 17 18 19 20 / 5 4 3 2 1

The author and the publisher of this Work have made every effort to use sources believed to be reliable to provide information that is accurate and compatible with the standards generally accepted at the time of publication. Because medical science is continually advancing, our knowledge base continues to expand. Therefore, as new information becomes available, changes in procedures become necessary. We recommend that the reader always consult current research and specific institutional policies before performing any clinical procedure. The author and publisher shall not be liable for any special, consequential, or exemplary damages resulting, in whole or in part, from the readers' use of, or reliance on, the information contained in this book. The publisher has no responsibility for the persistence or accuracy of URLs for external or third-party Internet websites referred to in this publication and does not guarantee that any content on such websites is, or will remain, accurate or appropriate.

Library of Congress Cataloging-in-Publication Data

Names: Marshall, Elaine S., author, editor. | Broome, Marion, author, editor.
Title: Transformational leadership in nursing: from expert clinician to
   influential leader / Elaine S. Marshall, Marion E. Broome, editors.
Description: Second edition. | New York, NY: Springer Publishing Company,
   [2017] | Includes bibliographical references and index.
Identifiers: LCCN 2016024065 | ISBN 9780826193988 | ISBN 9780826193995 (e-book)
Subjects: | MESH: Nurse Administrators | Leadership | Nursing, Supervisory
Classification: LCC RT89 | NLM WY 105 | DDC 362.17/3068—dc23 LC record available at
   https://lccn.loc.gov/2016024065

Printed in the United States of America by Bradford & Bigelow.

To Margaret Zuccarini, for her continued support, trust, and patience.

*To the authors who graciously contributed their expertise to
the chapters of this work.*

To John, my children, and my sweet grandchildren—for everything!

—Elaine Marshall

*I would first like to thank Elaine Marshall for giving me this unique
opportunity to work with her on the second edition of this book. It has been a
wonderful experience. I would also like to thank the many mentors and mentees
I have had throughout my career. I learned something unique about leadership
from each of them—particularly about the "strength it takes." As always, my
deepest gratitude goes to my best cheerleader, my husband, Carroll, who has
given of his time for me to complete this new adventure.*

—Marion Broome

CONTENTS

CONTRIBUTORS

Margaret (Midge) T. Bowers, DNP, RN, FNBP-BC, CHFN, AACC, FAANP
Associate Professor
Duke University School of Nursing
Durham, North Carolina

Marion E. Broome, PhD, RN, FAAN
Dean and Ruby Wilson Professor of Nursing
Vice Chancellor for Nursing Affairs, Duke University
Associate Vice President for Academic Affairs for Nursing
Duke University Health System
Durham, North Carolina

Elaine Sorensen Marshall, PhD, RN, FAAN
Professor and Chair (retired)
Department of Health Restoration and Care Systems Management
University Health Science Center School of Nursing
San Antonio, Texas

Katherine C. Pereira, DNP, RN, FNP-BC, ADM-BC, FAAN, FAANP
Associate Professor
Duke University School of Nursing
Durham, North Carolina

Mary Cathryn Sitterding, PhD, RN, CNS
Vice President, Patient Services
Center for Professional Excellence
Cincinnati Children's Hospital Medical Center
Cincinnati, Ohio

Brenda Talley, PhD, RN, NEA-BC
Clinical Associate Professor
The University of Alabama in Huntsville
Huntsville, Alabama

Megan Winkler, PhD, RNC-NIC, CPNP-PC
Postdoctoral fellow, Minnesota Obesity
Prevention Training Program
University of Minnesota

FOREWORD

Welcome to an amazing journey! The preface of *Transformational Leadership in Nursing: From Expert Clinician to Influential Leader* references the very personal journey one encounters in the process of becoming a transformational leader. The truth of that description could not be more relevant than when encountering the challenges faced by nurse leaders who impact the health of individuals, families, communities, and nations. As nurses, we have the ability to pass a daily exam I call the "Head on the Pillow Test." This is an evaluation we each face every night in those moments when our head first hits the pillow before we drift into sleep. In those moments, we evaluate our day and ask what we have accomplished in the past 24 hours that has made a meaningful difference. As nurses, regardless of our practice domain, we have the ability to pass that daily exam quite well. What is unique for nurses in leadership roles is the ability to reflect not only on our own impact, but also on the impact of those we lead. The ability to pass the pillow test by recognizing ways we have impacted others as a leader can ease us into rest. The crucial questions we ask ourselves during that daily self-examination often revolve around an assessment of aspects of the "who, what, why, how, and when" of leadership.

Who is a leader? All nurses are leaders. We are certainly viewed as leaders among professions for which trust is measured, according to a Gallup poll on honesty and ethics in professions. If you look at organizations in which nurses practice, you will see nurses leading in informal and formal ways. An organization in my community refers to their staff nurses as "bedside leaders" in recognition of the role of nurses as leaders, whether they do or do not have formal or line authority. I believe many, perhaps most, nurses are driven by a desire to make a meaningful difference. Given the vacuum of leadership in our country, nurses often become leaders whether or not they intend to do so. When asked to serve as a member of a hospital board of trustees, for example, a nurse might move into a different realm of leadership by becoming chair of the board. In that role, the nurse leader becomes a source of knowledge for other members of the board who do not have a background in health care. In this subtle way, nurses take on the informal role of *knowledge brokers* as part of this more formal leadership role.

What are the essential characteristics of leaders? This text about transformational leadership explores critical characteristics of leadership that are described as the ability to inspire a vision from a foundation of ethical values, to encourage the ability to view problems in new ways, and to communicate a humility that values the mission of the organization above self. Of course, there are many personal and professional characteristics that are useful for nurses in leadership roles. One of my favorites is a trait I have come to call *Sudoku thinking* (Weeks, 2012). The term refers to the ability not only to predict the desired impact of a decision, but to predict the unintended consequences. An important aspect of this trait is knowing those you are leading well enough to understand their possible reactions to your decisions, which can help you make wiser choices.

Why would you want to be a leader? Many individuals tend to believe the purpose of leadership is to accomplish the work of an organization. While the identified work to be done in any organization is a needed outcome, true leadership accomplishes more than simply generating outcomes. True leadership transforms an organization so that it exists and functions in a different way. As a result, your desire to be a leader may not only be a desire to accomplish an identified set of goals and objectives. Additionally, you may desire to leave the organization you are leading in a better state. Leadership journeys also transform you as an individual. The character traits one acquires and hones during the course of being a leader serve to develop you both personally and professionally. Your own character will be deepened and refined throughout your leadership journey.

How should you lead? Many texts share the activities in which excellent leaders engage. *Transformational Leadership in Nursing* provides a new viewpoint and context for leadership activities. What I would add is a note of encouragement to you to take action as a leader. As nurses, we sometimes are hesitant to take bold action and may wait for others to give us cues or clues that the time is right to act. The many nurses who do not live up to a leadership challenge may lack courage and perhaps are fearful of being viewed in a negative light, of being viewed as pushy, or of being the recipient of adverse comments. Bold leadership requires courage—courage to keep moving forward regardless of fear. As nurse leaders, we must keep pushing forward boldly!

Another "how" of leadership is how to lead in a collaborative manner. Our world is complex and the needs we face will rarely be sufficiently addressed by one individual or even by an individual discipline. If we do not learn to function as collaborative leaders, and as leaders of collaboration, our value will be diminished. One of the more challenging aspects of collaboration may be that of collaborating with our competitors. Learning to function as both collaborating competitors and competing collaborators is essential to our effectiveness as leaders.

When should you lead? Nurses will inevitably find themselves in situations where they have an opportunity to lead, but how do we know when we should take on a leadership role or when we should empower someone else to lead? The best formula I have found to help me decide when to lead is this: need + passion + opportunity. As nurses, we tend to notice needs all around us: needs of individuals, families, groups, organizations, and communities. Pay attention to needs that stir your passion, keep you awake at night, catch not only your mind, but also your heart. Looking for open doors providing opportunity will guide you in making wise decisions on where to invest time, abilities, and resources. When this coalescence of need + passion + opportunity occurs, you have found an experience that will create meaning, add value, and give you the ability to navigate the previously described pillow test.

These reflections on the who, what, why, how, and when of leadership may have raised some additional questions in your mind, such as:

- Who, or what organizations, will value my leadership?
- What skills should I acquire to be an effective leader?
- How can I prepare myself to be a leader?
- When should I exert my leadership through a formal leadership role?
- Where, or in what venues, can I best succeed as a leader?

I have good news to share. The second edition of *Transformational Leadership in Nursing* will help you explore and answer each of those questions, and more! The chapters on complexity will help you understand the "where," or the settings, where your leadership is most needed. The chapters on strategic planning will help you understand "when" to exert your leadership. The chapters on budgeting will provide essential "how" skills for leadership. I could go chapter by chapter to connect the contents of this book to needs of both established and emerging leaders. Rather than provide that litany, let me simply say that this text will prepare you for the challenging, yet rewarding, role of serving as a nurse leader. The contents of this text are congruent with my own observations as a nurse leader. As a result of your choice to be a nurse leader, you will find yourself enriched. Absorbing the insights offered in this text will allow you to answer each of the questions I have posed, as well as pass the nightly pillow test, in a way that will leave you more fulfilled. Will you choose to demonstrate courageous leadership? I hope so!

Susan Mace Weeks, DNP, RN, CNS, FNAP, FAAN
Dean and Professor, Harris College of Nursing and Health Sciences
Director, Center for Evidence Based Practice and Research
Texas Christian University
Fort Worth, Texas

REFERENCE

Weeks, S. M. (2012). Preface. *Critical Care Nursing Clinics, 24*(1), xi–xii.

PREFACE

The most important change to this second edition is the welcome addition of coauthor Marion E. Broome, PhD, RN. In a time of my own overwhelming personal challenge, Dr. Broome accepted an enormous responsibility to help create this edition. She has played a most significant role in the revision and refreshing of the book. She is highly respected and brings a lifetime of experience and expertise to this work on leadership. Her fine contributions will be recognized throughout the work.

This book is for leaders of the future. It speaks to clinicians who are expert in patient care and are now on a path toward leadership. It is offered as a resource as you embark on your own journey toward transformational leadership. You are needed to lead in the setting where you practice: from solo practice clinic to the most complex system, from an isolated rural community to an urban health sciences center. If you are reading this book, you are likely already prepared for clinical practice. You may be an expert in patient care, or work as a manager in administration, or you teach clinical nursing. Your challenge now is to enhance your skills and stature to become an influential leader. If that "becoming" is not a transforming experience, it will not be enough to prepare you to lead in a future of enormous challenges. The future of health care in the United States and throughout the world requires leaders who are transformational in the best and broadest sense. It requires a thoughtful, robust sense of self as a leader. It requires an intellectual, practical, and spiritual commitment to improve clinical practice and lead others toward their own transformation. It requires courage, knowledge, and a foundation in clinical practice. It requires an interdisciplinary fluency and ability to listen, understand, and influence others across a variety of disciplines. It requires vision and creativity.

Many who use this book are students in programs of study for a clinical practice doctorate. The book specifically references the *Essentials of Doctoral Education for Advanced Nursing Practice* (known as *DNP Essentials*, American Association of Colleges of Nursing [AACN], 2006). A decade ago, the doctor of nursing practice (DNP) emerged as the credential for leaders in clinical practice. The *DNP Essentials* and the position statement on the DNP of the AACN (2004) call for a "transformational change in the education required for professional nurses who will practice at the most advanced level of nursing" (AACN, 2006, p. 4) and "enhanced leadership skills to strengthen practice and health care delivery" (AACN, 2006, p. 5). Such transformational leaders focus not only on settings of direct patient care, but also on health care for entire communities.

This work is neither a comprehensive encyclopedia for health care leadership nor a traditional text in nursing management. Rather, its purpose is to identify some key issues related to leadership development and contexts for transformational leaders in health care. The book is meant to introduce you, as a clinical expert, to important issues in your own aspirations toward becoming a leader. It is offered as a text and supplement to your own study of the literature, experts, and important experiences in the transition to leadership. It is meant to accompany and guide you to more focused current literature and experts on a variety of issues that health care leaders face. It is an aid to launch or guide you on your own journey to become a leader.

You will read about transformational leadership, which needs some clarification. Although there are some formal theories and definitions of *transformational leadership,* this work refers to the concept in its best and broadest sense without adhering only to a specific theoretical perspective. This book is heavily referenced not only to provide citation, but also to lead you to a vast range of literature.

In this second edition, we have made some changes to update the messages for present-day and future readers. Since the previous edition, the Affordable Care Act has been enacted in the United States, and other developed countries of the world have continued to provide universal health care. Because a global view of health care is essential to today's leader, global perspectives have been added throughout the book. The focus on the context of complex health care organizations has been sharpened, with attention given to current legislation and concepts such as the triple aims to increase access, decrease costs, and improve quality; seamless care delivery; and competencies of the American Organization of Nurse Executives. There is also increased attention to national patient safety benchmarks, issues in health disparities, workforce issues, and patient and consumer satisfaction. We have invited experts to contribute on important issues of interprofessional collaboration, creating and shaping diverse environments for care, health care economics, and other significant areas of leadership development. *Qualified instructors may obtain access to ancillary PowerPoints by e-mailing textbook@springerpub.com.*

The messages of this book are to be taken personally. If your journey toward transformational leadership is not a deeply personal one, then you will not be the leader you must be or the leader for which the future pleads. Throughout the book, you will find occasional personal stories and opportunities for your own personal reflection.

Elaine Sorensen Marshall

REFERENCES

American Association of Colleges of Nursing. (2004). *AACN position statement on the practice doctorate in nursing.* Washington, DC: Author.

American Association of Colleges of Nursing. (2006). *The essentials of doctoral education for advanced nursing practice.* Washington, DC: Author.

PART I

CONTEXTS FOR TRANSFORMATIONAL LEADERSHIP

CHAPTER 1

Expert Clinician to Transformational Leader in a Complex Health Care Organization: Foundations

Marion E. Broome and Elaine Sorensen Marshall

The very essence of leadership is [that] you have to have a vision.
It has to be a vision you articulate clearly and forcefully on every occasion.
You cannot blow an uncertain trumpet.
—Theodore Hesburgh

OBJECTIVES

- *To provide an overview of the challenges facing today's leaders in health care systems and the need for leaders who can transform these challenges into opportunities*
- *To review foundational historical and theoretical contexts for leadership*
- *To discuss the evolution and envisioned role of doctorally prepared nurses in health care systems and how they can exert positive influence as leaders within these systems*
- *To explore theoretical contexts in nursing for transformational leadership*
- *To describe how the content and activities within this book can assist learners to develop leadership skills, assess current and preferred future environments where they can make a difference, and shape the future of nursing and health care*

HEALTH CARE ENVIRONMENTS: OPPORTUNITIES FOR NURSE LEADERS

The world needs visionary, effective, and wise leaders. Never has this statement been truer than it is in the world of health care today. Leadership matters. It matters in every organization, not just to survive but to thrive. The current state and pace of health care change create unprecedented challenges for individuals, families, the nation, and the world. Health care continues to grow more complex, corporate, costly, and expansive. In the United States, we face urgent problems of system complexity, financial instability, and poor distribution of resources; shortages of clinicians and provider expertise; issues of errors and patient safety; and controversy about who will pay for what, and at what level of quality and what cost for services (Institute of Medicine [IOM], 2000, 2001, 2003, 2010). Furthermore, we must address a host of health problems such as greater incidence of chronic illnesses, epidemics of new infectious diseases, and growing numbers of vulnerable, underserved, and aging populations. Meanwhile, society impatiently waits with waning confidence in the current health care system. Dialogue becomes more strident and positions become more polarized in legislatures, the federal government, private industry insurers, and within health systems themselves. Where are the leaders who can take us through these turbulent times?

The health care issues of past decades focused on clinical practice and educational preparation for practice. Society demanded clinical experts to master the burgeoning body of knowledge, research, clinical information, and skills. Nurses and physicians responded to that challenge; they became clinical experts. They devoted many years of learning and practice to clinical excellence. Despite years of intermittent shortages, the nursing profession continues to provide registered nurses at the bedside, advanced clinical specialists who work in acute care settings providing and managing care for patients, advanced practice nurses (APNs) who practice in primary care to provide health promotion and management of chronic conditions, and administrators who lead health systems through these turbulent times. These graduates effectively meet health care needs for thousands of individuals and families. If you are reading this book you are one of those nursing professionals who have made major contributions to care delivery. And the profession and society will continue to need expert nurse clinicians like you.

But our greatest need now is for leaders throughout our systems. Your clinical expertise, whether it is in direct patient care, clinical education, or administration, is now needed as a foundation for your emerging leadership. We need nurse leaders who can draw from their roots in clinical practice to collaborate with leaders in other disciplines, with policy makers, and with members of the community to create new solutions to the problems facing

REFLECTION QUESTIONS

1. Think about your current practice environment. Is it organized in such a way that patients and staff feel safe, cared for, ready to give voice to problems that arise for them?
2. Can you think of individuals in the environment who you expect to help others think about those problems and propose meaningful solutions?
3. How often do you find yourself in the position of being expected (or expecting yourself) to help others define problems and shape some solutions?

health care, to improve quality of life, to transform health care systems, and to inspire the next generation of leaders.

Preparation at the highest level of practice must include preparation for leadership. The world needs expert clinicians to become transformational leaders. The world needs you to become the leader to transform health care for the next generation.

HERITAGE AND LEGACY: HISTORICAL PERSPECTIVES ON LEADERS IN NURSING

The story of modern Western nursing began with little noted but no less great leaders, and traditionally starts with Florence Nightingale. Although her contributions are not usually described from a purely leadership perspective, the inspiration and effectiveness of her leadership have been celebrated for over 150 years. Her work in Scutari, Turkey, designing safer health care environments and hospital structures, training nurses, and using epidemiological data to improve health can only be described as "transformational." The list of transformational leaders in the history of nursing practice is daunting, including some who are unrecognized today. It includes people like Mary Ann Bickerdyke, who cared for men of the Union army in the American War Between the States. Kalisch and Kalisch (1995, pp. 46–47) quoted her authoritative words in 1861 as she agreed to carry medical supplies: "I'll go to Cairo [Illinois], and I'll clean things up there. You don't have to worry about that, neither. Them generals and all ain't going to stop me" (Baker, 1952, p. 11). In the South, volunteer nurse Kate Cummings recorded the courageous efforts of women who cared for Confederate troops: "We are going for the purpose of taking care of the sick and wounded of the army . . . for a while I wavered about the propriety of it; but when I remembered the suffering I had witnessed, and the relief I had given, my mind was made up to go . . ." (Harwell, 1959, pp. 9, 169; Kalisch & Kalisch, 1995, p. 51). Other well-known charismatic leaders in nursing of the 19th century were Clara Barton, who founded the American Red Cross; Dorothea Dix, who championed advocacy for patients and prisoners and ruled her staff nurses with an iron fist; and, perhaps, even Walt Whitman, the celebrated poet who was a volunteer nurse in the American Civil War.

Best known and revered models for the heritage of leadership in nursing include the handful of women in North America at the dawn of the 20th century who are credited with the vision of professional nursing: Isabel Hampton Robb, Mary Adelaide Nutting, Lavinia Lloyd Dock, and Lillian Wald.

- Robb led the nurse training school at Johns Hopkins in Baltimore. She envisioned standardized education for nurses and nursing teachers.
- Nutting was Robb's student at Johns Hopkins and was among the first visionaries to foresee academic nursing education, rather than apprentice nurse training solely in hospitals. She led efforts to develop the first university

nursing programs at Teachers College of Columbia University, and to secure funding for such programs (Gosline, 2004; Marshall, 1972; Nutting, 1926).

- Dock was a strong woman who was involved in many "firsts" that influenced the profession for years. She worked with Robb at Johns Hopkins when Nutting was a student. Dock firmly believed in self-governance for nurses and called for them to unite and stand together to achieve professional status. She was among the founders of the Society for Superintendents of Nursing and an author of one of the first textbooks for nurses and a history of nursing. She encouraged nurses and all women to become educated, to engage in social issues, and to expand their views internationally (Lewenson, 1996). She was known as a "militant suffragist" and champion for a broad range of social reforms, always fighting valiantly for nurses' right to self-governance and for women's right to vote.
- Wald, who modeled the notion of independent practice a century before it became a regulatory issue, founded the first independent public health nursing practice at Henry Street in New York. She not only devoted her life to caring for the poor people of the Henry Street tenements, but also was the first to offer clinical experience in public health to nursing students. She worked for the rights of immigrants, for women's right to vote, for ethnic minorities, and for the establishment of the federal Children's Bureau (Brown, 2014).

Modern leadership for advanced practice, ultimately leading to the development of the doctor of nursing practice (DNP) degree, must also recognize the vision, courage, and leadership of Loretta Ford and Henry Silver at the University of Colorado, who began the first nurse practitioner program in the United States in 1965. Early certificate programs did not award an academic degree. By the 1990s, advanced nursing practice had moved to the master's degree. Now, in the face of increasing complexity of health care, the trends among other health care disciplines toward the practice doctorate, and the urgent need for knowledge workers and wise leaders, the practice doctorate is becoming the required preparation for advanced practice. You are among the pioneer leaders to move health care forward to better serve those in need.

Today's health care leaders inherit courage, vision, and grit that must not be disregarded. We stand on the shoulders of a handful of valiant nursing leaders of the past who left a foundation that cries for study of its meaning and legacy for leadership today. They were visionary champions for causes that at present seem

REFLECTION QUESTIONS

Lurking in the archives of your own community are the stories of other exemplary leaders in nursing and health care.

1. Who were/are they?
2. What can you/we learn from them?

so essential, but were only dreams at their time. They dared to think beyond the habits and traditions of the time. These leaders were *truly transformational!*

FOUNDATIONAL THEORIES OF LEADERSHIP

Although a theme of this book is transformational leadership, it is important to understand that the purpose, content, and principles of this book are not confined to the tenets of a specific theory of transformational leadership. To become a full citizen of the discipline, it is important that the transformational leader in health care understand the history, culture, and theoretical language of the science and practice of the discipline of leadership.

The attraction of any particular theory for leadership may wax or wane, but some leadership principles are timeless. Any truly transformational leader will have a solid foundation of understanding many theories and will employ and integrate aspects of a variety of theories most appropriate to leadership in practice.

The first principle among theories recognized today is that leaders be grounded in some set of ethics or core values that guide human behaviors and actions. No matter how brilliant the strategy or how productive the actions, if leaders do not carry the trust or best interests of those they represent, there is no true leadership.

Leaders in today's health care and academic settings will deal with a variety of ethical issues and must ground themselves in values that will enable them to lead with grace and effectiveness when facing these and reaching some solutions. Nurse leaders have a responsibility to shape ethical cultures (Broome, 2015) using knowledge of ethical standards in the field (American Nurses Association, 2015) and expert guidelines (Johns Hopkins Berman Institute of Bioethics, 2014). Yoder-Wise and Kowalski (2006, p. 62) outlined the following principles for ethical leadership: respect for others, beneficence (promoting good), veracity (telling the truth), fidelity (keeping promises), nonmaleficence (doing no harm), justice (treating others fairly), and autonomy (having and promoting personal freedom and the right to choose). Such principles are stipulated among the theories reviewed here.

Traditional Management Theories and Methods

Traditional management theories were developed during the industrial revolution and, thus, reflected the factory environment of worker productivity. They moved away from the prevailing "great man" theories toward the idea that common people with skill and competence might gain power and a position of leadership (Clawson, 1999; Stone & Patterson, 2005). Such theories included classic and scientific management theory. They emphasized the organization and formal processes of the organization rather than the characteristics or behaviors of the individual. Primary concepts included hierarchical lines of authority, chain-of-command decision making, division of labor, and rules and regulations. Such theories were originated by early 20th-century industrial thinkers such as Max Weber,

Frederick W. Taylor, F. W. Mooney, and Henri Fayol. Approaches focused on organization and processes. They included time-and-motion studies, mechanisms, and bureaucracy. Advantages of such theories were clear organizational boundaries and efficiency. Disadvantages included rigid rules, slow decision making, authoritarianism, and bureaucracy (Garrison, Morgan, & Johnson, 2004). Ironically, an advantage of such theories was their setting the stage for modern theories of management by objectives (Stone & Patterson, 2005). Although we may think we have moved beyond the industrial age, you might still recognize some of the elements of traditional management theories in some organizations today.

Environment and Worker Needs Theories. In the mid-20th century, management focus turned away from the organization and moved toward people within the organization. This was the time of the well-known Hawthorne studies that sought to enhance human productivity and pride in work accomplished. Tables 1.1 and 1.2 outline other major theorists who influenced leadership theories in the last half of the 20th century.

Nevertheless, even with a new focus on people rather than organizations, both traditional industrial theories and behavioral theories promoted linear thinking, compartmentalization, functional work, process orientation, clear and fixed job requirements, and predictable effects (Capra, 1997; Cook, 2001; Wheatley, 1994).

TABLE 1.1 Examples of Behavioral and Trait Theories for Leadership

THEORY	MAJOR PRECEPTS	CONTRIBUTIONS TO OUR KNOWLEDGE ABOUT LEADERSHIP
Humans in an industrial environment (Mayo, 1953)	Leader promotes follower productivity and pride in work. Known for Hawthorne studies.	Basic assumptions of human nature in leading people.
Maslow's hierarchy of needs (1954)	Leader promotes follower (and leader) self-actualization.	Foundational theory in leadership and human development.
Theory X, Theory Y (McGregor, 1960)	Theory X (directive style) leader makes decisions, gives directions, and expects compliance. Follower productivity is related to incentives and punishments. Theory Y (participative style) leader seeks consensus, followers focus on quality and productivity, and are rewarded for problem solving.	Assert that leader is motivator and role model for follower behavior.
Herzberg's motivation-hygiene theory (1966)	Leader meets follower's intrinsic and extrinsic needs.	Continues to be foundational in organizations where productivity is critical.

(continued)

TABLE 1.1 Examples of Behavioral and Trait Theories for Leadership (*continued*)

THEORY	MAJOR PRECEPTS	CONTRIBUTIONS TO OUR KNOWLEDGE ABOUT LEADERSHIP
Theory Z (Ouchi, 1981)	Theory Z leader promotes employee/follower well-being on and off job to promote high morale, satisfaction, stable personnel employment, high productivity.	
Leadership tasks (Gardner, 1986a, 1986b, 1987a, 1987b)	Leadership tasks include envisioning goals, affirming values, motivating, managing, achieving workable unity, explaining, serving as a symbol, representing the group, renewing.	Less "theory," with associated concepts and propositions, and more "lists" of preferred characteristics or activities. Extends list of concepts that promote effective leadership.
Leadership attributes (Gardner, 1989)	Leadership attributes include physical vitality and stamina, intelligence and action-oriented judgment, eagerness to accept responsibility, task competence, understanding of followers and their needs, skill in dealing with people, need for achievement, capacity to motivate people, courage and resolution, trustworthiness, decisiveness, self-confidence, assertiveness, adaptability.	
Eight habits (Covey, 1989, 2004)	Eight habits of successful leaders: • Be proactive and take goal-directed action rather than reacting to circumstances • Begin with the end in mind—goal oriented • Put first things first—distinguish important versus urgent • Think win–win—negotiate to mutual benefit • Seek first to understand, then to be understood—listen • Synergize—engage in activities that amplify most effective aspects of all leadership habits • Sharpen the saw—attend to personal maintenance and renewal • Find and express your voice in vision, discipline, passion, conscience	First seven habits codified common-sense principles in a national bestseller of the popular business literature. Later added the eighth habit. Continues to influence business executives.

(continued)

TABLE 1.1 Examples of Behavioral and Trait Theories for Leadership (*continued*)

THEORY	MAJOR PRECEPTS	CONTRIBUTIONS TO OUR KNOWLEDGE ABOUT LEADERSHIP
Three leader styles (Pitcher, 1997)	Three styles: • Artist: "imaginative, inspiring, visionary, entrepreneurial, intuitive, daring, emotional" • Craftsman: "well-balanced, steady, reasonable, sensible, predictable, trustworthy" • Technocrat: "cerebral, detail-oriented, fastidious, uncompromising, hard-headed"	A particular leader style may be preferred, depending on situation.
Leadership attributes (George, 2003; Shirey, 2006, 2009)	Leadership attributes: genuineness, trustworthiness, reliability, compassion, believability.	Provides another list of common-sense effective characteristics.

TABLE 1.2 Examples of Situational and Constituent Interaction Theories for Leadership

THEORY	MAJOR PRECEPTS	CONTRIBUTIONS TO OUR KNOWLEDGE ABOUT LEADERSHIP
Contingency theory (Fiedler, 1967, 1997; Fiedler & Garcia, 1987)	Leadership effectiveness is interaction between style and extent to which situation allows leader's influence. Factors: • Nature and quality of relationship between leader and followers • Nature of task or goal • Formal and informal power of leader	Relationship-oriented and task-oriented styles with no favored *style*; rather, *situations* in which a specific style may be effective.
Path–goal theory (House, 1971)	Leader responds to follower motives in working relationship. Leader identifies and removes barriers, gives support and direction, secures resources, and facilitates goal or task achievement of followers. Leader focuses on follower needs for affiliation and control by promoting clarity of expectations and supportive structure. Describes transactional leader behaviors as achievement oriented, directive,	Leader influences follower's perceptions of work and goals, and paths to attain goals, and creates expectancies for goal attainment.

(continued)

TABLE 1.2 Examples of Situational and Constituent Interaction Theories for Leadership (*continued*)

THEORY	MAJOR PRECEPTS	CONTRIBUTIONS TO OUR KNOWLEDGE ABOUT LEADERSHIP
	participative, or suppressive. These are connected to environmental and follower afactors or situations.	
Situational contingency theory (Vroom & Yetton, 1973)	Taxonomy of leadership situations used in a decision-making model. Proposed that leaders allow followers to participate in decision making according to situational factors.	Expanded notion of leaders engaging followers in decision making.
Leader–member exchange theory (Graen, 1976; Miner, 2007)	Mutual responsibility for interaction between leader and follower. Concepts: "in-group" and "out-group" relationships	Leadership is portrayed as guidance of human interactions or relationships. Work productivity and outcomes are improved in an environment of optimal human relationships.
Situational leadership theory (Hersey & Blanchard, 1977; Hersey, Blanchard, & Johnson, 2008)	Four leadership styles and associated situations: • Telling, or giving direction • Selling, or participatory coaching • Participating, or sharing decision making • Delegating, or assigning responsibility for task or goal achievement	Expands scenario in which leadership occurs to include follower and situational needs.
Leader in context of quanta and chaos theory (Porter-O'Grady, 1992; Porter-O'Grady & Malloch, 2007; Wheatley, 1994)	Recognition of phenomena of disequilibrium, disorganization, or chaos to lead a natural course to new orders. Constant change is a way of being. Leadership and organizations can thrive on the paradox that order can emerge from disorder. Principles: • Partnership • Accountability • Equity • Ownership	Application of "New Age" theories from physics to leadership. Allowance for phenomena beyond the control of the leader to evolve and emerge.

(*continued*)

TABLE 1.2 Examples of Situational and Constituent Interaction Theories for Leadership (*continued*)

THEORY	MAJOR PRECEPTS	CONTRIBUTIONS TO OUR KNOWLEDGE ABOUT LEADERSHIP
Emotional intelligence (Goleman, 1995; Goleman, Boyatzis, & McKee, 2002)	Monitoring of emotional perceptions of self and others. Domains: • Self-awareness • Self-management • Social-awareness • Relationship management Five steps to advance as leader: • Identify "ideal self" • Identify "real self" • Create plan to build on strengths • Practice the plan • Develop trust and encourage others	Expands concepts of social–emotional aspects of human relationships to complement traditional business management/leadership competencies.
Servant leadership (Covey, 2004; Greenleaf, 1977; Jaworski, 1998; Senge, 1990)	Leader's motivation is to serve and meet needs of others. Rather than directing followers, leader inspires, motivates, influences, and empowers. Ten characteristics: • Listener first • Empathy through framing questions • Heal to make whole • Awareness • User of persuasion • Conceptualization • Foresight • Stewardship • Commitment to the growth of people • Co-builder of learning/working communities	Allows a type of spiritual focus and offers opportunities to create meaning in leadership and followership in health care settings.

Behavioral and Worker Style Theories. Other early behavioral theorists moved the focus from people, or even leaders themselves, to an emphasis on the *concept* of leadership. Thus, the ideas of leadership behaviors and styles emerged. Styles were considered people based, task based, or a combination. Such styles include authoritarian, democratic, and laissez-faire (Lewin, Lippitt, & White, 1939). Leaders were expected to determine objectives, initiate action, and coordinate the efforts of workers. Over the next two decades, executives and managers found themselves responsible for motivating workers and working with teams to accomplish goals and outcomes.

Problems with behavior or style theories are related to the issue of context. For example, in the heat of a crisis, such as pandemic influenza, which style is most effective? The artist or the craftsman? Produce-or-perish or middle-of-the-road? Theory X or Theory Y? Do the styles describe all aspects of the personality, character, motivation, or behavior of the leader? Do the behavioral styles account for all situations? Which, if any, style is uniquely applicable to leaders in health care? Another important question is, "Do all individuals respond to certain styles or do followers require some tailoring or combination of styles?"

Leader Trait Theories. Current trait theories seem, in some respects, to return to the "great person" approach as they target the intellectual, emotional, physical, and personal characteristics of the leader. The difference is that trait theories propose that desirable characteristics of successful leaders may be learned or developed. Trait theories continue to be popular. Just pass by the bookstore in any airport to find shelves full of business or leadership self-help books based on some list of qualities, behaviors, or habits marketed for success. The notion of successful leadership traits cannot be denied, but the science of predicting optimal traits under differing circumstances has still not matured.

Situation/Contingency and Constituent Relationship Theories

Situational theories grew largely as a reaction to trait theories, with the opposite premise that the characteristics of the situation, not the personal traits of the person, produced the leader. Theorists called for a repertoire of leadership traits or styles, and defined the appropriate style for specific types of situations. Building on the work of Lewin et al. (1939), situational theory would propose that authoritarian leadership may be required in a time of crisis, a democratic style in situations for team or consensus building, and laissez-faire style in traditional single-purpose, well-established organizations. Thus, the leader would adjust behaviors according to circumstances of worker experience, maturity, and motivation. Less-motivated workers

REFLECTION QUESTIONS

1. Is it possible to teach or learn successful traits?
2. Which traits are cultivated as behaviors or habits?
3. Does the leader of a state public health department need the same traits as the chief nursing officer of a large hospital system?
4. What traits are most predictive of effectiveness in a particular role?

would require a directive task focus, and more highly motivated workers would require a focus on support and relationships. For instance, according to ideas of emotional intelligence theory, the leader must be sensitive to the appropriate style and circumstance, largely by empathic listening to self and others.

Situational/contingency theories represented valiant attempts to consider both the leader and the situation. However, the situations examined were often typical American middle-class male organizations with little regard for situations or styles that considered gender, culture, or political climate, or for specific types of organizations such as those of health care. Relationship-based theories, which evolved later, paved the way for more transformational theories in the 21st century that are believed to be critical to the success of any organization and leader. They also expanded thinking to incorporate the notion that engaged followers are an essential part of any leader's effectiveness.

WHAT *IS* TRANSFORMATIONAL LEADERSHIP?

As you thought about your answers to the earlier reflection questions, did you think of certain individuals who were more effective than others in providing leadership for solution seeking? Or did you ask yourself some basic questions such as, "What is leadership?" and "Who are the leaders we need?" Leadership is one of those difficult concepts that is sometimes readily identified but never easily defined. Simply put, leadership is the discipline and art of guiding, directing, motivating, and inspiring a group or organization toward the achievement of common goals. It includes the engaging and management of people, information, and resources. It requires energy, commitment, communication, creativity, and credibility. It demands the wise use of power. Leadership has been defined by many people over the years. In Table 1.1, we described several leadership theories, which are explored in more depth in the chapters that follow. You will want to review some of the contemporary leadership frameworks to see which one resonates with you and your view of the world.

Leadership is the ability to guide others, whether they are colleagues, peers, clients, or patients, toward desired outcomes. A leader uses good judgment, wise decision making, knowledge, intuitive wisdom, and compassionate sensitivity to the human condition—to suffering, pain, illness, anxiety, and grief. A nursing leader is engaged and professional, and acts as an advocate for health and dignity.

You might ask at this point, "But what does a leader *do*, specifically?" Leaders "are people who have a clear idea of what they want to achieve and why" (Doyle & Smith, 2009, p. 1). They are usually identified by a title or position and are often associated with a particular organization—but not always. Leaders are the resource for confidence, assurance, and guidance. Renowned leadership guru Peter Drucker (2011) listed the following things leaders must *do* to be effective:

• Ask what needs to be done
• Ask what's right for the enterprise
• Develop action plans
• Take responsibility for decisions
• Take responsibility for communicating
• Focus on opportunities, not problems
• Run productive meetings
• Think and say "we" not "I"

These are very pragmatic but highly effective strategies to motivate others, improve the organization, and empower followers to achieve excellence. Not a single item on the list is easy or straightforward, but each provokes thinking and action. All can be learned behaviors if one is open to learning.

Leaders are seldom born, made, or found by luck, but rather emerge when preparation, character, experience, and circumstance come together at a time of need. Those leaders build on strong leadership characteristics they always had. Leaders are most often ordinary people demonstrating extraordinary courage, skill, and "spirit to make a significant difference" (Kouzes & Posner, 2007, p. xiv).

So, you can prepare yourself and you can learn to be a leader. That is one reason you returned for additional education. Others in your environment can and will support, coach, and mentor you as you learn to know yourself and your strengths, try on new behaviors, and own your future. The purpose of this book is to help you as an advanced clinician to prepare to become a transformational leader.

Transformational Leadership

Simply defined, transformational leadership is a process through which leaders influence others by changing the understanding of others of what is important (Broome, 2013; Collins, 2001; Eagly, Johannesen-Schmidt, & van Engen, 2003). An operative word here is *process*. It is not just a list of attributes or characteristics but a dynamic and ever-evolving style that is focused on self, others, the situation, and the larger context. Transformational leaders inspire others to achieve what might be considered extraordinary results. Leaders and followers engage with each other, raise each other, and inspire each other. Transformational leadership includes value systems, emotional intelligence, and attention to each individual's spiritual side. It connects with the very soul of the organization and honors its humanity. It raises "human conduct and ethical aspirations of both the leader and the led and, thus has a transforming effect on both" (Burns, 1978, pp. 4, 20). Transformational leaders are energetic, committed, visionary, and inspiring. They are role models for trust. Their leadership is based on commitment to shared values. For over a decade, nurses have discussed the need for transformational leaders. Where and how leadership is truly "transformational" in nursing and health care may still not be clear (McKenna, Keeney, & Bradley, 2004), but there is no question that such leadership is now much needed.

The original concept and foundational theory for transformational leadership are attributed to James MacGregor Burns, who proposed the idea in 1978. Other leadership scholars continue to build on the principle. Bass (1985) developed the idea of a continuum between transactional and transformational leadership, and Robert Kegan added a list of developmental stages of leadership traits toward transformational leadership (Kegan & Lahey, 1984). Goleman, Boyatzis, and McKee (2002) further advanced the perspective to include aspects of emotional intelligence, such as self-awareness, self-management, social awareness, and relationship management. Bass, Avolio, and Jung (2010) created an instrument to measure transformational leadership, and many studies have been conducted in diverse settings and disciplines to examine leadership among various groups. Since this book does not embrace a sole theoretical perspective, transformational leadership is considered here in its best and broadest sense, as a context and backdrop for leadership development.

Components of Transformational Leadership

The transformational leader must make the conscious decision to lead. Often, competent nurses are given opportunities to supervise or manage, but successful leaders *choose* to lead. And some individuals find they learn a great deal, very quickly, and go on to build on that experience and become transformational leaders, while others find the emotional costs and time investment of leadership not to be congruent with where they see themselves making a contribution. In Boxes 1.1 and 1.2 we share our personal leadership stories.

Though we refer to transformational leadership in its broadest sense, without strict adherence to a specific theoretical framework, it is important to recognize and review the foundational seminal work on the concept. Some of the core concepts of transformational leadership, as developed by theorists Burns (1978) and Bass (1985, 1990), Bass, Avolio, Jung, and Berson (2003), Bass et al. (2010), Bass and Riggio (2006), are outlined in the following paragraphs.

BOX 1.1 PERSONAL REFLECTION ON LEADERSHIP

Elaine Sorensen Marshall, PhD, RN, FAAN

I remember the first "official" day I was required to be a leader. I had been out of nursing school for less than a year, working at a job I loved as a staff nurse on a medical–surgical unit in a large flagship hospital. The nurse manager, then referred to as the team leader, called in sick. One by one, calls to all the other usual suspects to take her

(continued)

BOX 1.1 PERSONAL REFLECTION ON LEADERSHIP (*continued*)

place were in vain. The house supervisor came to me and said, "You are *it* today, you are in charge. I will be available if you need anything." I was left in charge of a unit staff of one other registered nurse, two practical nurses with more bedside experience than I had in years of life, two nursing assistants, and 22 very sick patients. My heart raced simultaneously with the surge of excitement and panic. I will not violate privacy regulations here to tell you all the near-death adventures that day, but I can say that it was probably not the ideal first step on a path toward transformational leadership. I did learn, almost immediately, what worked and what did not work to inspire or influence others. Eventually, over a lifetime, I gained knowledge, insight, and experience as a transformational leader, but I always return to that summer day when I learned the "sink or swim" theory of leadership. I learned that my heart was in the right place, that I wanted to care for others, that I had some innate abilities to influence others for good, that I was a natural goal setter, that I had fairly good judgment in making decisions, and that others trusted me. But I had no specific knowledge of how to lead, no preparation for leadership, no coach or mentor, little confidence, and not much insight on organization of resources to meet what came next. I knew only that I was in a situation that needed a leader, and on that day I was recruited and stepped up to it.

BOX 1.2 PERSONAL REFLECTION ON LEADERSHIP

Marion E. Broome, PhD, RN, FAAN

I spent my early career learning how to be a competent nurse, then nursing educator, and then nurse researcher—always focused on improving the care of children and their families. Twelve years after I graduated with my BSN, and 2 years after completing my PhD, I assumed my first administrative role, as an associate dean for research. For the first time in my nursing career I found myself on the "side" of hearing the complaints, issues, and needs of nurses in the organization, in this case related to support for faculty research development. I must admit I was not entirely prepared for the responsibility of "fixing the problems" faculty brought to me. However, once I began to reframe the issues—as problems to be solved, systems to be put in place so faculty could be successful—and honed my listening skills to focus intently on what a person was really asking for, my enthusiasm for the job increased. I began to see myself as a problem solver and someone who needed to have a vision for how things could be. To my amazement, I enjoyed solving problems, and I enjoyed thinking about how to make the systems we had in place work better. I also learned quickly that while you could tell others their issue was solved, it was not until they actually worked with the office (to submit a grant, to develop an institutional review board [IRB] proposal, or to hire personnel), and things went smoothly, that they became true believers. It seemed so easy (and fun). I found the real satisfaction of leadership, for me, was seeing others be able to achieve their goals with the least amount of hassle and the most amount of perceived support. Then they could dream bigger and better and move the whole organization ahead!

Charisma or Idealized Influence. A transformational leader is a role model of values and aspirations for followers. He or she inspires trust and commitment to a cause. Charisma refers to the ability to inspire a vision. Unlike narcissistic charisma, which focuses on self, the charisma of idealized influence finds its effectiveness stemming from a strong belief in others. Charisma is the ability to influence others, to inspire not only a willingness to follow, but also an expectation of success, an anticipation of becoming part of something greater than self. Charismatic leaders know who they are and where the organizational unit they are leading has the potential to go. They have themes and personal mantras in their lives. One leader keeps a file called "Dream" that holds ideas about future opportunities, and another keeps a hand-drawn diagram of her "Tree of Life" showing the roots, trunk, and branches of her life and future. Charismatic leaders, grounded in a commitment to values, influence others to make a positive difference in the world. Health care needs such leaders. Indeed, one study demonstrated higher satisfaction and greater happiness among workers who follow a charismatic leader (Erez, Misangyi, Johnson, LePine, & Halverson, 2008).

Charismatic leaders often emerge in times of crisis. They exhibit personal qualities that draw people to believe and follow them. If they are wise, they inspire followers in a synergistic manner that provides safety, direction, beliefs, and actions that exceed the expectations of either follower or leader.

To be charismatic does not mean to be flamboyant. Indeed, the most successful leaders "blend extreme personal humility with intense professional will"; they are often "self-effacing individuals who display the fierce resolve to do whatever needs to be done to make the [organization] great" (Collins, 2001, p. 21). In their seminal study of 28 elite companies (i.e., those who moved from "good to great"), Collins and colleagues found that level 5 (transformational) leaders channeled their ego away from themselves to the larger goal of building a great company. They were ambitious—but more for their organization than for themselves. One charismatic leader shared, "I want to look out from my porch at one of the greatest companies in the world someday and be able to say 'I used to work here'" (Collins, 2001, p. 26).

Charisma may refer to a quality of authenticity, transparency, and trust that draws others to you to share the vision and the will to work toward the goal. Kouzes and Posner (2007) noted that such leaders may be ordinary people who accomplish extraordinary results by being role models, being examples, and leading by behavior that authentically reflects the behaviors expected of and admired by others.

Inspiration and Vision. Bass (1985, 1990), Bass and Riggio (2006), Seltzer and Bass (1990) noted that authentic transformational leadership must be grounded in the moral character of the leader, a foundation of ethical values, and collective ethical processes. From an ethical foundation, transformational leaders create a compelling vision of a desired future. Kouzes and Posner (2007, p. 17) explained, "Every organization, every social movement, begins with a dream. The dream or vision is the force that invents the future." Transformational leaders influence others by high expectations with a sight toward the desired future. They set standards and instill others with optimism, a sense of meaning, and commitment to a dream, goal, or cause. They extend a sense of purpose and purposeful meaning that provides the energy to achieve goals. They inspire from a foundation of truth.

Intellectual Stimulation. The transformational leader is a broadly educated, well-informed individual who looks at old problems in new ways. He or she challenges boundaries, promotes creativity, and applies a range of disciplines, ideas, and approaches to find solutions. This involves fearlessness and risk taking. The transformational leader in health care reads broadly, takes lessons from many disciplines beyond clinical practice, and engages as an interested citizen in public discourse on a full range of topics. The transformational leader may find strategies from the arts and literature, humanities, business, or other sciences. And he or she consults experts from a variety of fields and settings to weigh in on complex problems faced by the organization. Such leaders ask questions. Asking questions about problems, large and small, allows leaders to understand the landscape in which the problem "lives," and they can pull together teams to work on the problem and encourage, expect, and nurture independent and critical thinking. The transformational leader assumes that people are willing and eager to learn and test new ideas.

Individual Consideration. The transformational leader has a kind of humility that looks beyond self to the mission of the organization and the value of the work of others as individuals. He or she uses many professional skills, including listening, coaching, empathy, support, and recognition of the contributions of followers. The transformational leader enables others to act toward a shared vision. The effective leader recognizes and promotes the contributions of others and creates a culture of sharing, celebration, and unity within the entire team. Who gets the credit is less important than how team members affirm each other's work.

Transformational leaders effectively build on these characteristics and integrate principles from a variety of leadership theories and pragmatic approaches to advance, enhance, and expand clinical expertise from a focus on direct individual patient care to a focus on the care of groups, aggregates, and entire populations in a variety of environments. They consider the individual and the aggregate at once.

In the past 5 years, in addition to a plethora of reviews about transformational leadership and leadership in general, there have been some studies of how leaders in nursing demonstrate transformative leadership and influences on followers. Yet, we still know little beyond the description of actions of such leaders (Broome, 2013; Disch, Edwardson, & Adwan, 2004). Of particular interest to the nursing discipline is a meta-analysis of gender differences of men and women in their enactment of transformational, transactional, and laissez-faire styles. In that analysis women were more likely than men to engage in transformational behaviors than men, and men relied more often on transactional and laissez-faire styles (Eagly et al., 2003). However, we still know little about how transformational leadership actually works, or what it ultimately means to followers and to patients. Such research and role models must emerge from the next generation of leaders. It is your job to envision and articulate the prototypes for transformational leadership in health care for the future.

MANAGEMENT AND LEADERSHIP: IS THERE REALLY A DIFFERENCE?

In their zeal to promote charismatic transformational leadership, some writers make unfortunate distinctions between managers and leaders, as though managers are undesirable and leaders are more effective across all situations. Jennings, Scalzi, Rodgers, and Keane (2007) reviewed the literature to find a growing lack of discrimination between nursing leadership and management competencies.

Nevertheless, Bennis (2003) asserted that managers "do things right," and leaders "do the right things" (p. 9). Managers are thought to control and maintain processes with a focus on the short term, relying on authority rather than influence, while leaders are visionary, insightful, and influential. Managers minimize risk, and leaders maximize opportunity. In reality, most leaders will tell you it is important to know enough about processes in one's organization to be able to decide what new directions to take and how to assess the efficiencies of a unit to preserve or redirect resources. It is likely a matter of balance between the two sets of competencies of manager or leader that is crucial to master.

Transformational leadership theorists refer to the manager style as transactional leadership (Bass et al., 2010). Transactional leaders primarily motivate others by systems of rewards and punishments. Their power lies largely in the authority of their position. A manager may be referred to as the "laissez-faire" supervisor who provides little direction or motivation for change, leaving most decision making to the followers. Transformational leaders, on the other hand, develop, innovate, focus on developing others, inspire and create trust, and hold a long-term, big-picture, futuristic view.

The reality is that anyone in charge of a group of people working toward effective goal achievement needs the wisdom to develop and use the qualities of both manager and leader in different situations. Indeed, Millward and Bryan (2005, p. xii) proposed that "the reality of clinical leadership must involve a judicious blend of effective management in the conventional sense with skill in transformational change in order to make real difference to the care delivery process." Thus, the terms *manager* and *leader* may be used interchangeably, as appropriate, in this book, not for lack of precision, but with the view that the characteristics of each are needed in effective leadership. Effective leaders (and managers) rely on a broad repertoire of style, rather than specialization of techniques. And neither should rely on their position to motivate or reward others. You must be able to distinguish when incentive/punishment motivation is needed versus when charismatic inspiration will achieve the desired results, or even when "well enough" is left alone. The next generation of leaders will be required to blend techniques of artistic management and wise leadership, all "on the run," in a rapidly changing health care environment (Bolman & Deal, 2013; Garrison et al., 2004). Indeed, some studies of military platoons in combat (the ultimate fast-paced and stressful environment) showed both transformational and transactional leadership to be positively related to group cohesion and performance (Bass et al., 2003). Researchers have compared the effects of transformational leadership with other leadership styles and have found high correlations among all styles with organizational outcomes and employee satisfaction (Molero, Cuadrado, Navas, & Morales, 2007), confirming the idea that a variety of leadership styles and approaches can be effective in differing roles and circumstances.

THE ROLE OF THE DNP IN ORGANIZATIONAL AND COMPLEX SYSTEMS LEADERSHIP

You have taken a step toward assuming leadership for the profession by pursuing the DNP degree. From the beginning of the development of the degree, leadership development has been a high priority (Lenz, 2005). Indeed, the need for leaders prepared in advanced clinical practice was a precipitating factor in the earliest discussions of the DNP. Carryer, Gardner, Dunn, and Gardner (2007) observed three role components of all advanced clinicians such as nurse practitioners: dynamic practice, professional efficacy, and clinical leadership. Draye, Acker, and Zimmer (2006, p. 123) called on DNP programs to prepare expert clinicians with "enhanced leadership" skills. Other leaders in the discipline (Marion et al., 2003; O'Sullivan, Carter, Marion, Pohl, & Werner, 2005, p. 6) have boldly announced that "educational programs need to prepare clinicians with increased leadership and management skills in order to better understand and master the emerging complex health care systems." Broome (2012) proposed that doctorally prepared nurses will bring unique expertise to a number of areas, including innovative educational approaches, patient management knowledge and expertise, theoretical expertise, research methods expertise (both qualitative and quantitative), statistical and analytical expertise, and political awareness. They will also open doors to new roles and positions to gain entry to care for specific patient populations at the highest levels.

When leaders in nursing education developed DNP programs in the early part of the 21st century, we joined other practice disciplines, such as medicine, optometry, pharmacy, physical therapy, and audiology, which had elevated their practices and leadership by preparing practitioners with the highest professional academic degree (Upvall & Ptachcinski, 2007). The American Association of Colleges of

Nursing (AACN, 2004, 2015) affirmed the fundamental need for DNP-prepared leaders, noting that "the knowledge required to provide leadership in the discipline of nursing is so complex and rapidly changing that additional or doctoral level education is needed" (2004, p. 7) and that "practice-focused doctoral nursing programs prepare leaders for nursing practice" (2004, p. 11).

One of the competencies listed in the *Essentials of Doctoral Education for Advanced Nursing Practice (DNP Essentials)* (AACN, 2006, p. 10) is "Organizational and systems leadership for quality improvement and systems thinking." Specifically, DNP graduates should be prepared to:

- Develop and evaluate care delivery approaches that meet the current and future needs of patient populations based on scientific findings in nursing and other clinical sciences, as well as organizational, political, and economic sciences.
- Ensure accountability for the quality of health care and patient safety for populations with whom they work.
  - Use advanced communication skills/processes to lead quality improvement and patient safety initiatives in health care systems.
  - Employ principles of business, finance, economics, and health policy to develop and implement effective plans for practice-level and/or system-wide practice initiatives that will improve the quality of care delivery.
  - Develop and/or monitor budgets for practice initiatives.
  - Analyze the cost-effectiveness of practice initiatives accounting for risk and improvement of health care outcomes.
  - Demonstrate sensitivity to diverse organizational cultures and populations, including patients and providers.
- Develop and/or evaluate effective strategies for managing the ethical dilemmas inherent in patient care, the health care organization, and research (AACN, 2006, pp. 10–11).

Although early in its development the DNP was met with controversy within the discipline of nursing (Chase & Pruitt, 2006; Dracup, Cronenwett, Meleis, & Benner, 2005; Joachim, 2008; Otterness, 2006; Webber, 2008), some leaders proclaim that "the question facing the nursing community is no longer whether the practice doctorate is 'future or fringe'" (Marion et al., 2003), but rather how do we move forward together (O'Sullivan et al., 2005). As of 2014, there were 264 DNP programs in the United States, with more than 18,000 enrolled students and over 3,000 graduates, and nursing education leaders in many other countries had indicated interest in developing DNP programs (AACN, 2015). Clearly the DNP degree has been embraced by many nurses in practice who want to take their careers as practitioners to a new level and provide leadership and expertise to shape care delivery. Graduates of DNP programs are fulfilling the hope for a new, more effective advanced practitioner and health care leader.

Taken together, the complexity of health care systems, emphasis on evidence-based practice and information management to improve patient outcomes, information explosions in science, advances in technology, and a new world of ethical issues only amplify the need for new leadership grounded in expert clinical practice. It is the hope of the profession that the DNP-prepared leader will offer the highest level of practice expertise "integrated with the ability to translate scientific knowledge into complex clinical interventions tailored to meet individual, family, and community health and illness needs" (Bellflower & Carter, 2006, p. 323). As a DNP-prepared leader, you will be expected to guide and inspire organizational systems, quality improvement, systems and analytical evaluations, and policy development and translation, and to forge intra- and interdisciplinary collaborations to improve patient health outcomes (Bellflower & Carter, 2006; Broome, 2012). Prepared at the highest level of practice, you will understand the broad perspective of resource management in a sociopolitical environment to influence policy decisions and use your influence to lead teams to develop and test new care models. There is every reason to hope that you will be able to invent systems of care yet unknown that will strengthen, correct, and transform health care systems as we know them today.

THE ROLE OF THE PhD-PREPARED NURSE IN PRACTICE

Many hospitals throughout the United States, especially those in academic health centers, also employ nurses prepared with the doctor of philosophy (PhD) degree to lead various sectors of the enterprise, including education, professional development, and research offices. PhD-prepared nurses are also most commonly employed in academic institutions. You might ask, "What is the difference between the two degrees? How will we work together?" The PhD is not a professional degree but rather the highest academic degree given across a variety of disciplines. The PhD program and degree require the student to understand the philosophy of science and the nature of knowledge, and to master, extend, and generate knowledge for the discipline through research. As of 2014, there were 136 PhD programs in nursing in the United States (AACN, 2014), whose students focus on developing research skills and expertise in a particular area of knowledge.

PhD programs provide graduates an understanding of the environment within which nurses practice and prepare graduates to advance the science of the discipline. The core of the PhD program is an understanding of nursing and the development of competencies to expand science that supports the discipline and practice of nursing (AACN, 2010). Since the mid-1990s, hospitals and health systems have employed nurse scientists to engage in the development and testing of interventions designed to improve patient outcomes. In addition, these nurse scientists collaborate with researchers in other practice disciplines to develop and evaluate evidence-based initiatives to improve care delivery. DNP- and PhD-prepared nurses will find themselves on teams of leaders or, in fact, leading teams of other providers to develop, test, and translate knowledge that has the potential to improve patient outcomes. The complementary in-depth skill base of both fields of study can maximize effectiveness and efficiency of any initiative.

BRINGING THE PERSPECTIVE OF DOCTORALLY PREPARED NURSES TO ENHANCE LEADERSHIP: ENVISIONING NEW ROLES

More than 20 years ago, Starck, Duffy, and Vogler (1993) pointed out that nursing would be dealing with many changes in the future and that we should devote more attention and resources to preparing leaders for clinical practice. Their statement remains true, and insightful clinicians are responding to the call. The professional background of the advanced clinician provides the unique opportunity for new eyes to examine the leadership tradition, including the vision of new roles for the leader and others. We cannot tell you what new roles you will envision or be expected to fill. We can only help you prepare to invent and to lead in those roles. You must find the fearlessness and creativity to envision the role. If you reach deep into your own knowledge and find the courage to step out of old habits, you will design and fulfill the models that will work.

To become a transformational leader requires both theoretical or conceptual understanding and the real-world practice of leadership. Leadership is a discipline in itself, with a body of knowledge, theories, culture, and practice expertise. By learning from theories and principles of leadership, then applying vision and courage, you will become a citizen of the community of leaders who will solve the problems of the future.

One of your major challenges as an advanced clinician and leader at the organizational level will be to shift the perspective of care from the individual patient to that of entire populations of professionals, peers, patients, and other stakeholders. Your world will broaden. This will mean you must learn new skills—especially the ability to "zoom in and zoom out" (Kanter, 2011) in the face of challenges. The ability to zoom out cannot be overestimated.

The viewpoint of the expert clinician is critical to leadership for the future of health care, but it also requires that nurses specifically "transition from the operational (doing) aspect of work to the strategic (reflective) element" (Savage, 2003, p. 2). Evidence is mounting that links the influence of transformational leaders to both improved nursing practice at the bedside and positive patient outcomes in the aggregate (Gifford, Davies, Edwards, Griffin, & Lybanon, 2007; Merrill, 2015; Wong & Cummings, 2007). There continues to be a need for more research and practice results in this area, particularly those aimed at examining how effective leaders influence both patient and staff outcomes.

The expertise of the advanced clinician in the position of the organizational leader offers a treasure trove of perspective, professional and personal knowledge, and in-the-trenches experience that is frequently missing in health care today. For example, in settings where the chief executive officer is not a clinician (which is frequently the case), it is often the chief nursing officer who provides the insight, experience, and model for clinical leadership. Clinical expertise brings context, credibility, and a dose of reality to a leadership position. So many areas of health care will benefit from the clinical leadership roles yet to be invented.

Such roles are currently needed to achieve the triple aim (Berwick, Nolan, & Whittingdon, 2008) of increased access to care, improved quality,

REFLECTION QUESTIONS

1. Do the expectations of and hopes for the DNP-prepared nurse in today's health care system align with those you have for your career?
2. What are your greatest concerns about assuming the mantle of leader? What resources can you take advantage of now and in the near future to address those concerns?
3. Identify your own goals and strengths. Consult any of the numerous free strength aptitude tests online. Then respond to the following:
   a. What are your greatest strengths?
   b. How can you use these strengths in the practice setting?
   c. How will they be useful to you while in this graduate program?

and decreased cost. New leaders are needed in clinical areas of child health and risk reduction for chronic conditions, transitions of aging, symptom management, and palliative and end-of-life care. They are needed in settings of primary and acute care, as well as community and home care. We need leaders for new kinds of comprehensive preventive screening centers, immigrant health, Internet and telehealth care, and other settings and practice areas as yet unimagined. In the environment of fast-paced complex systems, the bold and creative expert clinician will invent the new roles needed to lead care teams, patient groups, public interest groups, and organizations that may better manage challenges, solve problems, and take advantages of opportunities.

BECOMING A TRANSFORMATIONAL LEADER

We have moved from the "great person" era to an age of information, with the explosion of knowledge of facts and complexity of systems. You were likely trained as a clinician to meet the challenges of simply keeping up with growing information. Futurists predict with hope that the next generation will be the age of wisdom. What will be needed next are vision and wisdom regarding how to best employ information, resources, and people to meet health care needs within complex systems. Leadership can be learned and practiced, and you are in the right time and place to do it. Critical clinical skills and judgment, amplified and enriched by thoughtful, wise decision making and leadership, are what are most needed now.

Transformational Leader Theories

As noted at the beginning of this chapter, the theory of transformational leadership, as originated and advanced by Burns (1978, 2003) and Bass (1985), argued for a distinction between transactional and transformational leaders. Transactional leadership implies a transaction or exchange of actions by followers for rewards or punishments by the leader. Bass (1985) further refined the theory to diminish the idea of polar concepts between the two types of leadership, instead emphasizing how the transformational leader employs and transforms the transactional needs of the organization. There is a current surge of interest in transformational theory, and many authors promote some aspects of it, although not always explicitly. Doyle and Smith (2009) proposed that the works of such authors and thinkers as Bennis (2003), Kouzes and Posner (2007), and Covey (1989, 2004) on leader as a catalyst for change, and Senge (1990) on leader as a strategic visionary, might be considered transformational theories.

Transformational leadership is increasingly the focus of empirical study among health care organizations. For instance, one study examined the relationships among transformational leadership, knowledge management, and quality improvement initiatives among various departments in 370 hospitals in all 50 states. Results demonstrated that transformational leadership and quality management improve knowledge management. Researchers concluded that transformational leadership skills among health care executives promote effective knowledge of management initiatives that enhance quality improvement programs. Furthermore, the integration of transformational leadership, knowledge management, and quality improvement was closely associated with organizational and patient outcomes, including patient safety (Gowen, Henagan, & McFadden, 2009). There is particular hope for transformational leadership paradigms to energize human resources and optimize intellectual capital in health care organizations more than current "traditional hierarchical organizations that are team driven and mission oriented" (Schwartz & Tumblin, 2002, p. 1419). The idea of transformational theories sometimes refers to a group of several different approaches that focus on "positive constructs such as hope, resiliency, efficacy, optimism, happiness, and well-being as they apply to organizations" (Avolio, Walumbwa, & Weber, 2009, p. 423), rather than on traditional models, some of which focus on deficit reduction, or working on what is wrong with a leader.

From an empirical and theoretical perspective, evidence for the effectiveness of transformational theories remains to be demonstrated. Such theories continue to secure a major place in contemporary literature on leadership. There seems to be a hunger in society for the positive hope and promise of the transformational leader. The discipline of nursing offers a welcome laboratory to test the promise of transformational leadership. Nursing practice is grounded in concepts of caring and altruism; it already attracts people motivated toward self-actualization, achievement, and helping; and it embraces tenets of holism (Jackson, Clements, Averill, & Zimbro, 2009). Such principles are highly consistent with those of transformational leadership.

Related Theories Guiding Nursing Leadership

Much of the empirical literature about leadership in nursing is descriptive, with only a few studies focused on transformational leadership. McDaniel and

Wolfe (1992) examined the characteristics of transformational leadership among nurses in executive, midlevel, and staff positions, confirming transformational leadership scores among nurse executives, with a cascading effect to higher transactional leadership scores among staff nurses. Ohman (2000, p. 46) found critical care nurse managers to be highly transformational, "using inspiration, motivation, and vision to empower staff." Dunham-Taylor (2000) sampled 396 hospital nurse executives. Scores on transformational leadership were positively related to staff satisfaction and work group effectiveness. Leach (2005) also studied nurses in hospitals, examining the relationship between nurse executive leadership and nurse manager leadership, and between nurse executive leadership and organizational commitment among staff nurses. Management styles between nurse executives and nurse managers were highly related. Nurse executives who scored high as transformational leaders were more likely to promote an environment that fostered employee commitment.

Cummings et al. (2008) reviewed research on leadership in nursing and identified four groups of studies: behaviors and practices of individual leaders, traits and characteristics of individual leaders, influences of context and practice settings, and leader participation in educational activities. They also noted relatively weak designs among the studies and a need for robust theory and research on the development of nursing leaders needed for the future. Jennings et al. (2007) also reviewed works on nursing leadership and management from the perspective of competencies, noting little distinction between nurse managers and nurse leaders.

Jumaa (2008, p. 997) examined prevalent "myths" in the literature of leadership in nursing: "everyone can be a leader," "leaders deliver business (service) results," "people who get to the top are leaders," and that "leaders are great coaches" (Goffee & Jones, 2000). She chided, in confirming the need for models in nursing leadership, that such myths need to become realities. And Malloch and Melnyk (2013) described competencies and challenges for executive leaders. Their competencies included:

- Evidence-driven consciousness
- Cross-generation communication competence
- Innovation leadership expertise
- Work–life balance
- Commitment to lifelong learning
- Transdisciplinary teamwork and inspiring teams
- Management of dynamic time pressures
- Shaping policy

A growing number of leadership theories are grounded specifically in nursing. Jooste (2004, p. 220) proposed an "Arch of Leadership" model, composed of five key dimensions:

- Clarity: Are workers clear about their tasks?
- Commitment: What do followers need from their leader?

- Self-image: Do followers know their own abilities, what they can and cannot accomplish?
- Price: What is the price they pay or receive for working hard?
- Behavior: Does the leadership style promote positive and effective behavior among followers?

Although Jooste discussed issues of past, present, and future leadership settings, the role of authority, power, and influence in leadership, and the need for solutions in a future dimension, the actual model appears to be drawn from other traditional leadership theories, largely transactional in style, and with little specific distinction for clinical leadership.

One intriguing proposal is the "nursing leadership knowing" theory adapted from patterns of knowing in nursing (Jackson et al., 2009). The authors attempted to apply their theoretical ideas to various areas, including history and pedagogy (Averill & Clements, 2007; Clements & Averill, 2006). Borrowing from previous thinkers (see Carper, 1978; Heath, 1998; Munhall, 1993; White, 1995), Jackson et al. (2009) listed well-known ways of knowing for nursing as ways of leadership knowing—empirical, aesthetic, personal, sociopolitical, ethical, and unknowing—for which they outlined descriptions and qualities, as well as examples. Their theory seems to resonate with nursing, but its actual application to clinical leadership remains to be demonstrated.

The challenge of the next decade for nurse leaders is to create an empirical foundation of evidence for best practices in leadership in complex health care organizations. Such leadership needs to work for nursing practice but must invite interprofessional engagement in the bigger picture of health care. Perhaps the initiative of the advanced clinician in the organizational leadership role will launch that discovery. It is especially important to note that a working theory, empirically tested and specific to clinical leadership in complex health care systems, is yet to be developed, discovered, or invented.

Many impressive theories explain or guide leadership of people and organizations, but few have included environment or setting as much more than an artifact or a backdrop, implying that context may not be relevant. As a health care provider, you know that the context of health care is uniquely challenging and complex. The innovative leader is able to think in terms of multiprofessional caregivers, patients, community, and context from a systems perspective. He or she understands not only leadership theory but also theories of complexity and complex adaptive systems. The new transformational leader will design new environments and systems for care—some we have not dared to imagine. Perhaps, theories of the past will be revised or proven altogether irrelevant. The world is waiting for your creativity to care for those in need, and to inspire other leaders to come together in new ways of thinking and practice.

Transformational leaders of the future will see the world with a new vision, break old rules, discover or create new rules, and thrive in the paradoxes of complexity. Porter-O'Grady and Malloch (2007, p. 27) listed a few of the contradictions that inspire innovation: "Chaos and order, creativity and tension, conflict and peace, difference and similarity, complexity and simplicity." Innovation requires the space for creativity and the courage to be wrong. Mistakes teach as much as success. The truth is, there is often no right or wrong but, rather, change, diversity, and helping people come together to solve problems and help others.

Johnson (2006) told the story of London's worst epidemic of cholera in the mid-1850s, which persisted as a result of hundreds of years of conventional thinking that disease was caused by smells in the air. That idea was held by the most distinguished scientists and physicians of the time. Johnson called it the "sociology of error," when bad ideas stay around too long. What are those errors in our own world? When we were young graduate nurses, "science" required that we treat stomach ulcers with round-the-clock alternate doses of dairy cream and liquid antacid through a nasogastric tube. We would not have believed that any ulcer might be treated or cured by an antibiotic. Patients in the intensive care unit were not fed and became malnourished as a result. Neonates underwent surgery for repair of heart defects (e.g., patent ductus arteriosus) without the benefit of anesthesia because of their "instability." What other non–evidence-based assumptions ask for correction by creative thinking and testing? What bad ideas do we practice in leadership? What new miracles do we need to invite?

Innovation is a paradox that requires a willingness to learn all you can, bring your clinical experience to bear, and then eagerly suspend previous learning and experience to welcome the new idea, recognize a different point of view, embrace chaos, winnow what must remain and what must change, and set a new course. These are not easy things to do, but leaders must encourage those in their environment to ask questions and seek out new and different solutions to challenges that present themselves over and over in health care.

THE PATH FORWARD IN THIS BOOK

The chapters that follow will expose you to information and learning activities, cases, and sharing of expertise from key leaders in the field. You will learn about health care as a context in which the transformative leader must not just adapt but lead others to shape a preferred future. We discuss current theoretical perspectives about change management, chaos, and complex organizations. We consider contemporary challenges related to technology, quality and safety, health care workforce issues, and consumer and provider satisfaction. And we note other issues related to success in achieving the triple aim of increasing access, decreasing cost, and increasing quality with the goal of improving the health status of all.

You will learn how finance models influence care models and understand how financial complexities and solutions are the work of the successful leader. We also discuss the criticality of intra- and interprofessional team growth and management to help achieve an organization's goals, as well as how leaders can influence teamwork. Creating and shaping environments in which diversity is not just valued but embraced and used to maximize all individuals' contributions is the focus of one chapter and truly the primary job of any transformative leader. We close with the view forward for your career and provide some guidance for you to consider as you are required to work with others outside of professional provider contexts, including boards of trustees, community boards, and policy makers. In sum, we hope this book serves you as you begin your next leadership journey. The authors and editors in this book have provided you with their best knowledge and wisdom about leadership, an overview of the evidence to support leadership development, and opportunities to reflect on where you have been, where you are now, and where you hope to be in the future.

REFERENCES

American Association of Colleges of Nursing. (2004). *AACN position statement on the practice doctorate in nursing*. Washington, DC: Author.

American Association of Colleges of Nursing. (2006). *The essentials of doctoral education for advanced nursing practice*. Washington, DC: Author.

American Association of Colleges of Nursing. (2010). *The research focused doctoral program in nursing: Pathways to excellence*. Washington, DC: Author.

American Association of Colleges of Nursing. (2014). *Building a framework for the future: Advancing higher education in nursing*. Retrieved from http://www.aacn.nche.edu/aacn-publications/annual-reports/AnnualReport14.pdf

American Association of Colleges of Nursing. (2015). *The DNP fact sheet: June, 2015*. Retrieved from http://www.aacn.nche.edu/media-relations/fact-sheets/dnp

American Nurses Association. (2015). *Code of ethics with interpretive statements*. Silver Spring, MD: Author.

Averill, J. B., & Clements, P. T. (2007). Patterns of knowing as a foundation for action-sensitive pedagogy. *Qualitative Health Research, 17*(3), 386–399.

Avolio, B. J., Walumbwa, F. O., & Weber, T. J. (2009). Leadership: Current theories, research, and future directions. *Annual Review of Psychology, 60*, 421–449.

Baker, N. B. (1952). *Cyclone in calico: The story of Mary Ann Bickerdyke*. Boston, MA: Little, Brown, & Company.

Bass, B. M. (1985). *Leadership and performance beyond expectations*. New York, NY: Free Press.

Bass, B. M. (1990). From transactional to transformational leadership: Learning to share the vision. *Organizational Dynamics, Winter*, 19–31.

Bass, B. M., Avolio, B. J., & Jung, D. I. (2010). Re-examining the components of transformational leadership using the Multifactorial Leadership Questionnaire. *Journal of Occupational and Organizational Psychology, 72*(4), 441–462.

Bass, B. M., Avolio, B. J., Jung, D. I., & Berson, Y. (2003). Predicting unit performance by assessing transformational and transactional leadership. *Journal of Applied Psychology, 88*(2), 207–218.

Bass, B. M., & Riggio, R. E. (2006). *Transformational leadership* (2nd ed.). Mahwah, NJ: Lawrence Erlbaum.

Bellflower, B., & Carter, M. A. (2006). Primer on the practice doctorate for neonatal nurse practitioners. *Advances in Neonatal Care, 6*(6), 323–332.

Bennis, W. (2003). *Learning to lead: A workbook on becoming a leader* (3rd ed.). Cambridge, MA: Basic Books.

Berwick, D., Nolan, T., & Whittingdon, J. (2008). The triple aim: Care, health, and cost. *Health Affairs, 27*(3), 769–779.

Bolman, L. G., & Deal, T. F. (2013). *Reframing organizations: Artistry, choice, and leadership*. San Francisco, CA: Jossey-Bass.

Broome, M. (2012) Doubling the number of doctorally prepared nurses. *Nursing Outlook, 60*(3), 111–113.

Broome, M. (2013). Self-reported leadership styles of deans of baccalaureate and higher degree programs in the United States. *Journal of Professional Nursing, 29*(3), 323–329.

Broome, M. (2015). Nurse leaders can shape ethical cultures. *Nursing Outlook, 63*(4), 377–378.

Brown, A. (2014). *Brief history of the Federal Children's Bureau (1912–1935).* The Social Welfare History Project. Retrieved from http://www.socialwelfarehistory.com/programs/child-welfarechild-labor/childrens-bureau-a-brief-history-resources/

Burns, J. M. (1978). *Leadership.* New York, NY: Harper & Row.

Burns, J. M. (2003). *Transforming leadership: The pursuit of happiness.* New York, NY: Atlantic Monthly Press.

Capra, F. (1997). *The web of life: A new synthesis of mind and matter.* London, UK: HarperCollins.

Carper, B. (1978). Fundamental patterns of knowing in nursing. *Advances in Nursing Science, 1*(1), 13–23.

Carryer, J., Gardner, G., Dunn, S., & Gardner, A. (2007). The core role of the nurse practitioner: Practice, professionalism, and clinical leadership. *Journal of Clinical Nursing, 16*(10), 1818–1825.

Chase, S. K., & Pruitt, R. H. (2006). The practice doctorate: Innovation or disruption? *Journal of Nursing Education, 45*(5), 155–157.

Clawson, J. G. (1999). *Level three leadership: Getting below the surface.* Upper Saddle River, NJ: Prentice-Hall.

Clements, P. T., & Averill, J. B. (2006). Finding patterns of knowing in the work of Florence Nightingale. *Nursing Outlook, 54*(5), 268–274.

Collins, J. (2001). *Good to great.* New York, NY: HarperCollins.

Cook, M. J. (2001). The renaissance of clinical leadership. *International Nursing Review, 48*(1), 38–46.

Covey, S. R. (1989). *The seven habits of highly effective people.* New York, NY: Simon & Schuster.

Covey, S. R. (2004). *The eighth habit: From effectiveness to greatness.* New York, NY: Simon & Schuster.

Cummings, G., Lee, H., Macgregor, T., Davey, M., Wong, C., Paul, L., & Stafford, E. (2008). Factors contributing to nursing leadership: A systematic review. *Journal of Health Services Research & Policy, 13*(4), 240–248.

Disch, J., Edwardson, S., & Adwan, J. (2004). Nursing faculty satisfaction with individual, institutional, and leadership factors. *Journal of Professional Nursing, 20*(5), 323–332.

Doyle, M. E., & Smith, M. K. (2009). Classical leadership. *The Encyclopedia of Informal Education.* Retrieved from http://www.infed.org/leadership/traditional_leadership.htm

Dracup, K., Cronenwett, L., Meleis, A. I., & Benner, P. E. (2005). Reflections on the doctorate of nursing practice. *Nursing Outlook, 53*, 177–182.

Draye, M. A., Acker, M., & Zimmer, P. A. (2006). The practice doctorate in nursing: Approaches to transform nurse practitioner education and practice. *Nursing Outlook, 54*(3), 123–129.

Drucker, P. (2011). What makes an effective executive? In *On leadership* (pp. 23–36). Boston, MA: Harvard Business Review.

Dunham-Taylor, J. (2000). Nurse executive transformational leadership found in participative organizations. *Journal of Nursing Administration, 30*(5), 241–250.

Eagly, A. H., Johannesen-Schmidt, M. C., & van Engen, M. L. (2003). Transformational, transactional and laissez-faire leadership styles: A meta-analysis comparing women and men. *Psychological Bulletin, 129*(4), 569–591.

Erez, A., Misangyi, V. F., Johnson, D. E., LePine, M. A., & Halverson, K. C. (2008). Stirring the hearts of followers: Charismatic leadership as the transferal of affect. *Journal of Applied Psychology, 93*(3), 602–616.

Fiedler, F. E. (1967). *A theory of leadership effectiveness.* New York, NY: Harper & Row.

Fiedler, F. E. (1997). Situational control and a dynamic theory of leadership. In K. Grint (Ed.), *Leadership: Classical, contemporary, and critical approaches* (pp. 126–148). Oxford, UK: Oxford University Press.

Fiedler, F. E., & Garcia, J. E. (1987). *New approaches to effective leadership.* New York, NY: John Wiley & Sons.

Gardner, J. W. (1986a). *Leadership and power. Leadership papers/5.* Washington, DC: Independent Sector.

Gardner, J. W. (1986b). *The tasks of leadership. Leadership papers/2.* Washington, DC: Independent Sector.

Gardner, J. W. (1987a). *The heart of the matter: Leader–constituent interaction. Leadership papers/3.* Washington, DC: Independent Sector.

Gardner, J. W. (1987b). *Leadership development.* Washington, DC: Independent Sector.

Gardner, J. W. (1989). *On leadership.* New York, NY: HarperCollins.

Garrison, D. R., Morgan, D. A., & Johnson, J. G. (2004). Thriving in chaos: Educating the nurse leaders of the future. *Nursing Leadership Forum, 9*(1), 23–27.

George, B. (2003). *Authentic leadership: Rediscovering the secrets to creating lasting value.* San Francisco, CA: Jossey-Bass.

Gifford, W., Davies, B., Edwards, N, Griffin, P., & Lybanon, V. (2007). Managerial leadership for nurses' use of research evidence: An integrative review of the literature. *Worldviews of Evidence Based Nursing, 4*(3), 126–145.

Goffee, R., & Jones, G. (2000). Why should anyone be led by you? *Harvard Business Review, 78*(5), 62–69.

Goleman, D. (1995). *Emotional intelligence.* New York, NY: Bantam Books.

Goleman, D., Boyatzis, R., & McKee, A. (2002). *Primal leadership.* Boston, MA: Business School Press.

Gosline, M. B. (2004). Leadership in nursing education: Voices from the past. *Nursing Leadership Forum, 9*(2), 51–58.

Gowen, C. R., Henagan, S. C., & McFadden, K. L. (2009). Knowledge management as a mediator for the efficacy of transformational leadership and quality management initiatives in U.S. health care. *Health Care Management Review, 34*(3), 129–140.

Graen, G. B. (1976). Role-making process within complex organizations. In M. D. Dinette (Ed.), *Handbook of industrial and organizational psychology* (pp. 1201–1245). Chicago, IL: Rand-McNally.

Greenleaf, R. (1977). *Servant leadership.* Mahwah, NJ: Paulist Press.

Harwell, R. B. (Ed.) (1959). *Kate: The journal of a confederate nurse.* Baton Rouge, LA: Louisiana State University Press.

Heath, H. (1998). Refection and patterns of knowing in nursing. *Journal of Advanced Nursing, 27*(5), 1054–1059.

Hersey, P., & Blanchard, K. (1977). *The management of organizational behavior.* Upper Saddle River, NJ: Pearson Education.

Hersey, P., Blanchard, K., & Johnson, D. (2008). *Management of organizational behavior: Leading human resources* (9th ed.). Upper Saddle River, NJ: Pearson Education.

Herzberg, F. (1966). *Work and the nature of man*. New York, NY: World.

House, R. (1971). A path–goal theory of leader effectiveness. *Administrative Science Quarterly, 16*, 321–339.

Institute of Medicine. (2000). *To err is human: Building a safer health system*. Washington, DC: National Academies Press.

Institute of Medicine. (2001). *Crossing the quality chasm: A new health system for the 21st century*. Washington, DC: National Academies Press.

Institute of Medicine. (2003). *Health professions education: A bridge to quality*. Washington, DC: National Academies Press.

Institute of Medicine. (2010). *The future of nursing: Leading change, advancing health*. Washington, DC: National Academies Press.

Jackson, J. R., Clements, P. T., Averill, J. B., & Zimbro, K. (2009). Patterns of knowing: Proposing a theory for nursing leadership. *Nursing Economics, 27*(3), 149–159.

Jaworski, J. (1998). *Synchronicity: The inner path of leadership*. San Francisco, CA: Koehler.

Jennings, B. M., Scalzi, C. C, Rodgers, J. D., 3rd, & Keane, A. (2007). Differentiating nursing leadership and management competencies. *Nursing Outlook, 55*(4), 169–175.

Joachim, G. (2008). The practice doctorate: Where do Canadian nursing leaders stand? *Nursing Leadership, 21(4)*, 4251.

Johns Hopkins Berman Institute of Bioethics. (2014). *Report of the National Nursing Summit*. Retrieved from http://www.bioethicsinstitute.org/nursing-ethics-summit-report

Johnson, S. (2006). *The ghost map: The story of London's most terrifying epidemic—and how it changed science, cities, and the modern world*. New York, NY: Riverhead.

Jooste, K. (2004). Leadership: A new perspective. *Journal of Nursing Management, 12*, 217–223.

Jumaa, M. O. (2008). The "F.E.E.L." good factors in nursing leadership at board level through work-based learning. *Journal of Nursing Management, 16*(8), 992–999.

Kalisch, P. A., & Kalisch, B. J. (1995). *The advance of American nursing* (3rd ed.). Philadelphia, PA: J. B. Lippincott.

Kanter, R. M. (2011, March). "Zoom in, zoom out." *Harvard Business Review, 89*(3). Retrieved from http://www.hbs.edu/faculty/Pages/item.aspx?num=39994

Kegan, R., & Lahey, L. L. (1984). Adult leadership and adult development: A constructivist view. In B. Kellerman (Ed.), *Leadership: Multidisciplinary perspectives* (pp. 199–230). Englewood Cliffs, NJ: Prentice-Hall.

Kouzes, J. M., & Posner, B. Z. (2007). *The leadership challenge* (4th ed.). San Francisco, CA: Jossey-Bass.

Leach, L. S. (2005). Nurse executive transformational leadership and organizational commitment. *Journal of Nursing Administration, 35*(5), 228–237.

Lenz, E. R. (2005). The practice doctorate in nursing: An idea whose time has come. *Online Journal of Issues in Nursing, 10*(3). Retrieved from http://www.nursingworld.org/MainMenuCategories/ANAMarketplace/ANAPeriodicals/OJIN/TableofContents/Volume102005/No3Sept05/tpc28_116025.html

Lewenson, S. (1996). *Taking charge: Nursing, suffrage and feminism in America, 1873–1920*. New York, NY: National League for Nursing Press.

Lewin, K., Lippitt, R., & White, R. (1939). Patterns of aggressive behavior in experimentally created social climates. *Journal of Social Psychology, 10*(2), 271–301.

Malloch, K., & Melnyk, B. M. (2013). Developing high-level change and innovation agents: Competencies and challenges for executive leadership. *Nursing Administration Quarterly, 37*(1), 60–66.

Marion, L., Viens, D., O'Sullivan, A. L., Crabtree, K., Fontana, S., & Price, M. M. (2003). The practice doctorate in nursing: Future or fringe? *Topics in Advanced Practice Nursing E-Journal, 3*(2). Retrieved from http://www.medscape.com/viewarticle/453247_4

Marshall, H. (1972). *Mary Adelaide Nutting: Pioneer of modern nursing*. Baltimore, MD: Johns Hopkins University Press.

Maslow, A. H. (1954). *Motivation and personality*. Upper Saddle River, NJ: Prentice-Hall.

Mayo, E. (1953). *The human problems of an industrialized civilization*. New York, NY: Macmillan.

McDaniel, C, & Wolf, G. A. (1992). Transformational leadership in nursing service: A test of theory. *Journal of Nursing Administration, 22*(2), 60–65.

McGregor, D. (1960). *The human side of enterprise*. New York, NY: McGraw-Hill.

McKenna, H., Keeney, S., & Bradley, M. (2004). Nurse leadership within primary care: The perceptions of community nurses, GPs, policy makers, and members of the public. *Journal of Nursing Management, 12*(1), 69–76.

Merrill, K. D. (2015). Leadership style and patient safety: Implications for nurse managers. *Journal of Nursing Administration, 45*(6), 319–324.

Millward, L. J., & Bryan, K. (2005). Clinical leadership in health care: A position statement. *International Journal of Health Care Quality Assurance Including Leadership in Health Services, 18*(2/3), xiii–xxv.

Miner, J. B. (2007). *Organizational behavior 4: From theory to practice*. Armonk, NY: M. E. Sharpe.

Molero, F., Cuadrado, I., Navas, M., & Morales, J. F. (2007). Relations and effects of transformational leadership: A comparative analysis with traditional leadership styles. *Spanish Journal of Psychology, 10*(2), 358–368.

Munhall, P. (1993). "Unknowing": Toward another pattern of knowing in nursing. *Nursing Outlook, 41*(3), 125–128.

Nutting, M. A. (1926). *A sound economic basis for schools of nursing and other addresses*. New York, NY: G. P. Putnam's Sons.

Ohman, K. A. (2000). The transformational leadership of critical care nurse-managers. *Dimensions of Critical Care Nursing, 19*(1), 46–54.

O'Sullivan, A. L., Carter, M., Marion, L., Pohl, J. M., & Werner, K. E. (2005). Moving forward together: The practice doctorate in nursing. *Online Journal of Issues in Nursing, 20*(3). Retrieved from http://www.nursingworld.org/MainMenuCategories/ANAMarketplace/ANAPeriodicals/OJIN/TableofContents/Volume102005/No3Sept05/tpc28_416028.html

Otterness, S. (2006). Is the burden worth the benefit of the doctorate of nursing (DNP) for NPs? Implications of doctorate in nursing practice—still many unresolved issues for nurse practitioners. *Nephrology Nursing Journal, 33*(6), 685–687.

Ouchi, W. G. (1981). *Theory Z: How American management can meet the Japanese challenge*. Reading, MA: Addison-Wesley.

Pitcher, P. (1997). *The drama of leadership*. New York, NY: John Wiley & Sons.

Porter-O'Grady, T. (1992). Transformational leadership in an age of chaos. *Nursing Administration Quarterly, 17*, 17–24.

Porter-O'Grady, T., & Malloch, K. (2007). *Quantum leadership: A resource for health care innovation* (2nd ed.). Boston, MA: Jones & Bartlett.

Savage, C. (2003, July/August). Nursing leadership: Oxymoron or powerful force? *AAACN Viewpoint*, 1–8.

Schwartz, R. W., & Tumblin, T. F. (2002). The power of servant leadership to transform health care organizations for the 21st-century economy. *Archives of Surgery, 137*(12), 1419–1427.

Seltzer, J., & Bass, B. M. (1990). Transformational leadership: Beyond initiation and consideration. *Journal of Management, 16*(4), 693–703.

Senge, P. (1990). *The fifth discipline: The art and practice of the learning organization.* New York, NY: Doubleday.

Shirey, M. R. (2006). Authentic leaders creating healthy work environments for nursing practice. *American Journal of Critical Care, 15*, 256–267.

Shirey, M. R. (2009). Authentic leadership, organizational culture, and healthy work environments. *Critical Care Nursing Quarterly, 32*(3), 189–198.

Starck, P. L., Duffy, M. E., & Vogler, R. (1993). Developing a nursing doctorate for the 21st century. *Journal of Professional Nursing, 9*(4), 212–219.

Stone, A. G., & Patterson, K. (2005, August). *The history of leadership focus.* Paper presented at the Servant Leadership Research Roundtable, School of Leadership Studies, Regent University. Retrieved from https://www.regent.edu/acad/global/publications/sl_proceedings/2005/stone_history.pdf

Upvall, M. J., & Ptachcinski, R. J. (2007). The journey to the DNP program and beyond: What can we learn from pharmacy? *Journal of Professional Nursing, 23*(5), 316–321.

Vroom, V. H., & Yetton, P. W. (1973). *Leadership and decision-making.* Pittsburgh, PA: University of Pittsburgh Press.

Webber, P. B. (2008). The doctor of nursing practice degree and research: Are we making an epistemological mistake? *Journal of Nursing Education, 47*(10), 466–472.

Wheatley, M. J. (1994). *Leadership and the new science: Learning about organization from an orderly universe.* San Francisco, CA: Berrett-Koehler.

White, J. (1995). Patterns of knowing: Review, critique, and update. *Advances in Nursing Science, 17*(4), 73–86.

Wong, C. A., & Cummings, G. G. (2007). The relationship between nursing leadership and patient outcomes: A systematic review. *Journal of Nursing Management, 15*(5), 508–521.

Yoder-Wise, P. S., & Kowalski, K. E. (2006). *Beyond leading and managing: Nursing administration for the future.* St. Louis, MO: Mosby Elsevier.

CHAPTER 2

Understanding Contexts for Transformational Leadership: Complexity, Change, and Strategic Planning

Elaine Sorensen Marshall and Marion E. Broome

Change will not come if we wait for some other person or some other time. We are the ones we've been waiting for. We are the change that we seek.
—Barack Obama

OBJECTIVES

- *To describe how concepts in complexity and complex adaptive systems theories explain the context of today's health care environment*
- *To discuss how the individual leader takes a systems perspective to manage complexity*
- *To apply precepts of change theory to a case of implementation of a new model of care in a particular setting*
- *To describe the steps of strategic planning and how to mobilize talented individuals and teams to move selected initiatives through a system responding to continual change and new demands*

Leadership is never learned, developed, enacted, or evaluated outside the dynamic environment in which one actually works and leads. Although the context in which one leads can be constructed, that is rarely the situation in which most contemporary leaders must function. Instead most of us inherit an environment that we are expected to grow, improve, and enhance in effectiveness and work culture. Therefore, as a transformational leader, you must acquire an ability to understand and function effectively within the realities of the context and environment in which you work. Stichler (2006, p. 155) reminded:

> Today's [leader] is more challenged than ever to manage multiple, competing priorities in organizations with ever-diminishing financial and human resources. Accountability for ensuring positive patient outcomes, productivity goals, financial targets, retention quotas, customer and provider satisfaction goals, and other performance metrics demand that the contemporary [leader] possess and demonstrate well-developed leadership skills and organizational management competencies . . . [and] *excel in developing a culture and work environment that fosters professional models of care* [emphasis added], evidence-based practice, interdisciplinary and collaborative practice, professional autonomy and, quality nursing leadership.

Contemporary health care systems that survive and even thrive in today's market continue to evolve and change. Individuals in leadership positions are expected to help others assume new roles and models for doing their work, maintain high levels of employee satisfaction, and motivate others to "do their best"—even when it is not always clear what "best" would look like (Romley, Goldman, & Sood, 2015). The new jargon is all too familiar: complexity, cost-effectiveness, change, value, satisfaction, and populations. But what do these mean for the next generation of leaders?

These concepts all refer to context. In the past, the context of care was simple. It referred to *settings*, like hospital, clinic, or home—all with fairly simple linear and hierarchical models for care of the sick. Now the boundaries among these settings have blurred, and it is the transitions of what happens to patients (and providers) between and among such settings for which leaders are responsible. Now, and for the foreseeable future, context is everything. Context is the circumstance of your work as a leader. It refers to the multifaceted climate, background, domain, and terrain of care delivery. It is more than just the setting or environment, although it includes those. It comprises all systemic, physical, social, emotional, professional, informal, and formal aspects of care. The context for leadership has become as challenging as any aspect of leadership itself.

Beyond physical, social, or professional context, the context of our very thinking is challenged. The easy things have been done. All problems are more complex. Our old ways of thinking will not bring us to solutions. We must have the courage to think in new ways.

COMPLEXITY IN HEALTH CARE SYSTEMS

Nearly every discussion of current issues and contexts in health care begins with mention of the complexity of the problems we face and solutions we must implement. Complexity has become the introduction, the theoretical explanation, and the metaphor for the current and future state of health care. Consequently, chaos theory and complex adaptive systems are discussed in so many situations that they have become the catch phrases of the industry, with little general agreement on definitions and even less precision of application. Paley (2007, p. 234) chastised writers in health care literature for misuse and error in what he called "the over-hasty adoption of complexity ideas" as "essentially just one more intellectual fad." It is true that it has become fashionable to make "expansive claims" and "grand gestures" (Paley, 2007, pp. 233, 240) regarding chaos, complexity, and health care. Nevertheless, the references to complex states and issues continue to prevail, and it is difficult to argue that chaos and complexity have no real influence. Thus, it is helpful for any leader to have a basic awareness of such approaches to think-ing about and practicing in a new world of health care. Space is not adequate in this book to provide the quick-and-easy comprehensive discourse on chaos and complexity theory often desired by the emerging leader. The concepts cross a wide range of disciplines in their meanings and applications. Many of the ideas have been applied to areas as divergent as biology and art. Further, application of such theories to the daily practice of a leader can be daunting. Nevertheless, the com-plexity of the very concepts and theories of complexity should not intimidate you as a leader. These are topics that should be studied from a range of authors and perspectives. It is precisely because they are often discussed in areas far distant from health care that such theories provide an excellent opportunity for learning and practice for innovation in thinking and leading.

Chaos, Quanta, and Complexity Theory

Chaos theory arose in the 1960s in the fields of biology and physics. Meteorologist Edward Lorenz discovered that chaotic systems in weather forecasting appeared to be random, but actually eventually emerged as patterns. In other words, underlying natural phenomena that appear disordered, confused, or chaotic are actually processes of emerging order.

Quantum theory comes from the discipline of physics as a set of princi-ples that describe reality at the most fundamental level of the atom. The word *quantum* refers to a discrete unit (or "amount," which is the actual meaning) assigned to certain physical quantities, "such as the energy of an atom at rest" or discrete "energy packets" of wave ("Quantum Mechanics," 2016). In its most simplified sense, the idea of quantum refers to a kind of fluidity of the par-ticles of reality such that the state or velocity of the particles, or fundamental units, cannot be determined with certainty (Capra, 1982, 1997). Thus, the move-ment and relationships among the units are more significant than the individual nature of any particular particle. So quantum theory provides a metaphor for the integrated complex relationships among the numerous and varied elements of health care, as opposed to a focus on either the characteristics of any single element or the hierarchical linear building of individual parts. Quantum the-ory requires us to let go of traditional notions of *building blocks* of systems and instead adopt a perspective of ever-changing fluid integration of units as parts of a whole. Such a change of paradigm requires a new courageous leadership.

Complexity science is related to chaos theory and quantum perspectives. Complexity science is applicable in biology, physics, mathematics, economics, sociology, management, and the health care disciplines. It examines the nature and process of multiple interacting components of systems and the subsequent emergence of order and/or change (Lindberg, Nash, & Lindberg, 2008; Wall, 2013). Complexity science applies to living systems, examining the unpredictable, disorderly, nonlinear, and uncontrollable way. Unfortunately, this framework has sometimes led individuals to believe that complex systems and problems were not manageable or predictable (Goldstein, Hazy, & Lichtenstein, 2010). Importantly, leaders must understand that complex systems are in fact integrated and often predictable and support "emergence through novel behavior" (Pesut, 2008c, p. 123).

Complexity science focuses on the interacting elements of systems, seeking to identify principles and processes that explain how order emerges from change within the systems. Change is desirable and a natural way of being. Interacting elements of chaos may appear to be without order but actually occur in patterns, although these are not predictable in traditional ways of thinking. Key principles are diversity, emergence, self-organization, embeddedness, distributed control, the coexistence of order and disorder, nonlinearity, and inability to *predict in traditional ways of thinking* (Lindberg et al., 2008). Systems often have relationships among entities within them that reflect a high degree of systemic interdependence, which leads to nonlinear dynamics and outcomes (Goldstein et al., 2010).

Theory of Complex Adaptive Systems

The theory of complex adaptive systems, as one aspect of complexity science, adds a dimension that describes the ability of organizations to adapt in an ever-changing environment (Goldstein et al., 2010). This adaptability drives new and creative solutions to problems within the system. Complexity is the result of patterns of interactions that are a result of the ever-changing demands on the system, as well as the attempts of individuals and teams in the system to derive and test partial solutions to problems. When these partial solutions can be harnessed and individuals with different perspectives brought together to examine the problem from all angles, a synergistic effect often occurs that results in a creative approach that is much more likely to address the necessary changes and produce desired outcomes.

Most analysts of the contemporary health care scene mention complexity when referring to the complicated nature of all the structures, settings, and individuals. The term *health care system* has a variety of meanings itself. It may refer to the entire health care industry, including structures, processes, and personnel; or it may refer to a single hospital, ambulatory center, freestanding emergency department building, several hospitals under one organizational umbrella, or a system within any of those entities. Some may argue that although health care is complicated, it may not be the best example of a complex adaptive system. A complex adaptive system is characterized by flexibility and patterns of emerging change as opposed to predetermined change based on hierarchical or central control.

Any clinician can enumerate a long list of areas in health care that persist in the linear, hierarchical paradigm. They can also point to numerous evolutions in the care delivery model close to the point of service that are clearly adaptations to complex new regulations, compensation structures, or patient demographics that have mandated change in order for the organization to survive. Complexity frameworks offer models to frame the issues in the current realities of health care toward a hopeful transformation to a better future. Indeed, some of the current problems of health care may relate to the challenging transition from traditional thinking to a complexity perspective.

There are several key characteristics of complex systems:

- Emergence happens, or the idea that behaviors, patterns, and order develop as a result of nonlinear patterns of relationships and interactions among the elements or units of the organization.
- Relationships are short range, or interchanged from within a unit or near neighbors in a matrix of networks within the larger whole. The units, or parts, cannot contain, determine, or control the whole. Relationships are nonlinear, seldom cause-and-effect, and contain feedback loops.
- Feedback from those within the system may be damping (negative) or amplifying (positive), and a small stimulus may have a large powerful effect or none at all.
- Boundaries are open; energy and information constantly cross boundaries and create constant change.
- Coevolution is a "process of mutual transformation" for both smaller units and the larger organizational environment (Stroebel et al., 2005).

The "fitness landscape" is how an organization fits within an independent/dependent interaction with other agents, units, or organizations. Table 2.1 contains examples of these characteristics within the health care arena.

TABLE 2.1 Characteristics of Complex Adaptive Systems With Examples in Health Care Systems

CHARACTERISTICS OF COMPLEX ORGANIZATIONS	HEALTH CARE EXAMPLE
Emergence	Outpatient clinic systems, with components each serving patients with different care needs and illness states, require similar communication and monitoring systems across providers and patients.
Relationships: nonlinear, short range, within a matrix	Nurses on patient care units must interact with numerous people at various levels, including patients, families, other nurses, physicians, laboratory personnel, administrative staff, etc., on a daily basis.

(continued)

TABLE 2.1 Characteristics of Complex Adaptive Systems With Examples in
Health Care Systems (*continued*)

CHARACTERISTICS OF COMPLEX ORGANIZATIONS	HEALTH CARE EXAMPLE
Feedback loops	A small change in task of one role within a patient care model in one department reverberates across departments and must be acknowledged, communicated, and integrated.
Open boundaries	Continual changes in regulations governing care and systems improvements require flexible and evolving policies developed with a diversity of input.
Mutual transformation of units across system	Two small community hospitals merge with an academic health center hospital. Units within each original organization must change as an emerging new system replaces the original individual organizations.

The role of the leader in this system is to interact within the system such that those interactions help others to understand how they are expected to relate to other units or agents within the system in the future—all with the goal of creating solutions to complex problems arising in the system.

NURSE LEADERS WITHIN COMPLEX HEALTH CARE SYSTEMS

Many of the ingrained cultural aspects of large complex health care systems may originate in their history as hospitals. American hospitals are laden with history and cultural stories. Throughout most of the 20th century, hospitals were powerful symbols of progress and modern society's affinity for science, technical procedures, and efficiency. In midcentury Western cities, the edifice of the hospital served as a sort of temple in the center of the community where people came as disciples of the art and science of medicine and submitted to its secular–divine authority. Hospitals and health care systems are now much more corporate. But behind the reality of complex health care systems is the embellished nostalgia for the hospital we remember with fondness as an authoritarian but caring community landmark.

Penprase and Norris (2005, p. 128) provided a still relevant explanation of the complexity of a hospital environment:

As one unit makes changes, other nursing units are positively or negatively affected depending upon how each unit elects to adapt to that change. Because change cannot occur without its effects rippling into other competing areas or units, both competition and coevolution work together, as characterized by dynamic equilibrium and causing continuous changes in outcomes (Seel, 2008). Thus, each nursing unit is dependent on another nursing unit as each hospital is dependent on the actions of other hospitals and must adapt to change caused by internal and external factors in order to survive.

Leading within a complex health care organization requires a kind of "complex leadership" (Ford, 2009, p. 101), including facility and flexibility with business practices, beginning with an understanding of terminology. Leaders must be facile with issues of competition, payment models used in care delivery across settings, regulations, and social determinants of health as those factors together influence the effectiveness of the care delivery system.

The current focus on health care reform has revealed the growing trend toward integrated health care systems with boundaries that span emergency and acute care, chronic care management, primary care, and population care management. The evidence to support the effectiveness of this model of integration is yet to be determined. An integrated system may be the answer in one sector, but likely not the only solution for health care (Armitage, Suter, Oelke, & Adair, 2009). Generally, integrated systems link a variety of services and systems, potentially increasing value and reducing costs. Such systems are becoming increasingly competitive in a social environment that demands improved safety, quality, and values-based clinical performance (Englebright & Perlin, 2008). All providers will be expected to develop new competencies to thrive in the world of an integrated care model (Delany, Robinson, & Chafetz, 2013).

It is clear that now is the time for nursing leaders to be prepared to take key leadership roles at the highest levels of such systems in the following areas:

- Assuring quality and patient outcomes
- Promoting executive-level nursing leadership
- Empowering nurses' participation in clinical decision making and organization of clinical care systems
- Maintaining clinical advancement programs based on education, certification, and advanced preparation
- Demonstrating support for nurses in professional development
- Creating collaborative relationships among members of the health care provider team
- Utilizing technological advances in clinical care and information systems (American Association of Colleges of Nursing, 2016)

The complex environment of health care can provoke the development of new strategies to guide professionals and patients through chaos and uncertainty. It requires a clear vision, a few simple rules, and the extension of freedom to support adaptation, evolution, and emergence.

We would argue that in contemporary health systems, nurse leaders must be skilled in creating environments in which nurses can care for patients across boundaries within and outside hospital walls. However, any change in care delivery models will produce some ripple effect across the settings in which the patient receives care. Such interactions among various groups of people or units form feedback loops that move the organization toward new landscapes of care. It is important to understand that such feedback loops are not conceptualized in the same way as feedback loops of traditional systems or leadership theories, where such loops serve to support homeostasis. Rather, feedback loops in complexity theory support communication within the larger organization, feeding new information and creative thinking throughout the organization (Penprase & Norris, 2005). Think of them as webs of informal communication networks interconnected across and within all levels of the organization. Therefore, it is the leader's job to interact across settings and to be clear about expectations for linkages among various units. Proficient leaders can then influence optimal care delivery. Tradition-bound clinicians and leaders accustomed to predictable and controlled systems where change initiatives are based on top-down implementation of prescribed protocols or "best practices" will struggle with new expectations for organizational effectiveness.

Leaders of the next generation will embrace complexity and promote positive emergence. Sitterding and Broome (2015) described the challenges inherent in contemporary health care in which clinicians are continually bombarded with information and changing expectations and conditions, all of which influence care delivery with potential consequences for errors and omissions. In this environment Sitterding and Broome described a "new nurse." This nurse leader is expected to be a knowledge-worker managing competing demands within a very dynamic work environment whose architecture is not always configured in a way to reduce complexity (Sitterding & Broome, 2015). Such new leaders are expected to help nurses to manage the complexities of information overload. They can do this by (a) supporting nurses to tunnel their attention during high-risk or error-prone situations (e.g., medication administration); (b) reminding nurses to avoid relying on memory, but instead to use the tools in the environment to prompt memory (e.g., technology); (c) identifying and eliminating factors that increase fatigue and workload in caregivers at the point of care; and (d) determining which data points and information are critical for nurses to manage and which other data points would be more useful for others to manage.

Complexity in the environments in which we work promotes the opportunity for integrated independent autonomy, accountability, and action to prevent (rather than cause) errors in real time. We must move beyond the idea that complexity promotes error. Inherent in the challenges of complexity are opportunities for creativity and power to make critical immediate decisions and actions that change lives for the better. But seizing these opportunities requires personal integrity, accountability, commitment, and creative leadership.

REFLECTION QUESTIONS

1. Think about your current work environment. Identify a recurring challenge in care delivery that results in frustration, increased cost, fragmented care, or potential for errors. Identify the various factors that influence every aspect of the situation (personnel, process, etc.).

(continued)

REFLECTION QUESTIONS (*continued*)

2. Generate several solutions to the problem you have identified. Now choose one of those and map out what relationships would need to be explored, strengthened, or connected to begin to plan the implementation of your solution.

3. Now rate, using a three-option system, how time consuming (not at all, a little, a lot) that solution or connection would be. How many other relationships would need to be included to gather information, generate ideas about factors impinging on the problem, and so on, and how much energy and time might that take?

4. As you examine your plan, where would you begin to address the challenge you have identified if you were the leader of the area in which the challenge presents itself?

TAKING AN ORGANIZATIONAL AND SYSTEMS PERSPECTIVE

Clinicians who are accustomed to focusing on the care of individual patients often find it a challenge to acquire the larger organization and systems perspective. It is like learning a new language or culture. To gain the perspective of the entire organization or system requires a different way of thinking. It includes an emphasis on how people and processes are related, how they work, and how they are connected. As you have learned after completing the reflection exercise, rather than thinking of a procedure or problem in a one step-at-a-time linear fashion, organization or systems thinking considers multiple ideas, activities, and people connecting in a matrix of processes. Many dimensions are at play at the same time.

Systems thinking is the only hope to solve some of the most entangled problems. Cipriano (2008, p. 6) explained why systems thinking is critical for leaders in current health care settings:

> A systems thinker sees how the parts of an organization interact
> and how effectively people are working together. This new way of
> thinking permits us to see things we didn't see before. Expanded
> thinking allows us to recognize and imagine ways of solving problems
> by grasping entire processes and systems. Such thinking also
> reinforces the idea that the whole is greater than the sum of its parts.

Systems thinking is not simply moving the focus from the individual patient to the unit, organization, or even the institution. It requires an ability to begin with the big picture and to live in the world of an entire system. Most scientists and clinicians have been socialized according to a Descartian reductionist approach to deductively see the parts of the whole. Systems thinking is based on the opposite idea that the parts are best understood, and problems are best solved, as they relate to the whole system.

A system is a dynamic and complex whole. Porter-O'Grady and Malloch (2011) explained the difference between elements of the institution and the system as a whole by emphasizing that within institutions, most of the operational work is compartmentalized and organized vertically and distal from the administrators. To lead any one element, a leader must direct his or her vision from the whole to the part.

The leader who is a systems thinker understands that systems are about relationships, matrices of connections, community, and culture. It is often a challenging dance to lead both the individual at the point of service, who is focused on getting a discrete job done, and the larger system of connections and relationships related to the health, thriving, and future of the organization or constituency of organizations. It is also somewhat of an act of faith to understand that complex social systems self-organize within a context of chaos.

There are multiple advantages to a systems view. Systems thinking facilitates the analysis of structures, patterns, and cycles rather than a series of isolated events. From this perspective, problem solving becomes more systematic, and the solution to one problem can be seen to affect the solution to others within the system. The leader may think in terms of "leverage points" or positive change in one element of the system that subsequently improves another part (McNamara, 2009). Not only does systems problem solving show immediate or subsequent synergistic effects, but often, the positive effects are also long term rather than short lived.

Drucker (2004, p. 59) further outlined eight practices that distinguishes effective executives and enhance systems thinking. Such leaders see the big picture and take action from the perspective of entire systems. According to Drucker, the leader:

- Asks, "What needs to be done?"
- Asks, "What is right for the enterprise?"
- Develops action plans
- Takes responsibility for decisions
- Takes responsibility for communicating
- Focuses on opportunities rather than problems
- Runs productive meetings
- Thinks and says "we" rather than "I"

This list of behaviors of executive leaders may seem simple. However, within complex systems, such behaviors require much intentional thought and planning to achieve.

COMPLEX ENVIRONMENTS AND CONTINUAL CHANGE

Living and Working in Change

Continual change in our work environments is a reality of life. It is a necessary way of life for leaders to learn how to help themselves and others to live effectively with continual change and succeed in contexts of uncertainty and complexity. Effective change deeply affects the culture, structure, and processes in an organization. Change efforts can be planned or unplanned, tactical or strategic, evolutionary or revolutionary.

Modern human societies have developed across several distinct ages. The transitions, or change, between each era have been marked with turmoil. Between each age is a mix of thrill and concern, excitement and fear, energy and resistance, prophets and doomsayers. And there is always some chaos. Likely, there was strife as villages were born when farming communities moved from the era of hunter-gatherers to the agricultural age. Harder still were the disruption of family life and the eruption of whole new diseases, public health issues, and new economic paradigms when society moved from the farm to the industrial age. Individuals eventually learned how to live and love the industrial age with its rules, its linear thinking, and its focus on efficiency and production. Until the late 20th century, we also became comfortable as a society with hierarchical leadership and regulation of our lives. There were few sources for answers or information: the person in charge, an expert sage, or a book in a library. There were few choices of products and, usually, no or limited choices for public services. We were simply happy to have dependable public services.

We have left the industrial age and are now deep into an information/technology age. All the rules have changed. Those over age 30 learned about sources of information in completely different ways from those under 30 ("digital natives"), who grew up in the digital age. All information, and in fact perhaps too much information, is always available within minutes. Sources of information are vast and highly accessible, and the range of choices has exploded. Just a couple of decades ago, who would have thought you might listen to music, access e-mail, play a game, or even watch a movie on your telephone. We have more avenues for more information than any individual can accommodate. Drucker (2000, p. 8) predicted:

> In a few hundred years, when the history of our time is written
> from a long-term perspective, it is likely that the most important
> event historians will see is not technology, not the internet, not
> e-commerce. It is an unprecedented change in the human condition.
> For the first time—literally—substantial and rapidly growing
> numbers of people have choices. For the first time, they will have to
> manage themselves. And society is totally unprepared for it.

Drucker's observations continue to be relevant. In fact, given the shifts in health care, with much responsibility for self-management of chronic illness placed on individuals and families, it seems people still struggle with how to manage information and their responsibility for self-care.

We are now seeing the outcomes and effects of that continual change and information overload on health care workers. Many observers thought multitasking was the answer to managing the overload, but evidence has made it clear that the human organism, while capable of multitasking, is not efficient or effective when doing so (Sitterding & Broome, 2015). This has major implications for how leaders lead. Change is constant, but some changes in the environment that the leader must initiate to improve outcomes are fast paced, abrupt, and disruptive. So effective leaders must think not only about how change affects people but also about how execution of change can make all the difference in their responses and performance.

Supporting Others During Change. Recent fiscal realities have brought unforeseen change to nursing employment, practice, and leadership. Like other major industries, hospitals and some other health care facilities have engaged in restructuring to manage costs (Hewner, Seo, Gothard, & Johnson, 2014; Tsai, Joynt, Wild, Orav, & Jha, 2015). For the first time in recent memory, positions in nursing have decreased in abundance. This is largely due to restructuring of care delivery models that now include more diverse teams of care providers ranging from physicians to supportive care assistants. In a recent study (Pittman & Forrest, 2015) of the perceptions of leaders from 18 of the original 32 pioneer accountable care organizations, leaders believed that payment models were clearly affecting the roles of nurses in their organizations. These role changes required that teams of professional nurses and other nonprofessional but well-trained employees work together to provide care across settings. These roles will require new knowledge and skills for the professional nurse and nursing leader. This kind of role change produces stress for most individuals who must now adapt and learn new ways of working with and providing care for their patients. As a leader you must be continually aware of and responsive to how others perceive change and then provide strategies to support them.

Leading Change. Change means to transform or to become something different. To lead change is to generate and mobilize resources toward innovation and improvement. Change is described in terms of first order and second order. First-order change is an adjustment within an existing structure, doing more or less of something, and is reversible. Second-order change, on the other hand, is transformational. It requires new ways of perceiving and doing things, new learning, and it is irreversible. The rules are different in second-order change. Such change requires new learning and creates a new story (Pesut, 2008a). Pesut (2008a) further explained that problem-oriented change looks at what is wrong or why and how are we limited by the problem. Alternatively, an appreciative approach directs change toward identifying what is good, what is already working, what is desired, and what resources exist to achieve the desired result (Cooperrider, Whitney, & Stavros, 2008). Planned change often emerges from review of the meaning and relevancy of the organizational mission statement, from facing new systems or technology, and from recognition of the need for new ways of decision making, practice, and policies.

Change agents lead and support others in change by creating environments that promote desired change. They use their power to support and influence others toward change. Effective leaders are change agents. Change agents must:

- Be trustworthy, reliable, honest, competent, and credible
- Possess persuasion, negotiation, and effective listening skills
- Embody leadership through demonstration of a strong work ethic
- Be enthusiastic and demonstrate respect for individual differences
- Have the ability to think conceptually and organize thoughts logically
- Have the skill to plan and most importantly execute activities and plans
- Have good judgment and strong communication skills
- Be able to coach and facilitate others (Pesut, 2008b, pp. 103–104)

In environments of change, effective leaders are early adapters of innovation. They are able to see change as an opportunity to learn and improve. Leaders do not hand down mandates for change. Instead, they wisely identify needs or directions on the horizon; then they support, encourage, and feed local inclinations and movements toward change. Nevertheless, leaders in health care are often required by administrative mandate to implement change.

Change management experts believe *how* change is led makes all the difference in the organization's ability to negotiate change. Powerful principles of leading change are reflected in Kotter's (2007) well-known eight steps for organizational transformation:

1. Establish a sense of urgency
2. Form a powerful guiding coalition
3. Create a vision
4. Communicate the vision
5. Empower others to act on that vision
6. Plan for and create short-term wins
7. Consolidate improvements and produce more change
8. Institutionalize new approaches

However, many leaders forget that if one step in the list is skipped (e.g., communicate the vision), then later efforts to regain momentum and the clarity and engagement of others will be very difficult. It is impossible to empower others to act on a vision for the outcomes of the change occurring if they are not clear what the vison or outcome will be. In Box 2.1, read about how one leader successfully implemented a scale change in her department.

Change can happen through power, by empowering others to engage and contribute to the change. It can happen through reason, by appealing to logic and rationales, and by education and reeducation to provide knowledge and skills. Change also happens by altering structures and processes. The leader must identify which approach is the most appropriate. For example, if workers already *know* information or have skills but feel powerless to make decisions, then development of education or training programs will not produce

BOX 2.1. CASE STUDY: IMPROVING END-OF-LIFE CARE FOR PATIENTS ON A SURGICAL ONCOLOGY UNIT

Mary Simmons is the director for surgical services. She has been a director for 4 years and has four units that report to her, including oncology surgical services. The hospital system administration has been discussing a new model of care for two units in Mary's area. This new care model, called "An Integrated Learning Unit for Palliative Care," will be implemented in September. At that point the 20 baccalaureate-prepared registered nurses will lead 10 teams with three home care workers each, who will care for six to eight patients or families across both hospital and home care settings, 24 hours a day. The system expects to hire and train 20 new home care workers, who will work across the settings under the supervision of the professional nurses.

The unit manager, Sam Werley, MSN, just graduated with his degree in nursing administration in May. He first heard of this change in June after meeting with his director, Mary Simmons. Mary's leadership style, as a general rule, is transactional, and she expects her nurse managers to take charge of problems, come up with solutions, and present them to her for approval. In this case she assures Sam he will do fine with implementing the change, saying, "You have just learned all the new ways of managing change and people." But she also reminds him that he has only 3 months to prepare his unit for the change, hire new home care workers, prepare the professional nurses to assume leadership of teams, and develop a plan to monitor and evaluate the effectiveness of the care delivery model on patient and family satisfaction and other outcomes, such as return of patients to the emergency department, rehospitalizations, or adverse events.

1. What should Sam think is "the sense of urgency" in this situation? What would be a reasonable approach to communicate the sense of urgency to others? How do you think staff on the unit will respond?
2. Who should Sam assemble to create the coalition that will help him guide the unit personnel through this dramatic change in their roles? What is the best size for this kind of coalition?
3. Who should be primarily responsible for creating and communicating the vision for the change? What might the outcome look like? How is the vision connected to the evaluation plan?
4. What specific strategies could Sam and the coalition members enact that would build a sense of empowerment in those working on the unit? What should they do first? Second? What might be some short term "wins" for the employees that would encourage them?
5. When the hiring begins who should be involved? What kind of person do you think would be a "best fit" with the new model?
6. What kinds of criteria would you use to evaluate the effectiveness of the change model? The care model? The delivery of care and employee satisfaction?

desired changes. Rather, workers may need more independence, autonomy, and accountability in decision making.

Change is a journey taken together with those with whom you work. Each change process is unique. And it is important to remember that as nimble as your organization may be, change usually takes longer than you expect.

Change and Reflective Adaptation. The effective leader is well aware that not all organizations are necessarily ready for, or even need, immediate transformation at any given moment. It is often wise to watch and wait. Sometimes, resistance to change can be so strong as to defeat even the most charismatic leader. Even if it is your perception that immediate change is needed, particularly in a new role, take some time for assessment—be the chief listening officer for a while. Sometimes, no action is better than the full court press, at least for assessment. A sensitive systems thinker, especially in a new position, may be well advised to take time to simply watch.

One of the most effective strategies to launch change used by the authors of this book is that of appreciative inquiry (AI). Once a challenge is identified, it is helpful to engage the stakeholders who will guide the change in the four phases of AI (see Figure 2.1). AI builds on existing strength and success. It is based on the idea that those who focus on problems will continue to find and build on more problems, but organizations in which there is a sense of pride and appreciation will build on what is good or positive.

The model includes four concepts: discovery, dream, design, and delivery. Discovery represents the "positive core," based on the idea that in the heart of the organization something is working well. The dream concept invites imagination and envisioning of what can be better. Design means to articulate the values, propositions, and plans of the desired future; and delivery means to act on the dream, to implement the plan, and to create "what will be" (Cooperrider & Sravasta, 1987; Cooperrider & Whitney, 2005, p. 30; Keefe & Pesut, 2004, p. 104; Whitney & Schau, 1998). This positive and constructive approach to working with groups to promote and implement change allows them to be highly

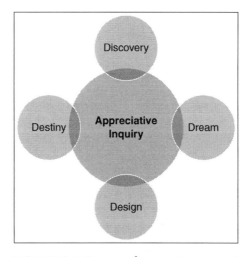

FIGURE 2.1 Stages of appreciative inquiry.
Adapted from Broome visualization of concepts and Cooperrider, Whitney, and Stavros (2008, p. 102).

involved in and identified with what the unit is doing well *now*, to identify the preferred future related to this challenge, to create a process and procedure for making the desired future a reality, and to engage in thinking about how to sustain the change and empower others.

The process of reflective adaptation is a helpful method to conceptualize and facilitate local change. Using the AI process can help others to adapt to a necessary change using a positive framework by structuring the conversations toward the mindset, "What good do we do, what good can we create?"

Although complexity and emergent change may be attractive and exciting for the new transformational leader, some planning, strategy, and a place for reflection must accompany such change initiatives. Five guiding principles support a successful, reflective adaptation process:

1. Vision, mission, and shared values are fundamental in guiding ongoing change processes in a complex adaptive system.
2. Creating time and space for learning and reflection is necessary for a complex adaptive system to adapt to and plan change.
3. Tension and discomfort are essential and normal during complex adaptive systems change.
4. Improvement teams should include a variety of the system's agents with different perspectives of the system and its environment.
5. System change requires supportive leadership that is actively involved in the change process, ensuring full participation from all members, and protecting time for reflection (Daly, Hill, & Jackson, 2014).

Using the reflective adaptive process, the leader models "reflection–action" cycles and encourages team members to reflect on change and learning. The leader guides the team to strengthen relationships and improve self-organization processes, provides images of adapting processes rather than a sole focus on outcomes, and facilitates the team in creating new "stories" or different ways to perceive, understand, and work in new conceptual environments (Stroebel et al., 2005, p. 442). The sensitive leader, even in the midst of chaos, plans, reflects, and allows the group involved in change to plan, practice change, and reflect on learning from the experience.

Change as a Personal Challenge for the Leader. Most leadership texts address change as something that leaders are not only involved in but also encourage and manage. Wheatley (2009, p. 81) described a state of "groundlessness," when nothing seems to be working. She reminded, "Groundlessness is a frightening place . . . , at least at first, but as the old culture turns to mush, we would feel stronger if we stopped searching for ground, if we sought only to locate ourselves in the present and do our work from *here*."

It is important to manage your own time and stress when you find yourself in the midst of a big change initiative. Identify a confidant (often the best choice is someone outside of the organization who can be objective) who will support you through the challenges of your work. That person can help you to recognize the effects of your own nature on others during the change process. Stand strong to your own values and maintain the image of your change model from in your mind, recognizing that your image likely will not be exactly what eventually evolves. Resist the temptation to either overcontrol or "do the work yourself." Allow others to put their own marks on the initiative while you ensure that the change activities support the mission of the organization. Identify and share early successes. Remember that you are changing processes or products, not people or personalities. Build on strengths where you can. Build in accountabilities and be careful to monitor the process at regular intervals. Stay close to and touch base often with those experiencing the change. Identify opportunities for learning for everyone and celebrate small and large accomplishments along the way.

Facing the uncertainty of change is a personal challenge, particularly if you are in charge of the lives and work of others. Realities in health care sometimes bring mandates for change and the requirement for you as a leader to move it forward. Although the temptation may be to resist or stall, often, the best way to find a sense of power or security is to simply step forward and engage yourself and others in change processes. Gilbert and Broome (2015) outlined several strategies to be used by managers and clinical leaders expected to negotiate change. These are:

- Learn to let go of your position to control. This is risky as one then has to depend on others to effect the changes you think you want and things may not occur on your timetable.
- Learn to be comfortable with life on the edge, requiring you to build on strong networks of relationships, communication channels, and trust in others.
- Get out of the data trap. Use your skills to identify what data are really important to help the participants you work with to understand the situation. Communicate clearly how long-range goals are related to the data.

Clinical leaders must develop a sense of timing and a willingness to engage in the rhythm of change processes. It requires anticipation, responsiveness, nimble action, and the willingness to lead others into a new reality. You can become the model of change for others and, thereby, can communicate the invitation and urgency for transformation.

One of the most critical and least discussed aspects of change leadership is the fundamental principle of trust. Such trust is earned only by consistent ethical behavior and clearly defined values. Regardless of our rhetoric on embracing complexity and relishing change as a way of life, usually change is difficult for people to accept. Subordinates often fear that change will "happen" to them, and there is sometimes an uneasy expectation that change will threaten control, autonomy, habit, or comfort. The wise leader who has grounded his or her leadership in relationships will be honest and transparent. Furthermore, the successful leader will remember that "*truth* is more important during periods of change and uncertainty than good news" (Rogerson, n.d.). Such a leader will always consider perceptions and the dynamics of human relationships when launching change.

REFLECTION QUESTIONS

1. How do you find yourself thinking and feeling in the midst of change in your organization? What are your biggest concerns?
2. What are your greatest strengths from which you draw in times of change?
3. Do you have a personal ritual (e.g., exercise, meditation, reading) that you find useful in reducing your stress?
4. Can you identify two people outside the organization who can listen to your thoughts and feelings as you negotiate and support others during a major change?
5. Can you mobilize resources within the organization to help you support others (e.g., facilitators in human resources)?

Real change will happen only when each individual makes the decision to implement the change. If people trust you as the leader, and you share a clear direction and vision and extend meaningful opportunity for input and contribution into the change planning and processes, followers will help to define the most effective path to change and improve quality as a matter of their own personal integrity and commitment to the mission of the organization and the work.

Drawing on the Wisdom of All Experts During Change. Effective change does not happen within the purview of a solitary leader. In the position of leader, you have the freedom and opportunity to network with experts from all disciplines. The world of leadership in health care practice is wide. The effective leader learns the language, reads the literature, and becomes interested and informed about the inside view of a vast variety of disciplines, both within and outside health care. Successful organizations owe their success to the dedication and inventiveness of their people. At the end of the day, our progress and success depend on each other—as peers, colleagues, subordinates, and strangers. We are all explorers in the new world of the future. We must develop our own areas of expertise, respect the expertise of others, and acknowledge where we must come together when none of us has the answer.

In the context of complex adaptive systems, do not confine your thinking to working only with people you know inside the organization or even by the usual professional networking. Furthermore, do not be limited to collaboration only with health care professionals. One of the delights of being a leader is the ability to invite collegiality with a broad range of professional friends. It is amazing how people respond when you simply introduce yourself and ask them to help. In this age of websites and e-mail, when you admire the work of an expert, do not be afraid to send off a note or make a call. Be prepared, respectful, gracious, and specific in your need.

Think about including experts in business, politics, anthropology, geography, languages, and even the arts as you build your personal style and repertoire to lead the next generation. Read the works of other disciplines, including those of current great minds. Think about how their thoughts might contribute to your work. Imagine how your world might expand and how others will benefit from your renaissance approach to health care leadership. Among the most inspiring mentors in my own experiences [Marshall] in health care leadership have been a lawyer, a development officer, a musician, and a professor of Italian.

When you draw from a broad range of disciplines and communities, you create generative relationships (Rowe & Hogarth, 2005) that release energy, create ideas, and support change. When there is productive sharing of ideas, problems, responsibility for decisions, and a variety of viewpoints, your work becomes more fulfilling and productive. It generates goodwill, positive change, worker satisfaction, and a generative foundation for the next generation of leaders. Soon, you will be surprised how others will be drawn to your leadership and your organization. They will want to be part of your team.

STRATEGIC PLANNING IN THE MIDST OF CONTINUAL CHANGE

Effective strategy is built on the organization's vision, mission, and values. It is *not* operational efficiency (Porter, 2011), despite the focus in many health care organizations today. Vision, mission, and values have become the well-worn currency of strategic planning. First, remember that mission, vision, and values *represent* what you do. They are important symbols and expressions. They are the voice of your organization—but they are not what you actually do. Regardless of their overuse in today's corporate world, mission, vision, and values retain their position as the foundation for the strategic direction of organizations. They are the currency of the day. So they are reviewed here to help you avoid cynicism within your own organization. It is in your best interest as a leader to make them yours and make them live.

The vision should clearly identify *why* you do what you do. Vision provides people with a passion for what they do—it is the touchstone for every employee in the organization. It is the "why" we get up and go to work every day. Sinek (2010) spoke in a TED talk about "How great leaders inspire action," underscoring how critical it is that every leader examines the "why" of what he or she does before trying to work with others to develop a vision. Vision statements should be short and clearly inspire others as well as those within the organization. Some examples of vision statements for nonprofit organizations include:

- Our vision is a world without Alzheimer's (Alzheimer's Association)
- A world where everyone has a decent place to live (Habitat for Humanity)
- To become a world leader at connecting people to wildlife and conservation (San Diego Zoo)
- That the United States is a humane community in which all animals are treated with respect and kindness (ASPCA)
- A world free of breast cancer (Alamo Breast Cancer Foundation)

A vision is the picture of your ideal future. It is idealistic, elegant, and ambitious but reflects the work and mission of the organization. It sets a standard of excellence; it reflects the purpose, direction, and uniqueness of the organization; and it inspires.

The mission clearly identifies *what you do*, *what your purpose is*, and *why you do it* as an organization. It is your vision put to work. Keep it simple and to the basics of the essential activities of the organization. Following is a home-made example: "Shawfeld Community Care is a community-based agency of professional nurses and volunteers who provide compassionate home health and support services to Smith county adults and children suffering chronic or life-threatening illness." Another example is the mission statement of the Alamo Breast Cancer Foundation (2016): "To end breast cancer by assisting patients, informing health professionals and policymakers, and expanding knowledge through education and community outreach."

Values are the guides for conduct and principles of behavior in performing the mission and following the vision. Examples are compassion, caring, quality, respect. Values are easy for people to list, but less easy for them to reflect and enact in their behavior on a daily basis.

Strategic Planning Process

Strategic planning in the midst of continual change is somewhat akin to driving a car while the road is still under construction. Some of the uncertainties the future holds can make it difficult to dream about the future to create a meaning-ful vision statement. Strategic planning is a useful process to guide the organization into your *preferred future*, but it is just an exercise if you are not committed to it. It can only be effective if you are a strategic leader.

The strategic leader continually thinks of the organization with a perspective from higher levels, taking a larger perspective of analysis, and looking into the future. You must think conceptually and creatively, always examining internal applications in a context of the larger community. Strategic thinking looks forward. Thus, it always carries some challenges and risks. It is a challenge to think large and into the future while concurrently attending to the local immediate issues.

Strategic planning has been defined as a "process of identifying directions and facilitating the alignment of purpose, people, plans, and actions with the aim of serving a co-created, value driven, desired outcome" (Pesut, 2008b). It is not an option for the health care leader. It is a mandate. Strategic planning is one of your most important activities.

As organizations have become more complex, so has the process of strategic planning. But the basic steps are simple. Schaffner (2009, p. 152) encouraged, "Start simple, but start." Thoughtful planning, effective execution, and ongoing evaluation are critical for the strategic plan to be more than just a symbolic exercise.

Strategic planning refers to long-range visioning and planning for the entire organization. In today's health care systems, it is a critical exercise in order for the organization not just to survive but to thrive. Strategic planning is expansive and conceptual, whereas tactical or operational planning involves goal setting or objective development for shorter term, more targeted, or local plans that are part of the larger strategic plan. Both kinds of planning are necessary and critically important to ensure all stakeholders are included in the organization. Some kind of strategic planning is helpful at the team, group, unit, or system level. Strategic planning from a transformational perspective involves visioning, planning, and executing in the best possible manner to fulfill the purpose or principles for which the organization stands. Deliberate and careful planning helps the transformational leader to define and crystallize goals for the organization and the people involved. It allows the opportunity to affirm values, define principles, and break the path toward a more effective organization with high personal satisfaction for all involved in the enterprise. It requires precision of expression and innovative thinking.

A strategic plan is a roadmap to the desired future, so it may address a future of 1, 3, 5, or even more years, but it must project into the future. Baker et al. (2000, p. 98) outlined significant purposes of the strategic plan:

- Represents a long-range vision for improving organizational performance
- Provides a model for planning and implementing structures and processes for the management of outcomes
- Reflects and shapes the organizational culture and customer focus
- Provides decision support for difficult operational choices day by day
- Integrates and aligns the work of the organization

Schaffner (2009) outlined 10 steps for success in strategic planning for nursing, which we shall draw from and adapt to the larger health care perspective. Schaffner's work provides the framework and foundation for the following discussion:

1. Appoint a strategic planning steering committee. This team should include the appropriate number of key personnel and stakeholders of the organization. Think about who should be included. You need some visionary thinkers, some realists, and some representatives from all corners of your influence as an organization, and you must have the support of higher administration. Orient members of the committee to their roles and to the process of strategic planning itself.
2. Use strategic analysis to guide the planning, using key indicators. Schaffner proposed that this step may be done "behind the scenes" (p. 153). This is often done by external consultant teams who know the organization but who have the time to collect the data both internally and externally to present to the steering committee. The data may include information related to finances, personnel, satisfaction and quality metrics, community demographics, health care trends, competitors' scope of delivery and business, and whatever else is deemed important in planning.
3. Key stakeholder interviews are conducted to assess perceptions of the enterprise. This step is often overlooked in strategic planning activities and must be

done carefully to ensure that those interviewed believe their responses will be only reported in the aggregate. Schaffner suggested the use of a standard set of questions, but you should spread the net wide for the interviews. Include all who have any vested interested in your enterprise. Include computer-based surveys of the broader population. Most important is to develop a data-based picture of the perceptions of the current situation and visions of the future.

4. Share key stakeholder interview and analytical data. Everyone involved in planning needs the benefit of all baseline data.

5. Conduct a SWOT analysis. This is a critical step in any strategic planning process: examination of **S**trengths, **W**eaknesses, **O**pportunities, and **T**hreats related to effective performance or to the fulfillment of the vision of the organization. The SWOT analysis can be valid only to the degree that all players are involved at some point in the process. Using data from the interviews, the steering committee can create a SWOT analysis and then vet it widely for feedback at town halls with a broad representation of employees. Evaluation of strengths and weaknesses must be honest, performed within an environment where all discussion is safe. This helps the leader and members of the organization to identify internal capabilities and challenges. Evaluation of opportunities and threats includes consideration of possibilities and challenges outside the organization. It requires analysis of issues within the community and the entire industry, and identification of signs of future or emerging issues outside the realm of the organization. Use of the term *threats* is not always accurate in this context because this component of the analysis often does not refer to actual threats to the mission or success of the organization. Threats may include challenges in the community, changes in the external environment, or technological innovations that the organization should consider.

6. Brainstorm potential strategies. The first part of this step needs to be wide open and free. Allow time and space for dreaming. Record all possibilities; let no idea be withheld or precluded. The next step is to narrow the strategies to less than half a dozen strategic actions or goals that are aligned with the mission and goals of the organization and speak to its vision. This can be done by a smaller group and then presented back to the larger group for voting and prioritizing. Strategies are stated within a framework of a roadmap or goals for the future. The strategies need to imply that their accomplishment will change the organization toward its desired future.

7. Complete a gap analysis around the strategies. Analyze the difference between the newly designed strategies and the current state of the organization. This helps the group to develop tactical goals or objectives.

8. Develop a tactical plan. Usually, a handful of specific tactical objectives are identified under each strategy.

9. Develop metrics for the strategic plan. Metrics are the measures that reflect success or failure on each objective and strategy. They need to produce outcome data. In addition to specific measures, an evaluation plan needs to outline what the data sources are, when and how often measurements are taken, who is responsible, and to whom the results will be reported.

10. Communicate a strategic plan. The plan should be broadly communicated at all stages. It can become a vehicle for sharing your mission and direction as well as eliciting internal and external support.

The strategic plan is launched from the vision, which is the inspiring banner that reflects the loftiest identity and dream of the organization. The plan begins with broad but achievable and measurable goals. They may relate to strategic leadership, systems, and specific aspects of the work of the organization. Under each of the strategic goals are listed more local, specific, and measurable objectives. In addition, the responsible team or person who is accountable for the achievement of the objectives is identified. The process to achieve the objectives is usually mapped out by some sort of timeline or logic model.

Moving the Plan Into Action

Once the strategic planning process is in place, obviously, it will do no good if it is put on the shelf until the next committee meeting, annual retreat, or accreditation visit. It really is possible for a well-developed strategic plan to guide the direction of the organization. But it is up to you as the leader to make it work. This will require that you, as a leader, ask for quarterly reports verbally and annual reports in writing, using the framework of the strategic plan. Evaluating people is a special case. Invite workers to articulate their performance goals alongside your expectations for their performance. Document and measure achievement of expectations. Track progress with data. Provide opportunities for improvement and follow-up. Use personnel evaluations not only as performance reviews for retention or advancement, but also for teaching and growth.

To implement the strategic plan, begin by communicating it broadly. It is helpful to outline the plan in a specific format or template (Schaffner, 2009). Templates are likely available within your organization and certainly can be found by looking at the strategic plans of other organizations. It is also a good idea to assign a champion for each section of the plan who can monitor implementation and achievement of goals. In addition, it is critical that the plan be evaluated annually so that if new initiatives surface they can be integrated into the existing plan and not ignored.

Effective Evaluation of the Strategic Plan

Achievement of goals of the strategic plan is documented by an evaluation plan. Most evaluation plans follow some sort of logic model that includes inputs, activities, outputs, intermediate outcomes, and end outcomes. End outcomes must reflect tangible results that represent the success or failure of the organization. In other words, evaluation requires data, and the results of data and analyses should reflect the mission and purpose of the work. Intermediate outcomes reflect the success of strategies to achieve the end outcomes. In addition to the strategic plan, evaluation plans may map performance plans, accountability tracking, or other data collection and data-tracking plans. All major aspects of the organization should be included somewhere on the overall organizational evaluation plan.

Components of the plan may include performance management, financial management, information technology and management, and management of activities related to the mission of the organization. Mission activities include patient outcome and satisfaction data.

Each objective should be measurable, and the evaluation plan should include specific tools or measures with accountability and designated time intervals for taking measurements on each objective. Avoid too many tools or a plan that measures process instead of outcomes. If there is general resistance to an outcomes orientation or an evaluation plan, this component will be meaningless. Therefore, your evaluation activities should include motivation, clarification, and invitations to engagement. The organization must invest in evaluation and use the results to improve its work.

In today's culture of outcomes, evaluation encompasses much more than measures related to the strategic plan. Evaluation is a part of every activity of health care. Entire volumes, courses, and experts are available and should be consulted as you set out to develop and sustain an evaluation plan. We evaluate resources, personnel, patient outcomes, satisfaction, processes, and everything else we care about. As a leader, always think about how you will evaluate what you are doing, who is responsible for doing it, or both. Have an overall plan for data collection to provide evidence for the evaluation decisions you make. Evaluation should be done as systematically as research, with a plan, specific questions, data, analysis, and use of the data to make informed decisions. This pertains to processes, outcomes, and people. It is only when the loop of visioning, planning, implementing, and evaluating is closed that true progress can be made.

REFERENCES

Alamo Breast Cancer Foundation. (2016). *About us: Mission.* Retrieved from http://www.alamobreastcancer.org/about-us/mission/

American Association of Colleges of Nursing (2016). Hallmarks of the professional nursing practice environment. Washington DC: Author. Retrieved from http://www.aacn.nche.edu/publications/white-papers/hallmarks-practice-environment

Armitage, G. D., Suter, E., Oelke, N. D., & Adair, C. E. (2009). Health systems integration: State of the evidence. *International Journal of Integrative Care, 9*, e.82.

Baker, C., Beglinger, J., Bowles, K., Brandt, C., Brennan, K. M., Engelbaugh, S., . . . LaHam, M. (2000). Building a vision for the future: Strategic planning in a shared governance nursing organization. *Seminars in Nursing Management, 8*(2), 98–106.

Capra, F. (1982). *The turning point.* Toronto, ON, Canada: Bantam.

Capra, F. (1997). *The web of life.* New York, NY: Anchor.

Cipriano, P. F. (2008). Improving health care systems thinking. *American Nurse Today, 3*(9), 6.

Cooperrider, D., Whitney, D., & Stavros, J. (2008). *Appreciative inquiry handbook.* (2nd ed.). Brunswick, OH: Crown Custom.

Daly, J., Hill, M., & Jackson, D. (2014). Leadership and healthcare change management. In J. Daly, S. Speedy, & D. Jackson (Eds.), *Leadership and nursing* (2nd ed.). Sydney, Australia: Elsevier.

Delany, K., Robinson, K., & Chafez, L. (2013). Development of integrated mental health care: Critical workforce competencies. *Nursing Outlook, 61*(6), 384–391.

Drucker, P. (2000). Managing knowledge means managing oneself. *Leader to Leader, 16.* Retrieved from http://rlaexp.com/studio/biz/conceptual_resources/authors/peter_drucker/mkmmo_org.pdf

Drucker, P. (2004, June). What makes an effective executive. *Harvard Business Review, 82*(6), 58–63.

Englebright, J., & Perlin, J. (2008). The chief nurse executive role in large healthcare systems. *Nursing Administration Quarterly, 32*(3), 188–194.

Ford, R. (2009). Complex leadership competency in healthcare: Toward framing a theory of practice. *Health Services Management, 22*(3), 101–114.

Gilbert, J., & Broome, M. E. (2015). Leadership in a complex world. In M. Sitterding & M. E. Broome (Eds.), *Information overload: Framework, tips, and tools to manage in complex healthcare environments.* Washington, DC: American Nurses Association.

Goldstein, J., Hazy, J. L., & Lichtenstein, B. B. (2010). *Complexity and the nexus of leadership.* New York, NY: Palgrave Macmillan.

Hewner, S., Seo, J. Y., Gothard, S. E., & Johnson, B. J. (2014). Aligning population-based care management with chronic disease complexity. *Nursing Outlook, 62*(4), 250–258.

Keefe, M., & Pesut, D. (2004). Appreciative inquiry and leadership transitions. *Journal of Professional Nursing, 20*(2), 103–109.

Kotter, J. P. (2007, January 3–10). Leading change: Why transformation efforts fail. *Harvard Business Review,* 92–107.

Lindberg, C., Nash, S., & Lindberg, D. (2008). *On the edge: Nursing in the age of complexity.* Bordentown, NJ: Plexus Press.

McNamara, C. (2009). *Field guide to consulting and organizational development.* Minneapolis, MN: Authenticity Consulting.

Paley, J. (2007). Complex adaptive systems and nursing. *Nursing Inquiry, 14*(3), 233–242.

Penprase, B., & Norris, D. (2005). What nurse leaders should know about complex adaptive systems theory. *Nursing Leadership Forum, 9*(3), 127–132.

Pesut, D. J. (2008a). Change. In H. R. Feldman, M. Jadde-Ruiz, M. L. McClure, M. H. Greenberg, & T. D. Smith (Eds.), *Nursing leadership: A concise encyclopedia* (pp. 100–102). New York, NY: Springer Publishing Company.

Pesut, D. J. (2008b). Change agents and change agent strategies. In H. R. Feldman, M. Jaffe-Ruiz, L. McClure, J. M. Greenberg, & T. D. Smith (Eds.), *Nursing leadership: A concise encyclopedia* (pp. 103–105). New York, NY: Springer Publishing Company.

Pesut, D. J. (2008c). Complex adaptive systems (chaos theory). In H. R. Feldman, M. Jaffe-Ruiz, L. McClure, J. M. Greenberg, & T. D. Smith (Eds.), *Nursing leadership: A concise encyclopedia* (pp. 123–124). New York, NY: Springer Publishing Company.

Pittman, P., & Forrest, E. (2015). The changing roles of registered nurses in Pioneer Accountable Care Organizations. *Nursing Outlook, 63*(5), 554–565.

Porter, M. (2011). What is strategy? *Harvard Business Review,* November, 3–20.

Porter-O'Grady, T., & Malloch, K. (2011). *Quantum leadership: Advancing innovation, transforming health care* (3rd ed.). Sudbury, MA: Jones & Bartlett.

Quantum Mechanics. (2016). Retrieved from https://en.wikipedia.org/wiki/Quantum_mechanics

Rogerson, L. (n.d.). *Twelve principles of managing change.* Retrieved from http://www.lynco.com/12prin.html

Romley, J., Goldman, D., & Sood, N. (2015). US hospitals experienced substantial productivity growth during 2002–2011. *Health Affairs, 34*(3), 511–517.

Rowe, A., & Hogarth, A. (2005). Use of complex adaptive systems metaphor to achieve professional and organizational change. *Journal of Advanced Nursing, 51*(4), 396–405.

Schaffner, J. (2009). Roadmap for success: The 10-step nursing strategic plan. *Journal of Nursing Administration, 39*(4), 152–155.

Seel, R. (2008). *Complexity and organization development: An introduction.* Retrieved from http://www.new-paradigm.co.uk/complex-od.htm

Sinek, S. (2010, May 10). How great leaders inspire action. *TED talks.* Retrieved from https://www.ted.com/talks/simon_sinek_how_great_leaders_inspire_action?language=en

Sitterding, M., & Broome, M. E. (2015). *Information overload: Framework, tips, and tools to manage in complex healthcare environments.* Washington, DC: American Nurses Association.

Stichler, J. F. (2006). Skills and competencies for today's nurse executive. *AWHONN Lifelines: The Association of Women's Health, Obstetric and Neonatal Nurses, 10*(3), 155–157.

Stroebel, C. K., McDaniel, R. R., Jr., Crabtree, B. F., Miller W. L., Nutting, P. A, & Stange, K.C. (2005). How complexity science can inform a reflective process for improvement in primary care practices. *Joint Commission Journal on Quality & Patient Safety, 31*(8), 438–446.

Tsai, C. T., Joynt, K. E., Wild, R. C., Orav, E. J., & Jha, A. (2015, March). Medicare's bundled payment initiative: Most hospitals are focused on a few high-volume conditions. *Health Affairs, 34*(3), 371–380.

Wall, K. (2013). Complexity science and innovation: Interview with Curt Lindberg. *Innovation Management.se.* Retrieved from http://www.innovationmanagement.se/2010/06/14/complexity-science-and-innovation/

Wheatley, M. (2009, March). The place beyond fear and hope. *Shambhala Sun,* 79–83.

Whitney, D., & Schau, C. (1998). Appreciative inquiry: An innovative process for organization change. *Employment Relations Today, 25*(1), 11–21.

CHAPTER 3

Current Challenges in Complex Health Care Organizations: The Triple Aim

Katherine C. Pereira and Margaret T. Bowers

Culture does not change because we desire to change it. Culture changes when the organization is transformed—the culture reflects the realities of people working together every day.

—Frances Hesselbein

OBJECTIVES

- To *understand current forces driving health care delivery in the United States*
- To *appreciate the responsibility of the leader in facilitating a healthy workplace environment*
- To *identify the influence of technology in shaping health care worker satisfac*tion

Health care in the United States in the 21st century is a product of a multitude of factors, including legislation, public policy, and consumer mandates. Many of these factors coalesced in the implementation of the Patient Protection and Affordable Care Act (ACA) in 2010 and introduction of the triple aim (McClellan, McKethan, Lewis, Roski, & Fisher, 2010; Whittington, Nolan, Lewis, & Torres, 2015). In March 2010, the ACA was signed into law by President Obama, reforming American health insurance coverage (National Association of Insurance Commissioners & Center for Insurance Policy Research, 2010; U.S. Department of Health and Human Services, 2014). These reforms were intended to provide consumers and patients with more control over their health care by making it more accessible, affordable, and of higher quality. By mandating health insurance coverage overall, the ACA cast a broad net to capture people in the low- and middle-income categories. The most significant impact of the ACA was seen in two distinct areas: state adoption of Medicaid expansion and increased coverage of adults 18 to 30 years old (Long et al., 2015). On the downside, Medicaid expansion has had variable impact based on whether or not states adopted the option to expand coverage for those previously uninsured (Long et al., 2015). However, states with Medicaid expansion have seen a 38.3% reduction in the number of uninsured individuals. It has been assumed that providing insurance coverage to those who do not have it will improve health outcomes and reduce disparities. The next step in evaluating the effects of ACA implementation will be to analyze outcomes on population health and the impact on health care costs.

THE TRIPLE AIM

The ACA has implications for the delivery of health care in the United States, through a focus on "value over volume" and maximizing performance of health systems (Shirey & White-Williams, 2015). The triple aim, as defined by the Institute of Medicine (IOM), includes (a) population health, (b) management of health care costs, and (c) enhancement of the patient care experience, including quality and satisfaction (Whittington et al., 2015). In an effort to address these aims, leaders in health care must evolve and focus on new priorities for health care delivery. Transformational leadership is one strategy that focuses on motivating followers to achieve more than expected by looking beyond their own interests and challenging assumptions (Mitchell, 2014).

The successful implementation of the triple aim depends on several important factors influencing the context of health care. Among these are the success of emerging health care teams; improved health literacy of patient populations; effective implementation and use of the electronic health record (EHR); issues related to productivity, effectiveness, and safety; nursing workforce issues; and social determinants of health. Though this list is not exhaustive, it offers some important examples to be addressed here.

CURRENT FORCES INFLUENCING HEALTH CARE

In 2008, the Institute for Healthcare Improvement (IHI) introduced the concept of the triple aim in an effort to provide a framework to link multiple goals of health care (IHI, 2016; Whittington et al., 2015). By the time the ACA was passed in 2010, the triple aim was well integrated, and implementation and evaluation are now underway.

Kaplan (2015) provided a comprehensive overview of the influence of the triple aim on health care delivery. Efforts at measuring value should focus on the patient as the "unit of analysis." Kaplan proposed that measuring value includes looking at health outcomes in relation to costs. This model can be applied from wellness to illness and across a cycle of care. This process must be transparent, and health sectors must be accountable for their outcomes. Determining appropriate outcome measures must be done in a methodical manner and is not a swift process. Kaplan proposed value-based bundled payments as a strategy to address the triple aim by providing a single payment for a specific medical condition over a cycle of care. This payment amount considers individual patient risk factors and is contingent upon positive patient outcomes.

Several pioneer accountable care organizations (ACOs) were created as groundbreaking models for health care delivery in this new paradigm. Initially 32 pioneer institutions were selected because they were well developed and had the potential to succeed. Although 13 such organizations have chosen to leave the program, those remaining have emerged as innovators, improving quality of health care to Medicare beneficiaries while reducing costs (Nyweide et al., 2015). For ACOs to become effective on a broader scale there will need to be improved alignment across regulatory agencies, as well as incentives for both patients and providers to be fully engaged in the health care system (Noble & Casalino, 2013). Signs that the triple aim has been realized will include a healthier population with a focus on prevention rather than treatment of illness, reduced disparities in access to and quality of care, patient satisfaction and engagement with the community that provides health care, and reduced cost. Achieving these goals will require a team approach.

HEALTH CARE TEAMS AND MODELS

Multidisciplinary health care teams are part of a model that has demonstrated clinical effectiveness in a variety of settings (Okun et al., 2014). Core competencies for interprofessional collaborative practice have been developed and endorsed by key health professional organizations. These competencies focus on values and ethics, roles and responsibilities, interprofessional communication, and teams and teamwork (Mackintosh et al., 2011). Interprofessional teams function in dynamic ways across clinical situations as well as environments of care. For example, a social worker may be the team leader when facilitating a transition from an acute care setting to long-term care, or a pharmacist may emerge as the team leader in a critical care environment in the care of a medically complex patient. Successful teams balance individual strengths of their members with the needs of the entire team.

Another model that has been proposed more recently includes the patient and family caregivers as key members of the team in an effort to create effective health care partnerships (Okun et al., 2014). The addition of these key team members supports the tenets of the triple aim by focusing on partnering with patients to achieve a key value in health care: a satisfying experience with positive outcomes in a cost-effective manner. Future research will be necessary to evaluate the effectiveness of such dynamic health care teams.

Challenges arise when the composition of health care teams is affected by organizational downsizing of personnel. Organizational restructuring may lead to gaps in needed numbers of skilled personnel to provide direct care. In an era of dynamic health care systems, there are leadership opportunities to address these gaps. Kilpatrick, Lavoie-Tremblay, Ritchie, and Lamothe (2014) proposed that advanced practice nurses (APNs) take advantage of these leadership opportunities. As expert clinicians, educators, researchers, and leaders, APNs can positively influence health care teams in the context of both primary and acute care settings (Kilpatrick et al., 2014). In addition to the challenges posed by reduction in staff, APNs in acute care settings face barriers to integrating themselves into health care teams. Using effective leadership strategies, APNs can bridge communication across diverse members of the health care team as they focus on providing quality patient-centered care. Effective utilization of resources is one example of how APNs have demonstrated their leadership in clinical care (Kapu, Kleinpell, & Pilon, 2014). In a retrospective secondary analysis, Kapu and colleagues determined that the addition of nurse practitioners to an inpatient care team at a single site demonstrated enhanced revenue through gross collections and cost efficiency, reduced overall length of stay, and standardization of practices to improve quality care.

One example of a model focused on population health and cost reduction was described by Tetuan et al. (2014). The setting was a nurse-run clinic for annual wellness visits to promote adherence to mammogram and colonoscopy screening in a targeted Medicare population. The premise was that during an extended nurse visit, patients had the opportunity to express their personal health beliefs and discuss concerns about health screenings (Tetuan et al., 2014). The results of implementing this model of care demonstrated an increase in adherence to mammogram screening recommendations and a trend toward improvement in colonoscopy screenings. Through early detection and prevention of breast or colon cancer, mortality can be reduced, cure rates can increase, and total cost of care can be reduced. There are future opportunities for deploying nurse-run clinics to improve adherence to health maintenance recommendations in specific populations, such as patients with diabetes, hypertension, or dyslipidemia (Tetuan et al., 2014). These interventions have the potential to improve preventive health behaviors and reduce costs related to late detection of complex diseases.

APNs as transformational leaders have the potential to play a pivotal role in care redesign by addressing patient-specific needs that look beyond the domain of a traditional clinical practice site. APNs should be the leaders in coordinating care and identifying alternative methods of providing access to care. Amy Compton-Phillips, president and chief clinical officer of Providence Health & Services, has described opportunities to focus on caring, curing, and coordinating in future health care redesign in a specific setting (see Compton-Phillips, 2015).

REFLECTION QUESTIONS

1. How can APNs influence care redesign as transformational leaders?
2. What strategies or skills are needed for APNs to be successful in promoting the triple aim?

IMPROVING HEALTH LITERACY TO INCREASE PATIENT ENGAGEMENT IN HEALTH CARE

When increasing patient involvement in care, it is important to consider such factors as health literacy. Health literacy, along with health numeracy skills, can influence the quality of care delivery across the spectrum of settings and is vital to maintaining patients' engagement in their own health. Health literacy is defined as "the degree to which individuals have the capacity to obtain, process and understand basic health information needed to make appropriate health decisions and services needed to prevent or treat illness" (Health Resources and Services Administration [HRSA], 2015) and can promote understanding and safety in care delivery. Health numeracy is "the individual-level skills needed to understand and use quantitative health information, including basic computation skills, ability to use information in documents and non-text formats such as graphs, and ability to communicate orally" (Ancker & Kaufman, 2007). Both of these skills are crucial in addressing quality and safety concerns.

It is estimated that one-third of adults in the United States have low health literacy (Kutner, Greenburg, Jin, & Paulsen, 2006), meaning the inability to read medication label instructions. People with low health literacy skills are more likely to have poor health along with an associated risk for increased mortality (Bostock & Steptoe, 2012). Many individuals with functional literacy skills do not necessarily have functional numeracy skills. It is estimated that about 26% of all Americans have low numeracy skills (Kutner et al., 2006). Low numeracy skills are associated with poorer health outcomes, higher rates of hospitalization or rehospitalization, and inability to self-manage chronic disease (Sheridan et al., 2011). Poor numeracy skills can affect how patients are able to interpret risk for disease, read graphs and tables in their own EHRs, and perform practical calculations such as determining portion sizes, counting carbohydrates, and interpreting peak-flow readings. As patients are required to develop stronger self-management of chronic illness skills, numeracy skills must receive as much attention as literacy skills.

Low health literacy is more common in underserved and under-resourced populations, among elders, lower socioeconomic groups, and minority populations (HRSA, 2015). Thus, low health literacy is one cause of the health disparities seen in these populations. Another layer of literacy challenges for patients includes implementation of the EHR and the complexity of data available. Federal mandates related to EHR implementation include incentives for patient registration and interaction with agency electronic portals, such as viewing health information and communicating with health care providers through such portals. However, it has been recognized that racial and ethnic minorities and those with low health literacy are less likely to interact with health portals (Sarkar et al., 2010). As EHR adaptation becomes more widespread and oral communication is increasingly replaced with written communication, EHR design will need to employ novel strategies that assure widespread usability of this technology across literacy levels. Inclusion of various ethnic groups during usability testing, availability of EHR data in many languages, and the use of enhanced visual and video instructions would all increase patient comprehension of EHR data (Lyles, Schillinger, & Sarkar, 2015).

From a health care system perspective, removing barriers to understanding would allow more individuals to actively engage in health promotion activities. Initial research on health literacy focused on patient determinants of health literacy, but recently the movement is toward the skills needed by health care providers to facilitate accurate communication of health care information (Coleman, 2011). This goes beyond just providing written information at sixth grade reading level. The Plain Language Act, passed in 2000, mandated the use of easily understood language in government documents and materials as a move to enhance comprehension for those reading them. Since lower health literacy is more common in minority populations, health information and communication methods must also be constructed using concepts consistent with cultural competency.

Roter (2011) employed a successful model to increase patient comprehension of complex orally communicated information by three simple constructs. The first of these, "strip it down," involves restricting the use of medical jargon terms and intricate explanations. The second, "bring it home," means providing the patient with contextual relevance and personalization of the provided information. "Mix it up," the final construct, refers to avoiding monologues and long-winded explanations with patients, with a shift to conversational exchanges of information (Roter, 2011). Interventions to improve numeracy skills have been studied most frequently among patients with diabetes, an illness that requires multiple numeracy skills in order to successfully participate in self-care. Skills such as insulin titration, reading food labels, calculating serving sizes, and insulin pump therapy are particularly challenging for those with low numeracy skills. The Diabetes Literacy and Numeracy Toolkit, developed by researchers at Vanderbilt University and the University of North Carolina, provides 24 learning units that can be customized to individual patient skill level. Color-coded instructions, visual aids, and alternative methods for portion estimation and insulin titration are provided. The toolkit is also available in a Spanish language version (Wolff et al., 2009).

Health care providers may overestimate the understanding of health literacy challenges of their patients. Thus, increasing awareness of the problem may be the first step toward increasing competence in many organizations. A health literacy curriculum has been implemented into various health professional training programs as validation of the importance of this topic. Strategies that enhance knowledge include use of standardized patients in the simulated learning environment, practicing communication skills that avoid jargon, and use of the "teach-back" method (Coleman, 2011). Incorporation of the health literacy status into the patient assessment and plan of care teaches practitioners to consider this as an important part of every interaction. Other interventions have incorporated health literacy into the Chronic Care Model, stressing the importance of the team approach to maximizing every health care encounter. Continued challenges include health literacy obstacles that occur during emergency and crisis situations,

Several national organizations promote and provide resources to health care leaders to improve health literacy, including the American Medical Association

Foundation (2010) and the Centers for Disease Control and Prevention (2016). The IOM identified 10 attributes of a health literate health care organization (Brach et al., 2012) that can truly support patients as they navigate their engagement with the health care system.

A health literate health care organization:

1. Has leadership that makes health literacy integral to its mission, structure, and operations
2. Integrates health literacy into planning, evaluation measures, patient safety, and quality improvement
3. Prepares the workforce to be health literate and monitors progress
4. Includes populations served in the design, implementation, and evaluation of health information services
5. Meets the needs of populations with a range of health literacy skills while avoiding stigmatization
6. Uses health literacy strategies in interpersonal communications and confirms understanding at all points of contact
7. Provides easy access to health information and services and navigation assistance
8. Designs and distributes print, audiovisual, and social media content that is easy to understand and act on
9. Addresses health literacy in high-risk situations, including care transitions and communications about medicines
10. Communicates clearly what health plans cover and what individuals will have to pay for services

EHR IMPLEMENTATION: A PARADIGM SHIFT IN HEALTH CARE

The introduction of the Health Information Technology for Economic and Clinical Health (HITECH) Act in 2009 not only mandated transition to EHRs, but also included features that were imperative as contributors to "meaningful use" in the delivery of clinical care (Weeks, Keeney, Evans, Moore, & Conrad, 2015). The purpose of meaningful use documentation was to reduce disparities in care while improving quality and safety in delivery of care (Snyder & Oliver, 2014). Financial incentives for reporting meaningful use measures have been rolled out in stages as an incentive to promote adherence, and financial penalties were ascribed to those not meeting the meaningful use standard in the designated timeframe (Snyder & Oliver, 2014).

In an effort to centralize information related to the challenges of EHR implementation, the Office of the National Coordinator for Health Information Technology had regional extension centers collect information to evaluate specific issues related to implementing meaningful use (Heisey-Grove, Danehy, Consolazio, Lynch, & Mostashari, 2014). The most common themes that emerged were administrative issues and provider engagement, while the primary clinical meaningful use measure that posed a challenge was the clinical summary measure (Heisey-Grove et al., 2014).

An integrative review of evidence-based practice strategies provided a more detailed perspective on factors that promote successful implementation of meaningful use in EHRs (Snyder & Oliver, 2014). Provider training, including usability of the EHR within clinical workflow, emerged as a challenge which, when addressed prospectively, enhanced adoption of meaningful use. Ongoing challenges in stage 2 of meaningful use deployments include barriers to usage of patient portals. Although exchange of clinical information and communication with eligible health care professionals is the primary goal of patient portals, disparities persist among the patients who access these portals (Snyder & Oliver, 2014).

An academic health center conducted an evaluation of how meaningful use was implemented using a three-pronged approach: leadership, administration, and technology (Unger, Aldrich, Hefner, & Rizer, 2014). From a leadership perspective, multipronged communication strategies were used across the health system to encourage staff to use their EHR "meaningfully." From an administrative perspective, a centralized office was developed to manage credentialing and registration and attest for Medicaid and Medicare services. As for technological implementation, report building and validation were key components to track providers' progress and offer individualized feedback regarding meaningful use (Unger et al., 2014). These authors provide a thoughtful perspective on strategies for applying the multiple stages of meaningful use in an academic health center.

PRODUCTIVITY, EFFECTIVENESS, AND SAFETY: IMPACT ON QUALITY CARE

The scope of measuring productivity and effectiveness in the current health care climate has created new challenges for the entire health care industry. Insurers, providers, policy makers, and consumers all influence how productivity and effectiveness are measured and evaluated.

The American Heart Association and the American College of Cardiology published a statement on the cost and value of implementing clinical practice guidelines and performance measures in cardiology. The statement focuses on the introduction of cost-effectiveness and value assessments as integral components to be included in clinical practice guidelines (Anderson et al., 2014). This statement is in line with the premise of the triple aim, which focuses on measuring the value of health care in the context of patient satisfaction. Resource utilization and value are proposed as the nomenclature to ensure that the focus on cost is not the primary measure of performance. The inclusion of value in the context of medical decision making is a new concept and is only one aspect of implementing clinical guidelines (Anderson et al., 2014). Health care providers face clinical and ethical issues that may arise while balancing the value of a medical decision with resource utilization. Historically these issues arise when resources are scare, as in the case of organ transplantation. As value is considered, the implementation of clinical practice guidelines will require considerations of resource allocation.

Practice implications for implementing the triple aim affect both productivity and clinical effectiveness. EHR implementation has had a significant impact on clinical implementation projects aimed at reducing costs and patient complications. The aforementioned initiatives have focused on reducing hospital-acquired infections, including catheter-acquired urinary tract infections (CAUTI), catheter-acquired bloodstream infections, and ventilator-associated pneumonia.

In a study by Shepard et al. (2014), an EHR was used to surveil CAUTI in an adult population over a 5-month period. An electronic algorithm was developed to streamline the process for CAUTI surveillance. This single-site intervention included an analysis of over 6,000 positive urine cultures in a 6-month period. Through use of this electronic algorithm, the study site was able to reduce CAUTI surveillance requirements by 97% (Shepard et al., 2014). This type of intervention was low cost with a high yield in productivity and effectiveness and could be integrated in diverse EHR systems.

Introducing new models of care has implications for improving efficiency, reducing cost, and ultimately enhancing productivity. APNs do not consistently receive the same level of clinical support in primary care settings as their physician colleagues. For example, although medical assistants (MAs) are able to complete basic clinical tasks, they are often assigned to support only physicians and not APNs. Liu, Finkelstein, and Poghosyan (2014) created queuing models to analyze APN utilization in an effort to determine the provider service rate. By focusing on the provider service rate, they allowed for the variability among providers across practice settings. It is well known that APNs have longer consultation periods than physician colleagues and therefore lower service rates (Laurant et al., 2009). Liu et al. (2014) compared APN practice with and without MA support to determine which model was cost-effective and what ratio of MA to APN yielded the most cost-effective care while improving access to care. They found that APN productivity and cost efficiency improved significantly when the nurses had assistance from MAs. As the workforce embraces a significant increase in APN providers, health care systems will need to evaluate the workforce mix to determine which models maximize the scope of practice for all levels of providers. An increase in the number of APN providers should improve access to care; if supported by MAs, these APNs can maximize productivity in a cost-effective manner.

As a discipline, nursing is grounded in advancing knowledge focused on promoting health and addressing human responses in health and illness. Doctorally prepared APNs are poised to step into their role as change agents to examine systems of care and how they can be the leaders of new models of care. APNs bring a unique perspective as nurses and need to rise to the challenge to lead practice change initiatives, asserting themselves to be more than just token representatives on the health care team. The contributions of nursing to the implementation and study of care delivery models is crucial to the success of these models; therefore, APNs need to have an active voice in the process.

It is well known that U.S. health care spending has increased exponentially over the past three decades, yet morbidity and mortality rates exceed those of countries that spend less on health care (Kaplan & Witkowski, 2014). As models of health care delivery continue to evolve, so, too, do financial structures and payment models. Relative value units, which assign cost to patients based on procedures and diagnoses, do not provide a true accounting of how cost relates to patient outcomes.

Kaplan and Witkowski (2014) reiterated the changes in value-based health care and urged us to prepare for this new model of care, which includes bundled payments over a cycle of care while promoting provider and system accountability for measured outcomes. Care redesign is a significant component of this paradigm and relies on improving efficiency, developing standards of care, and consistently measuring outcomes across the cycle of care. Of increasing importance in such measurement of outcomes is the assurance of patient safety.

The passage of the ACA in 2010 included incentives and benchmarks for implementation of EHR technology. The implementation of EHRs has raised unique safety concerns and challenges, leading some observers to suggest the creation of EHR-specific patient safety goals (PSGs; Sittig & Singh, 2012). Since all care delivery documentation is now funneled through the EHR, system malfunction, computer virus infection, or unanticipated "down time" has the potential to severely disrupt care delivery in most health systems. For instance, one hospital system in Rhode Island was forced to cancel elective surgical procedures and divert non–life-threatening emergencies due to a glitch in an antivirus software update (Sittig & Singh, 2012). Three EHR-specific PSGs are (a) addressing patient safety concerns unique to EHRs, (b) mitigating safety concerns arising from failure to use EHRs appropriately, and (c) using EHRs to monitor and improve patient safety.

NURSING WORKFORCE ISSUES

Direct Care Nurses

Various factors may affect the appropriate number of nurses needed. The total U.S. nursing workforce supply increased substantially between 2003 and 2013, with a doubling of nursing graduates from 76,727 to 155,098. As a result, the nursing supply between 2013 and 2025 is expected to exceed demand, with a projected 3,849,000 nurses available for 3,509,000 positions—an excess of 340,000 nurses. Variations in the supply of registered nurses (RNs) could occur from state to state, depending on population trends and nurse retirement rates. On the other hand, the projected nursing faculty shortage could significantly reduce the supply of nurses, while implementation of newer models of care delivery may increase the need for nurses in nontraditional care settings. Additionally, implementation of the ACA has resulted in an increased number of individuals with health insurance (HRSA, 2013b), which translates to an increased need for nurses.

Advanced Practice Nurses

The national supply of APNs has steadily increased in the past few years, yet the projected need for primary care providers will continue to grow in the next decade due to an aging population, population growth, and an increase in insured patients with access to health care under the ACA. Current projections include a deficit of 20,400 primary care providers by 2020 (HRSA, 2013a). Nurse practitioners are poised to meet this need, yet many barriers exist to sustain the supply of APNs. The range of practice authority varies from state to state, hindering job mobility for many APNs. Also, the cost of APN education is prohibitive for many nurses wishing to pursue an advanced practice degree, and limited availability of clinical learning sites for APN students can limit enrollment capacity in many training programs (Broome, 2015).

The graduate nurse education (GNE) demonstration grant was initiated by the Centers for Medicare and Medicaid Services in 2012 as one solution to increase the supply of primary care providers nationwide, and will be in progress until 2017. The first of its kind, this 4-year, $200 million grant provides support to health systems that work with schools of nursing to increase the numbers of APN students. Graduate medical education support from HRSA has been a mainstay of educational support for physicians, funding 115,000 residency positions at a cost of $115,000 per resident per year (Goodman & Robertson, 2013). The primary goal of GNE is to increase the availability of qualified training for APN students, including nurse practitioners, certified RN anesthetists, and clinical nurse specialists. Five accredited schools of nursing partnering with nonhospital community-based care settings and university health systems were chosen to participate in this grant: Duke University Health System, Scottsdale Healthcare Medical System, Rush University Medical Center, Hospital of University of Pennsylvania, and Memorial Hermann–Texas Medical Center Hospital. A key feature of the grant involves collaboration between the selected schools of nursing and health systems to create novel strategies to increase the supply of preceptors for APN students, with a plan of payment for preceptors' services. Other important aspects of the grant include preceptor development, with an emphasis on teaching needs and preparation of APN students, giving feedback appropriately, and how to be a preceptor in a busy practice. The results of this demonstration will be reported to Congress and could serve as a model for other government-funded APN education support. Concerns include the sustainability of these innovations once the grant funding cycle concludes.

During this time of rapidly changing health care delivery, leaders must mobilize the nursing workforce while fostering innovative interprofessional partnerships and partnerships with other health care organizations. Nursing leaders will be crucial as part of the teams testing innovative and cost-saving models of care. Building strong teams with a strong likelihood of success, while facilitating nursing vision in shaping these innovations, will become an important role for the nurse leader. Many of these models include nurses as key players to facilitate success, and leaders must act as both change agents and advocates for those they lead.

Looming Faculty Shortages

In order for the profession to remain strong, nurses need to be prepared by expert faculty members who are leaders in shaping health policy, generating new knowledge, promoting knowledge translation, and advancing innovative curriculum design. One of the biggest threats to the nursing workforce is the declining number of nursing faculty to prepare students. In 2014–2015, nursing schools turned away 68,936 qualified applicants for baccalaureate and graduate programs due to faculty shortages and other resource shortfalls, including lack of clinical learning sites, poor budget support, and inadequate teaching facilities. During this same year, nursing schools identified 1,236 open faculty positions (American Association of Colleges of Nursing [AACN-a], 2014). Seventy-two percent of nursing faculty members are over the age of 50, while 14% are age 65 or older, working past the usual retirement age. The average age of doctorally prepared nursing faculty is 55 years, suggesting that many faculty will begin retiring from teaching within the next decade, worsening the shortage. In contrast, only 4% of nurses under the age of 40 work in academia (Budden, Zhong, Moulton, & Cimiotti, 2013). Maintaining faculty diversity is also a challenge, with minorities comprising only about 11% of faculty.

Most nursing faculty members (about two-thirds) report being of junior rank, with the majority holding the title of assistant professor, which reflects a deficit in faculty prepared to take on more complex leadership roles in schools of nursing. While many nursing faculty members find their work fulfilling, they report symptoms of emotional exhaustion from long working hours (averaging 48 hours a week). About half of currently employed faculty members younger than 50 are considering leaving teaching in the next 5 years (Yedidia, Chou, Brownlee, Flynn, & Tanner, 2014). The faculty shortage also creates a vicious cycle of faculty overwork and lack of teaching support, which may prompt decisions to leave teaching after only a few years.

One major cause of faculty shortages has been a lack of doctorally prepared faculty, although there is a trend toward increasing numbers of nurses enrolling in doctoral programs. In 2014 to 2015, there were 18,352 students enrolled in doctor of nursing practice (DNP) programs, which is a 26.2% increase from the previous year. Likewise, enrollment in research-focused doctoral programs in 2014 increased by 3.2% from the previous year to 5,290 students. Could this increasing enrollment mean an end to the looming shortage? The answer remains unclear. Many DNP graduates are interested in incorporating teaching into their clinical role after graduation (Loomis, Willard, & Cohen, 2006). The salaries in academia may be a hindrance to doctorally prepared APNs pursuing faculty opportunities. The average annual salary of an APN is $93,310 whereas the average salary of a doctorally prepared nursing faculty member is $73,333 for a 12-month appointment (AACN-a, 2014). Another barrier is that many universities preclude DNP-prepared faculty from participating in the tenure tracks, and only 11% of DNP programs offer formal training in curriculum design and educational concepts (Udlis & Mancuso, 2012). Also, the length of time required for doctorate completion, along with expense, continue to create barriers for many nurses interested in pursuing higher degrees. Finally, some schools do not provide formal practice opportunities for APNs to maintain professional certification, so these faculty often find themselves working at sites disconnected from the university on evenings and weekends, increasing role stress workload.

What would be effective strategies to address the nursing faculty shortage? With many faculty holding junior roles, there is a need for intentional efforts toward faculty development and succession planning in nursing schools. Succession planning has been overlooked by many institutions, with only 38% of nursing schools reporting strategies in place (Wyte-Lake, Tran, Bowman, Needleman, & Dobalian, 2013). There is also growing recognition of the need for formal professional leadership development of faculty members. National organizations are placing more emphasis on leadership development within both the profession itself and academia. Examples include the Robert Wood Johnson Foundation's (RWJF) *Future of Nurse Scholars* program, which aims to develop nurses pursuing a PhD through scholarships, mentoring, development of leadership skills, and postdoctoral research funding. Other organizations, including the National League for Nursing, AACN, Sigma Theta Tau International, American Academy of Nursing, and Johnson and Johnson Nurse Leadership Program, have developed nurse leadership programs for nurses at all levels. Academic–practice partnerships along with increased pay, other incentives, and increased faculty support have also been used to attract more nurses to pursue higher degrees within university health systems (Wyte-Lake et al., 2013). The federal Nurse Faculty Loan Program provides loans to nurses pursuing doctoral programs with 85% loan forgiveness if the graduate works in nursing education for 4 years after graduation.

Workplace Violence

Health care institutions are by definition stressful environments, and this situation has unfortunately been exacerbated by an escalation in incivility, bullying, and workplace violence. These phenomena are in direct opposition to the ethical principles innate in the nursing profession and the values of respect and acceptance. They are increasingly recognized as sources of significant stress for nurses and can be triggers for posttraumatic stress disorder, other mood disorders, and poor job performance (Lanctôt & Guay, 2014).

Workplace violence is any act or threat of physical violence, harassment, intimidation, or other threatening disruptive behavior that occurs on the job (Occupational Safety and Health Administration, n.d.). Violence can originate from patients, family members, visitors, or other community members. Estimates of verbal abuse aimed toward health care workers vary widely from 22% to 90%, with threats of physical violence occurring 12% to 64% of the time (Pompeii et al., 2013). In 2013, the U.S. Department of Labor noted that 13% of workplace absenteeism could be attributed to workplace violence (U.S. Department of Labor Bureau of Labor Statistics, 2014). Emergency departments, long-term care facilities, and psychiatric settings see a much higher incidence of violence than other health care settings (Gacki-Smith et al., 2009). Workplace violence also increases the likelihood that a nurse will leave the profession permanently, thus contributing to nursing workforce retention challenges.

In addition to workplace violence, the problem of incivility in nursing is well recognized. In contrast to civility (defined as participation in a respectful and considerate way), incivility is "behavior of low intensity that can include such behavior as being rude, discourteous, impolite or violating workplace norms of behavior." (Grimlsey, 2003–2016).

Incivility can take on many forms, from demeaning statements and rumors to refusal to acknowledge a coworker's need for assistance. This incivility is bidirectional, occurring between nurses, but also between subordinate nurses and those in leadership positions, and likewise from leaders toward nurses working in lower ranked positions. Incivility also occurs commonly in nursing academia, aimed by students toward faculty, and from faculty toward students (Gallo, 2012). Regardless of the direction, incivility can lead to burnout (Trépanier, Fernet, & Austin, 2013), higher absenteeism (Ortega, Christensen, Hogh, Rugulies, & Borg, 2011), and poor job satisfaction (Nielsen & Einarsen, 2012). Nurses may learn these behaviors in personal environments, educational settings, or nursing school and transfer them to the workplace after graduation. Incivility in academic settings can lead to an inability to attract new nurses and nursing faculty to the profession.

Bullying is "repeated, unwanted harmful actions intended to humiliate, offend and cause distress in the recipient" (American Nurses Association [ANA], 2015). When leaders bully their team members, it gives implicit permission for others to participate in this type of behavior. Others identify *workplace mobbing* as the form of bullying more frequently seen in the workplace. This term describes behaviors of "ganging up" on a targeted worker to demean and psychologically harass the individual. These behaviors can include isolation, refusing to work with someone, unfair assignments, eye rolling, gossip, name calling, intimidation, criticism, and fault finding. Bullying can occur in health care settings and also in nursing academia. Many times the bullied individual is one who is an exceptional employee or a newcomer, reflecting the elements of change theory that speak to the group desire for the status quo. Dealing with issues of workplace violence, incivility, and bullying may consume large amounts of a leader's time as attempts are made to resolve these conflicts and retain valued employees.

In response to these issues, the ANA released a position statement in 2015 addressing incivility, bullying, and workplace violence. Key features of the statement emphasize that violence of any kind from any source should not be tolerated by the nursing profession, and that nurses and employers must join forces to build a culture of respect in the workplace. The ANA Code of Ethics holds nurses to behaviors that treat colleagues, patients, and students with respect and dignity. The ANA position statement recommends preventive strategies against bullying and incivility for both nurses and nursing leaders or employees. These are summarized in Table 3.1 (ANA, 2015). Table 3.2 outlines examples of other resources from some national health care organizations.

TABLE 3.1 Recommendations to Reduce Workplace Violence and Incivility

RECOMMENDATIONS FOR NURSES	RECOMMENDATIONS FOR EMPLOYERS
Commit to establish healthy interpersonal relationships.	Create an organizational mission, vision, and values that include respect and safety.
Self-reflect on own interactions and communication patterns.	Orient new employees to organizational policies and encourage employee participation in policy development.
Participate in co-creation of civility standards for the workplace.	Create zero-tolerance policies regarding bullying and incivility. These should include reporting mechanisms, investigational procedures, assigned departmental responsibility for investigation, and nonretribution for reporting.
Take responsibility for knowledge and awareness of institutional codes of conduct, professional behavior, and antibullying/ incivility policies. If policies are not in place, then participate in their development with appropriate leadership.	Create mechanisms for employees to obtain assistance.
Practice using predetermined phrases and behaviors that will detract from and prevent incivility and bullying.	Educate employees about institutional policies defining incivility, bullying, and zero tolerance.
Use a predetermined code word to signal for support when feeling threatened.	Give clear details of consequences related to nonadherence to policies.
Advocate for antibullying/incivility initiatives in community and schools.	
Model respect and civility as workplace norms.	
Adhere to the ANA Code of Ethics.	
Academic leaders should integrate civility into curricula while modeling this behavior for students. Coaching and mentoring also model supportive behavior to students and other faculty. Incorporate crisis theory and intervention, conflict negotiation and resolution, and interprofessional communication into curricula.	
Nursing curricula should include opportunities for role play, problem-based learning, and simulation activities related to resolving incivility and bullying.	

TABLE 3.2 Examples of Resources to Prevent and Manage Issues Related to Workforce Violence or Incivility

ORGANIZATION	RESOURCE
American Nurses Association	Webinars on a variety of topics, including diversity, creating positive nursing culture, etc. (ANA, 2016)
American Association of Critical Care Nurses	*AACN Standards for Establishing and Sustaining Healthy Work Environments: A Journey to Excellence* (AACN-b, 2005)
Robert Wood Johnson Executive Nurse Fellows	*Civility Tool Kit: Resources to Empower Healthcare Leaders to Identify, Intervene, and Prevent Workplace Bullying* (RWJ ENF, 2012a) *Stop Bullying Nurses* (RWJ ENF, 2012b)
Centers for Disease Control and Prevention	*Workplace Violence Training for Nurses* (CDC, 2014)

In both health care institutions and academia, organizational culture must create intolerance for bullying and incivility. In addition, positive interventions such as mentoring, recognition of accomplishments, and appreciation of diversity can help foster a more supportive work environment (Clark, 2013). Nursing leaders have opportunities to serve as exemplary role models for ethical, honest, and positive behaviors. Whether formally appointed or an informal organizational leader, all leaders will influence behaviors and workplace norms through their behavior.

SOCIAL DETERMINANTS OF HEALTH

"The social determinants of health are mostly responsible for health inequities—the unfair and avoidable differences in health status seen between countries" (World Health Organization, 2011). Access to health care has been seen as an answer to improving population health in the United States, but access cannot be untangled from the issue of social determinants of health. Health is determined by an intricate interaction among individual lifestyle choices and the physical, social, and economic environments. Behaviors that are known to increase risk for disease, such as smoking, inactivity, poor diet, and alcohol use, differ across various social and ethnic groups. The chronic stressors of financial insecurity and poor social support systems also create physiological changes that have been proven to increase the likelihood of developing illnesses such as cardiovascular disease, mental health problems, and a hastened aging process. This chronic stress also reduces resiliency in the face of health problems (Adler & Stewart, 2010).

Preventive services are vital for improving the health of the nation, reducing health care costs, and sustaining individual productivity. Healthy behaviors and risk prevention are more likely to occur at higher incomes and education levels. Smoking rates are higher in individuals aged 18 and older who have not completed high school (Garrett, Dube, Winder, & Caraballo, 2013). Non-Hispanic

Blacks have a 50% higher chance of cardiovascular mortality prior to age 75 as compared to non-Hispanic Whites. Infant mortality rates for non-Hispanic Blacks are more than twice those for non-Hispanic Whites (Meyer et al., 2013). And poor education (particularly lack of high school completion) and low income are associated with populations and ethnic groups that have more chronic health problems, such as diabetes. Twenty-seven percent of Americans lack convenient access to healthy food retailers, and the likelihood of living in geographical areas referred to as "food deserts" is increased for seniors and neighborhoods comprising mostly non-Hispanic Blacks (Grimm, Moore, & Scanlon, 2013).

As the implementation of the ACA unfolds, focus is shifting toward creative approaches and health equity. The RWJF established the Commission to Build a Healthier America to identify why some Americans are healthier than others, and why health outcomes in the United States are worse than those in many other countries. The commission recommended government funding efforts to emphasize efforts to create healthier communities, enrich childhood development services, and establish safer communities. Priorities include enhancing early childhood development services, nutrition programs for food insecure families, and public–private partnerships that would provide for grocery stores with healthy choices in food deserts. Childhood education that includes required physical activity in grades K through 12 and healthy food choices in schools promote the idea that healthy children are more likely to be healthy adults. Other priorities, such as community health partnerships, initiatives that provide safe and healthy local housing, and employment opportunities, will increase the likelihood of healthy behaviors. Figure 3.1 illustrates how medical care is dependent on other direct and indirect influences on health (Braveman, Egerter, & Williams, 2011).

The city of Philadelphia offers an exciting illustration of the impact of widespread community–government–business partnerships. Crime, inadequate housing, poverty, low employment, suboptimal schools, and limited access to healthy foods were making parts of the city some of the unhealthiest places to live in the country. Get Healthy Philly is a citywide initiative and partnership with the Food Trust. Project leaders worked with over 900 retailers to increase

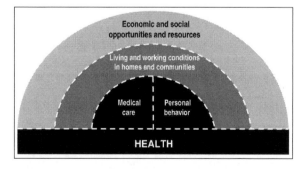

FIGURE 3.1 Social determinants of health.

Source: Braveman, P., Egerter, S., & Williams, D. R. (2011). The social determinants of health: Coming of age. *Annual Review of Public Health, 32,* 381–398. Reproduced with permission of Annual Review, © by Annual Reviews, http://www.annualreviews.org.

healthy food choices in restaurants, farmers' markets, and grocery stores. "Certified Healthy Food Stores" were designated for increasing their health food choices and advertising them. Other incentives included bonus food coupons for purchasing fresh fruits and vegetables, safer areas for exercise, cooking competitions, educational campaigns about sugared drinks, and healthier choices at all city supported activities. This multipronged approach has led to a 4.7% reduction in childhood obesity over 3 years (RWJF, 2015). Barriers to continued demonstration projects like this include needed political and economic support.

Some observers believe that better health care to underserved areas could be influenced by educating a more diverse nursing and health care workforce. Recent estimates note that minorities make up 19% of the nursing workforce, whereas ethnic and minority groups make up 37% of the U.S. population (AACN-a, 2013). An important trend is that ethnic minorities are now more likely to obtain a bachelor's degree or graduate degree in nursing than their White counterparts, although minorities are underrepresented on nursing school faculties. Individuals from areas that are racially, socioeconomically, and ethnically diverse are more likely to return to work in these areas after receiving training (HRSA, 2006). A nursing workforce that has the language skills needed to serve ethnically diverse populations can also enhance health teaching and understanding of health conditions while enhancing trust. Patients from various ethnic backgrounds may be more likely to trust a health care system that is not staffed by one exclusive ethnic or racial group.

No one would argue that challenges for APNs and other nursing leaders are abundant. As the past decade has evidenced the development and growth of leaders by DNP education, nurses are now armed with additional skills in leadership, scholarship, and change implementation that will make them pivotal team leaders able to bring solutions to these problems in health care. Solving these problems cannot be done in isolation and will require active engagement of nurses, APNs, and all health care leaders at all levels of health care delivery and policy creation.

Every nurse, particularly every APN, practices under high standards for providing patient-centered quality care while considering costs, access, and population health. APNs are more likely to practice in rural and underserved areas and focus on the needs of the community. They are poised to solve important problems and improve health care.

REFLECTION QUESTIONS

1. Assume that the nation has decided that all Americans should have access to care. As a leader, what do you think the care delivery system should look like, and what will your role in that care delivery system be?
2. How would you use your leadership skills as the nurse or APN member of an interprofessional health care team?

(continued)

REFLECTION QUESTIONS (*continued*)

3. As the United States approaches the goal of health insurance coverage for all citizens, how do you think this will change how nurse leaders function within organizations? How will social determinants of health challenge the ability to achieve the triple aim?
4. How do literacy skill challenges affect the successful implementation of the triple aim? How do organizations create and operationalize systems that consider health literacy?
5. What can leaders do to remove barriers to workplace incivility, bullying, and violence?
6. Have you experienced bullying or incivility in your workplace? If so, how has this affected the morale and productivity of the work environment?
7. Does the successful implementation of interprofessional teams and educational activities have the potential to contribute to reduced workplace incivility?
8. How do fluctuations in nursing workforce affect care delivery? What is one solution to attract and retain more nurses into faculty roles?

REFERENCES

Adler, N. E., & Stewart, J. (2010). Preface to the biology of disadvantage: Socioeconomic status and health. *Annals of the New York Academy of Sciences, 1186*(1), 1–4.

American Association of Colleges of Nursing (AACN-a). (2013). *Fact sheet: Enhancing diversity in the nursing workforce.* Washington, DC: Author. Retrieved from http://www.aacn.nche.edu/media-relations/fact-sheets/enhancing-diversity

American Association of Colleges of Nursing (AACN-a). (2014). *Nursing faculty shortage.* Washington, DC: Author. Retrieved from http://www.aacn.nche.edu/media-relations/fact-sheets/nursing-faculty-shortage

American Association of Critical Care Nurses (AACN-b). (2005). *AACN standards for establishing and sustaining healthy work environments: A journey to excellence.* Aliso Viejo, CA: Author. Retrieved from http://www.aacn.org/wd/hwe/docs/hwestandards.pdf

American Medical Association Foundation. (2010). *Health literacy and patient safety: Help patients understand.* Retrieved from https://www.youtube.com/watch?v=cGtTZ_vxjyA

American Nurses Association. (2015). *Position statement on incivility, bullying and workplace violence.* Silver Spring, MD: Author.

American Nurses Association. (2016). *Nursing knowledge center: ANA leadership institute.* Washington DC: Author. Retrieved from https://learn.ana-nursingknowledge.org/catalog?pagename=ANA-Leadership-Institute

Ancker, J. S., & Kaufman, D. (2007). Rethinking health numeracy: A multidisciplinary literature review. *Journal of the American Medical Informatics Association, 14*(6), 713–721.

Anderson, J., Heidenreich, P., Barnett, P., Creager, M., Fonarow, G., & Gibbons, R. (2014). A report of the American College of Cardiology/American Heart Association Task Force on Performance Measures and Task Force on Practice

Guidelines. ACC/AHA statement on cost/value methodology in clinical practice guidelines and performance measures. *Journal of the American College of Cardiology, 63*, 2304–2322.

Bostock, S., & Steptoe, A. (2012). Association between low functional health literacy and mortality in older adults: Longitudinal cohort study. *British Medical Journal, 344*, e1602.

Brach, C., Keller, D., Hernandez, L. M., Baur, C., Dreyer, B., Parker, R., . . . Schillinger, D. (2012). *Ten attributes of health literate health care organizations*. Washington, DC: Institute of Medicine. Retrieved from http://www.ahealthyunderstanding.org/Portals/0/Documents1/IOM_Ten_Attributes_HL_Paper.pdf

Braveman, P., Egerter, S., & Williams, D. R. (2011). The social determinants of health: Coming of age. *Annual Review of Public Health, 32*, 381–398.

Broome, M. E. (2015). Collective genius. *Nursing Outlook, 63(2)*, 105–107.

Budden, J. S., Zhong, E. H., Moulton, P., & Cimiotti, J. P. (2013). Highlights of the national workforce survey of registered nurses. *Journal of Nursing Regulation, 4(2)*, 5–14.

Centers for Disease Control and Prevention. (2014). *Occupational violence*. Atlanta, GA: CDC & National Institute for Occupational Safety and Health. Retrieved from http://www.cdc.gov/niosh/topics/violence/training_nurses.html

Centers for Disease Control and Prevention. (2016). *Health literacy*. Retrieved from http://www.cdc.gov/healthliteracy/index.html

Clark, C. M. (2013). National study on faculty-to-faculty incivility: Strategies to foster collegiality and civility. *Nurse Educator, 38*(3), 98–102.

Coleman, C. (2011). Teaching health care professionals about health literacy: A review of the literature. *Nursing Outlook, 59*(2), 70–78.

Compton-Phillips, A. (2015). Care redesign. *New England Journal of Medicine (NEJM) Catalyst.* Retrieved from Catalyst.nejm.org/videos/the-three-cs-of-care-redesign/

Gacki-Smith, J., Juarez, A. M., Boyett, L., Homeyer, C., Robinson, L., & MacLean, S. L. (2009). Violence against nurses working in US emergency departments. *Journal of Nursing Administration, 39*(7/8), 340–349.

Gallo, V. J. (2012). Incivility in nursing education: A review of the literature. *Teaching & Learning in Nursing, 7*(2), 62–66.

Garrett, B. E., Dube, S. R., Winder, C., & Caraballo, R. S. (2013). Cigarette smoking—United States, 2006–2008 and 2009–2010. *CDC Health Disparities and Inequalities Report—United States, 62*(3), 81.

Goodman, D. C., & Robertson, R. G. (2013). Accelerating physician workforce transformation through competitive graduate medical education funding. *Health Affairs, 32*, 111887–111892. Retrieved from http://content.healthaffairs.org/search?ck=nck&submit=yes&fulltext=Graduate+Medical+Education&x=24&y=7

Grimm, K. A., Moore, L. V., & Scanlon, K. S. (2013). Access to healthier food retailers—United States, 2011. *CDC Health Disparities and Inequalities Report—United States, 62*(3), 20.

Grimsley, S. (2003–2016). Workplace incivility: Definition and overview. Chapter 8, Lesson 31, Study.com. Retrieved from http://study.com/academy/lesson/workplace-incivility-definition-lesson-quiz.html

Health Resources and Services Administration. (2006). *The rationale for diversity in the health professions: A review of the evidence.* Washington, DC: Author. Retrieved from http://bhpr.hrsa.gov/healthworkforce/reports/diversityreviewevidence.pdf

Health Resources and Services Administration. (2013a, November). *Projecting the supply and demand for primary care practitioners through 2020.* Washington, DC:

Author. Retrieved from http://bhpr.hrsa.gov/healthworkforce/supplydemand/usworkforce/primarycare/projectingprimarycare.pdf

Health Resources and Services Administration. (2013b, April). *The U.S. nursing workforce: Trends in supply and education.* Washington, DC: Author. Retrieved from http://bhpr.hrsa.gov/healthworkforce/supplydemand/nursing/nursingworkforce/

Health Resources and Services Administration. (2015). *Health literacy.* Washington, DC: Author. Retrieved from http://www.hrsa.gov/publichealth/healthliteracy/

Heisey-Grove, D., Danehy, L. N., Consolazio, M., Lynch, K., & Mostashari, F. (2014). A national study of challenges to electronic health record adoption and meaningful use. *Medical Care, 52*(2), 144–148.

Institute for Health Improvement. (2016). *The IHI triple aim.* Retrieved from http://www.ihi.org/Engage/Initiatives/TripleAim/Pages/default.aspx

Kaplan, R. S. (2015, April). *Under the microscope: Advancing health care value through greater transparency.* Hewitt Health Care Lecture presented to Harvard Medical School, Boston, MA.

Kaplan, R. S., & Witkowski, M. L. (2014). Better accounting transforms health care delivery. *Accounting Horizons, 28*(2), 365–383.

Kapu, A. N., Kleinpell, R., & Pilon, B. (2014). Quality and financial impact of adding nurse practitioners to inpatient care teams. *Journal of Nursing Administration, 44*(2), 87–96.

Kilpatrick, K., Lavoie-Tremblay, M., Ritchie, J. A., & Lamothe, L. (2014). Advanced practice nursing, health care teams, and perceptions of team effectiveness. *Journal of Trauma Nursing, 21*(6), 291–299.

Kutner, M., Greenberg, E., Jin, Y., & Paulsen, C. (2006). *The health literacy of America's adults: Results from the 2003 National Assessment of Adult Literacy. NCES 2006-483.* Washington, DC: National Center for Education Statistics.

Lanctôt, N., & Guay, S. (2014). The aftermath of workplace violence among health care workers: A systematic literature review of the consequences. *Aggression and Violent Behavior, 19*(5), 492–501.

Laurant, M., Harmsen, M., Wollersheim, H., Grol, R., Faber, M., & Sibbald, B. (2009). The impact of nonphysician clinicians: Do they improve the quality and cost-effectiveness of health care services? *Medical Care Research & Review, 66*(6 Suppl.), 36S–89S.

Liu, N., Finkelstein, S. R., & Poghosyan, L. (2014). A new model for nurse practitioner utilization in primary care: Increased efficiency and implications. *Health Care Management Review, 39*(1), 10–20.

Long, S. K., Karpman, M., Kenney, G. M., Zuckerman, S., Wissoker, D., Shartzer, A., . . . Hempstead, K. (2015). *Taking stock: Gains in health insurance coverage under the ACA as of March 2015.* Washington, DC: Urban Institute, Health Policy Center. Retrieved from http://hrms.urban.org/briefs/Gains-in-Health-Insurance-Coverage-under-the-ACA-as-of-March-2015.html

Loomis, J. A., Willard, B., & Cohen, J. (2006, December 22). Difficult professional choices: Deciding between the PhD and the DNP in nursing. *Online Journal of Nursing Issues, 12,* 1. Retrieved from http://www.nursingworld.org/MainMenuCategories/ANAMarketplace/ANAPeriodicals/OJIN/TableofContents/Volume122007/No1Jan07/ArticlePreviousTopics/tpc28_816033.html

Lyles, C., Schillinger, D., & Sarkar, U. (2015). Connecting the dots: Health information technology expansion and health disparities. *PLOS Medicine, 12*(7), e1001852.

Mackintosh, S., Meyer, S. M., Robinson, D., Rouse, L. E., Sorensen, A. A., Viggiano, T. R., & Wathington, D. (2011). *Core competencies for interprofessional collaborative practice:*

Report of an expert panel. Washington, DC: Interprofessional Education Collaborative. Retrieved from http://www.aacn.nche.edu/education-resources/ipecreport.pdf

McClellan, M., McKethan, A. N., Lewis, J. L., Roski, J., & Fisher, E. S. (2010). A national strategy to put accountable care into practice. *Health Affairs, 29*(5), 982–990.

Meyer, P. A., Penman-Aquilar, A., Campbell, V. A., Graffunder, C., O'Connor, A. E., & Yoon, P. W. (2013). Conclusion and future directions: CDC health disparities and inequalities report—United States, 2013. *Morbidity & Mortality Weekly Report (MMWR), Supplements, 62(3),* 184–186. Retrieved from http://www.cdc.gov/mmwr/preview/mmwrhtml/su6203a32.htm.

Mitchell, R. (2014). Transformation through tension: The moderating impact of negative affect on transformational leadership in teams. *Human Relations, 67*(9), 1095–1121.

National Association of Insurance Commisioners & Center for Insurance Policy Research. (2010). *Patient Protection & Affordable Care Act: Section by section analysis.* Washington, DC: Author.

Nielsen, M. B., & Einarsen, S. (2012). Outcomes of exposure to workplace bullying: A meta-analytic review. *Work & Stress, 26*(4), 309–332.

Noble, D. J., & Casalino, L. P. (2013). Can accountable care organizations improve population health? Should they try? *Journal of the American Medical Association, 309*(11), 1119–1120.

Nyweide, D. J., Lee, W., Cuerdon, T. T., Pham, H. H., Cox, M., Rajkumar, R., & Conway, P. H. (2015). Association of Pioneer Accountable Care Organizations vs traditional Medicare fee for service with spending, utilization, and patient experience. *Journal of the American Medical Association, 313*(21), 2152–2161.

Occupational Safety and Health Administration. (n.d.). *Safety and health topics: Workplace violence.* Washington, DC: Author.

Okun, S., Schoenbaum, S. C., Andrews, D., Chidambaran, P., Chollette, V., Gruman, J., . . . Henderson, D. (2014). *Patients and health care teams forging effective partnerships.* Washington, DC: Institute of Medicine.

Ortega, A., Christensen, K. B., Hogh, A., Rugulies, R., & Borg, V. (2011). One-year prospective study on the effect of workplace bullying on long-term sickness absence. *Journal of Nursing Management, 19*(6), 752–759.

Pompeii, L., Dement, J., Schoenfisch, A., Lavery, A., Souder, M., Smith, C., & Lipscomb, H. (2013). Perpetrator, worker and workplace characteristics associated with patient and visitor perpetrated violence (type II) on hospital workers: A review of the literature and existing occupational injury data. *Journal of Safety Research, 44,* 57–64.

Robert Wood Johnson Executive Nurse Fellows. (2012a). *Civility toolkit.* Retrieved from http://stopbullyingtoolkit.org/

Robert Wood Johnson Executive Nurse Fellows. (2012b). *Stop bullying nurses: Nurse leader stop bullying tool kit launched by RWJ ENF.* Princeton, NJ: Author. Retrieved from http://www.stopbullyingnurses.com/blog/2014/6/23/nurse-leader-stop-bullying-tool-kit-launched-by-rwjf-enf.html

Robert Wood Johnson Foundation. (2015, February 5). *Philadelphia, Pennsylvania: City reports 4.7 percent decline in obesity among children in grades K through 12.* Retrieved from http://www.rwjf.org/en/library/articles-and-news/2013/07/philadelphia--signs-of-progress.html

Roter, D. L. (2011). Oral literacy demand of health care communication: Challenges and solutions. *Nursing Outlook, 59*(2), 79–84.

Sarkar, U., Karter, A. J., Liu, J. Y., Adler, N. E., Nguyen, R., López, A., & Schillinger, D. (2010). The literacy divide: Health literacy and the use of an Internet-based patient portal in an integrated health system—results from the Diabetes Study of Northern California (DISTANCE). *Journal of Health Communication, 15*(S2), 183–196.

Shepard, J., Hadhazy, E., Frederick, J., Nicol, S., Gade, P., Cardon, A., . . . Madison, S. (2014). Using electronic medical records to increase the efficiency of catheter-associated urinary tract infection surveillance for National Health and Safety Network reporting. *American Journal of Infection Control, 42*(3), e33–e36.

Sheridan, S. L., Halpern, D. J., Viera, A. J., Berkman, N. D., Donahue, K. E., & Crotty, K. (2011). Interventions for individuals with low health literacy: A systematic review. *Journal of Health Communication, 16*(Suppl. 3), 30–54.

Shirey, M. R., & White-Williams, C. (2015). Boundary spanning leadership practices for population health. *Journal of Nursing Administration, 45*(9), 411–415.

Sittig, D. F., & Singh, H. (2012). Electronic health records and national patient-safety goals. *New England Journal of Medicine, 367*(19), 1854–1860.

Snyder, E., & Oliver, J. (2014). Evidence based strategies for attesting to meaningful use of electronic health records: An integrative review. *Online Journal of Nursing Informatics, 18*(3).

Tetuan, T., Ohm, R., Herynk, M., Ebberts, M., Wendling, T., & Mosier, M. (2014). The Affordable Health Care Act annual wellness visits: The effectiveness of a nurse-run clinic in promoting adherence to mammogram and colonoscopy recommendations. *Journal of Nursing Administration, 44*(5), 270–275.

Trépanier, S. G., Fernet, C., & Austin, S. (2013). Workplace bullying and psychological health at work: The mediating role of satisfaction of needs for autonomy, competence and relatedness. *Work & Stress, 27*(2), 123–140.

Udlis, K. A., & Mancuso, J. M. (2012). Doctor of Nursing Practice programs across the United States: A benchmark of information: Part I: Program characteristics. *Journal of Professional Nursing, 28*(5), 265–273.

Unger, M. D., Aldrich, A. M., Hefner, J. L., & Rizer, M. K. (2014). A journey through meaningful use at a large academic medical center: Lessons of leadership, administration, and technical implementation. *Perspectives in Health Information Management, 11*(Fall).

U.S. Department of Health and Human Services. (2014). *Key features of the Affordable Care Act*. Retrieved from http://www.hhs.gov/healthcare/facts-and-features/key-features-of-aca/index.html

U.S. Department of Labor Bureau of Labor Statistics. (2014). *Nonfatal occupational injuries and illnesses requiring days away from work in 2013*. Washington, DC: Author.

Weeks, D. L., Keeney, B. J., Evans, P. C., Moore, Q. D., & Conrad, D. A. (2015). Provider perceptions of the electronic health record incentive programs: A survey of eligible professionals who have and have not attested to meaningful use. *Journal of General Internal Medicine, 30*(1), 123–130.

Whittington, J. W., Nolan, K., Lewis, N., & Torres, T. (2015). Pursuing the triple aim: The first seven years. *Milbank Quarterly, 93*(2), 263–300.

Wolff, K., Cavanaugh, K., Malone, R., Hawk, V., Gregory, B. P., Davis, D., . . . Rothman, R. L. (2009). The Diabetes Literacy and Numeracy Education Toolkit (DLNET) materials to facilitate diabetes education and management in patients with low literacy and numeracy skills. *Diabetes Educator, 35*(2), 233–245.

World Health Organization. (2011). *Closing the gap: Policy into practice on social determinants of health: Discussion Paper.* Geneva, Switzerland: Author. Retrieved from http://www.who.int/sdhconference/Discussion-paper-EN.pdf

Wyte-Lake, T., Tran, K., Bowman, C. C., Needleman, J., & Dobalian, A. (2013). A systematic review of strategies to address the clinical nursing faculty shortage. *Journal of Nursing Education, 52*(5), 245.

Yedidia, M. J., Chou, J., Brownlee, S., Flynn, L., & Tanner, C. A. (2014). Association of faculty perceptions of work-life with emotional exhaustion and intent to leave academic nursing: Report on a national survey of nurse faculty. *Journal of Nursing Education, 53*(10), 569.

CHAPTER 4

Economics and Finance

Brenda Talley

We are in a position of financial and social power, and we could be agents of change in our society. Without pretension, I believe we could be a nice little gardener who takes care of the garden, and hopefully our neighbor will do the same. Then, maybe we'll achieve a better world.

—Guy Laliberté

OBJECTIVES

- *To appreciate the power inherent in effective use of resources*
- *To articulate the interrelationship between quality of care (processes and outcomes) and health care finance models*
- *To utilize financial management tools, such as budgeting, to support the best use of resources*
- *To determine various means of revenue and resource generation for the delivery of health care*
- *To recognize opportunities related to emerging payment models for the provision of care*

Effectively dealing with scarce resources is a perennial concern and perhaps should be the first sentence in the job description of the health care leader. Financial pressures are among the most significant challenges that have provoked a recent wave of departures of leaders, particularly from hospitals (Carlson, 2009; Carlson, Evans, Lubell, Rhea, & Zigmond, 2009). This exodus marks an unfortunate loss of experience but offers the opportunity for new talent to introduce new ways of thinking about health care and finance. Additionally, recent changes in reimbursement methods have influenced clinical practice models. The expert practitioner must be an active participant in changes that affect both approaches to clinical care and the financial viability of practice.

This chapter introduces selected topics related to financial issues and essential concepts of financial management for those in the leadership role as well as clinicians who, as we will see, also carry a responsibility for the financial health of the organization. The relationships among power and influence, decision making, achieving goals, and leadership growth are related to finance. Entire texts, courses, and experts are devoted to teaching economics, finance, accounting, and budgeting. While no attempt is made here to include every aspect of financial management that you will need, effort is made to connect the skills of financial management to leadership, to change, and to emerging practice patterns and opportunities.

THE FINANCING OF HEALTH CARE

Early financing of health care was mainly provided by charitable, religious, ethnic, and women's organizations, and by philanthropists and others. As modern hospitals developed with advances in technology, treatment procedures, and the health care professions, models of fee-for-service governed payment for health care, leading to payment by third parties, insurance, and public sources (Halloran, 2008, pp. 229–230). The role of payers has emerged as more and more directive.

For much of the history of nursing education, budget and fiscal management were neither seriously considered nor taught. Never underestimate the power of the one who knows where the money is. Kibort (2005, p. 53) warned, "There is no doubt about it, the people who get the most response are the ones who create most of the wealth in the organization. . . . Because these groups generate the contribution margins for the system, they are the ones who get listened to first. It takes a lot of fortitude to balance this phenomenon and give heed to the smaller players."

In the traditional fee-for-service model of payment, providers were paid without regard to the outcome of care. Charges were submitted and in only more recent years were charges mitigated by payers' determination of "usual and customary charges" for a geographical area. Revenue was grounded in the volume of services provided. Other models of payment, such as health maintenance organizations (HMOs) and capitation approaches, eventually arose in which a set amount of compensation was provided for all care required for an individual. This step was the beginning of attaching the outcomes of care to financial net gain. Payment amounts did not differentiate according to quality, but there was increased liability for providers if services delivered less than optimal outcomes. These models remain active, but are slowly being replaced by other models.

THE PRESENT STATE OF HEALTH CARE FINANCE

The last decades of the 20th century brought a shift in reimbursement for health care services instigated by Medicare (and soon followed by other payers) that tied hospital reimbursement to outcomes related to individual patient experience. Using diagnosis-related groups (DRGs), reimbursements for services were determined by analysis of payment histories of certain conditions, beginning with inpatient acute care facilities, with adjustments related to individual patient characteristics, population mix, geography, and hospital types (Centers for Medicare and Medicaid Services [CMS], 2014). Volume-based reimbursement remains the focus, though services for complications related to patient safety indicators, such as falls and nosocomial infections, are ineligible for payment. The major difference lies with the uniform determination of reimbursement (with the described adjustments) based on "normalized" averages of the cost of care, rather charges for care (interim reimbursement rates) as determined by the submitted cost reports of facilities and related factors, which are then reconciled by judgment of allowable costs on the filed reports. Quality concerns focus on selected outcomes: the aforementioned patient safety indicators, mortality rates, and 30-day readmission rates (CMS, 2015, September).

The Patient Protection and Affordable Care Act (ACA) of 2010, known commonly as Obamacare, provided many people who had lacked coverage the opportunity to obtain health insurance. The payment of services for Medicare recipients also changed dramatically under this legislation. The influence of the ACA is pervasive in health care delivery, and no attempt will be made here to fully describe all aspects. Instead, the focus is on the relationship to financial concerns in the provision of care.

The ACA aims to reduce costs as well as improve the processes of care by supporting a value-based system. This calls for new designs for care that are consistent with new systems for payment. Practice issues and financial concerns are firmly linked in this health care reform movement (Harris, Holm, & Inniger, 2015). It is the expert clinician who will collaborate with financial leaders to ensure that both processes and outcomes of care are optimal in terms of patient needs and that financial well-being is achieved. Finding the exquisite balance between quality and efficiency will be the challenge for visionary leaders.

Since 2012, inpatient value-based reimbursement has been based on hospital performance scores. These scores are calculated annually and are compared to those of other hospitals and to a hospital's own year-to-year performance. Of the 34 quality indicators considered, seven are *outcomes* and 27 are *processes* (CMS, 2013). These measures, weighted, are calculated into the performance scores; top scorers are rewarded with financial incentives while poor performers are penalized. Although some measures will eventually "top out" (i.e., there is no room for improvement) and others be added, the rapidly changing and complex requirements require constant attention (Wilson, 2011). The Hospital Consumer Assessment of Healthcare Providers and Systems (HCAHPS) survey is a national, standardized survey of patients' perspectives of hospital care introduced by the CMS. Hospitals participating in Medicare are required to administer the survey to a sampling of patients soon after discharge. The results are reported to the public and are used as a scoring factor for reimbursements (CMS, 2014). This measure is currently limited to inpatient hospital settings, but some believe that a similar plan will be factored into reimbursement for other settings, including primary care (see Edwards & Landon, 2014; Ryan et al., 2015). Private insurance companies and other providers usually follow the lead of Medicare in determining policy and coverage changes.

Patient satisfaction scores represent one of the more controversial indicators of quality that are factored into ratings for reimbursement. Data analysis produces a strong correlation between patient satisfaction scores and more global indicators of quality (Issac, Zaslavsky, Cleary, & Landon, 2010; Jha, Orav, Zheng, & Epstein, 2008), though some argue that patient satisfaction scores are not reliable determinants of quality in care processes and, indeed, have the potential for harm (Nix, 2013; Ryan et al., 2015). One concern is that smaller, rural, and resource-poor facilities will fail to meet comparisons with other institutions due to financial constraints and other factors not within their control (Nix, 2013).

CULTIVATING CONFIDENCE IN FINANCIAL MATTERS

Because financial matters are not often emphasized in the educational preparation of nurses, some may be intimidated by financial management and may avoid engagement in activities that require knowledge of financial dynamics. But the days are long gone when nurses might come forward with good ideas simply because they are good for patients or clinicians. Transformational leaders always make a strong business case for new models of care.

Must a successful leader have the skills of a financial manager? While those who describe successful leaders cite their ability to create a vision, in order to communicate that vision, and to support and motivate others to accomplish it, managers must be able to control resources, interpret and implement policies, organize work, and focus on short-term goals (Yoder-Wise, 2011). Moseley (2009, p. 296) identified the critical connection between financial management and a leader's ability to meet strategic goals, pointing out that lack of such connection may result in the following:

- Failing to integrate the strategic planning and capital allocation process. This can result in inefficiency, missed opportunities, and failure to meet targets.
- Defaulting from a strategic financial planning process to a budgeting process. Budgets tend to be year to year, while strategic visions may require 3 to 5 years or more.
- Spending more on strategic initiatives than is justified by the strategies' financial prospects and the organization's credit rating. Strategic plans that are not appropriately budgeted and do not generate acceptable returns can expend critical capital reserves.
- Inadequately monitoring strategic financial performance. An effective mechanism for monitoring financial performance is necessary to avoid wasted capital, cash flow problems, and failure to reach objectives.

Power struggles over resources have consumed individuals' lives, divided families and friends, initiated wars and rebellions, and resulted in upheavals of

REFLECTION QUESTIONS

Caring is not restricted to nurses. Those in other roles, such as financial management, have concerns that, for nurses, may not be in the forefront of thought. Consider the statement: *Values may not differ so much as perspectives.*

1. What values may be held in common?
2. How might perceptions between those responsible for financial management and resources differ from clinicians?
3. How might caring be manifested from a *financial perspective*?
4. How might reaching an appreciation of the other's perceptions be a positive force in interdisciplinary collaboration?

social, political, and economic systems. It is no wonder, then, that conflict can erupt over how best to allocate an organization's resources. Priorities differ, and poor communication among disciplines and specialties exacerbates the problem. The considerations of the business manager can conflict with those of the clinician. Values may not differ so much as perspectives.

Effective leadership requires creativity and the ability to work with others to fulfill a vision. While doctorally prepared nurses may or may not actually be developing the budget, there is much to know about overseeing or supporting the process, validating the inputs, setting priorities, enabling evaluative mechanisms, or responding to variances and deviants from financial and output goals. Financial management and planning tools provide the vehicle by which vision can be realized. The ability to communicate effectively with health care providers *and* with financial experts on knowledgeable levels is a powerful means toward providing both efficient and effective health care.

UNDERSTANDING THE LANGUAGE OF FINANCE

While it is not necessary for you to *be* an accountant, in order to take the initiative in financial matters as the leader it may wise to seek the counsel of experts in finance. As in any profession, finance has its own terminology. Knowledge of basic terms used by financial officers demonstrates an ability and willingness to learn about finance and can convey an intention to be "hands on" in making decisions. Frankly speaking, knowledge of basic accounting concepts and terms is empowering. Once you learn the terminology, applications, and meanings, your confidence will soar and your role in the financial matters of the organization will become increasingly significant (see U.S. Small Business Administration, 2016).

Many resources are available online that explain the terminology of finance. More importantly, by keeping abreast of relevant, current literature you will be introduced to newly coined words and acronyms. Indeed, because of the increasing connections between approaches to health care delivery and reimbursement, some emerging terms reflect this very connection. New phrases arise related to collaborative practice arrangements and what is identified as improvement opportunities:

- Practice sustainability
- Clinical documentation
- Shared savings
- Employed practices; streamlined workflows; and enhanced patient access, quality, and satisfaction
- Transparent and equitable compensation methodology (Harris et al., 2015, p. 71)

Indeed, it may be the responsibility of the expert clinician to fully explain the meaning of these phrases *in the terms of* practice conditions, standards, and patient needs. You can be an important interpreter to those whose expertise lies solely within the financial framework as new practice models are explored in response to pervasive and innovative payment models. As you continue your adventure to learn more about financial matters, take advantage of every opportunity and resource. Table 4.1 provides online resources related to financial matters.

TABLE 4.1 Online Resources for Financial Management

ONLINE RESOURCES FOR THE HEALTH CARE LEADER	
Accounting principles for entrepreneurs	http://www.entrepreneur.com/money/moneymanagement/bookkeeping/article21908.html
Accounting principles for nonprofit organizations	http://managementhelp.org/finance/np_fnce/np_fnce.htm
Free online management library	http://www.managementhelp.org/aboutfml/what-it-is.htm
Mind tools	http://www.mindtools.com/pages/main/newMN_TED.htm
Centers for Disease Control and Prevention cost–benefit analysis	https://www.mindtools.com/pages/article/newTED_08.htm http://www.dummies.com/how-to/content/performing-a-costbenefit-analysis.html
Making grafts and charts using Microsoft Excel	http://www.excel-easy.com/data-analysis/charts.html http://www.wikihow.com/Create-a-Control-Chart http://www.internet4classrooms.com/excel_create_chart.htm
Strategic planning	http://work911.com/planningmaster/faq/scan.htm https://www.sba.gov/tools/sba-learning-center/training/strategic-planning

(continued)

TABLE 4.1 Online Resources for Financial Management (*continued*)

ONLINE RESOURCES FOR THE HEALTH CARE LEADER	
Developing business plans— Service Corp of Retired Executives (SCORE)	http://www.score.org/template_gallery. html?gclid=COm-57nLrpcCFQO5GgodagL_iQ
U.S. Small Business Administration Learning Center	https://www.sba.gov/tools/sba-learning-center/ search/training
Short courses on writing grant proposals	http://foundationcenter.org/getstarted/tutorials/ shortcourse/index.html http://www.mcf.org/mcf/grant/writing.htm
Searching for grants	http://grants.nih.gov/grants/guide/index.html http://nnlm.gov/funding/grants.html http://www.ahrq.gov/ http://www.grants.gov/

Comfort in Collaborative Financial Relationships

Rarely do individuals enter into business ventures totally alone. Even when an individual does not have business partners, he or she must collaborate with funding institutions, affiliated and associated agencies and providers, governmental agencies, or other members of the community. Nurses, especially, know the stories of health care and can make the need for services real to other collaborators. While standards of care and levels or types of services provided may not appear negotiable, they do warrant open discussion. In such negotiations, leaders must always examine and weigh the need to have control for control's sake and the need to maintain standards and employ expertise. Developing confidence in one's own ability to listen, to contemplate, and to make informed, collaborative decisions in areas such as practice or education will improve confidence in working with others on financial matters. Such collaboration can add to knowledge and confidence in all matters, including risks related to financial issues.

Rational Risk Taking

When resources are designated to produce a specific outcome, there is always a certain amount of inherent risk in reaching that outcome. Though you can develop skills to forecast changes affecting organizational, economic, and social environments, exact outcomes will always remain uncertain.

All decisions and actions are rife with risk. Risk cannot be eliminated and should not necessarily be decreased because courses of action that possess great value tend to be associated with higher risk.

REFLECTION QUESTIONS

The fact that you are a doctor of nursing practice (DNP) student says something about your propensity to take chances—you are approaching a new educational degree and new opportunities for practice.

1. How do you feel about risk?
2. Do you find energy in new adventures or does the "tried and true" support your strengths? In this time of rapid change, even the tried and true is bound to change as new opportunities arise.
3. Do your preferences in risk taking translate well into the learned skill of *rational risk taking*?
4. What decision-making skills would you employ to minimize risk and support success in a new financial venture?
5. As you continue to read the chapter, make notes on aspects of financial leadership that would support your success.

> What is important to determine is not whether the risk can be eliminated, but whether the level of risk is appropriate for the actions undertaken and, if so, what strategies can accommodate the risk. (Porter-O'Grady & Malloch, 2007, p. 28)

Fear of risk taking can paralyze decision making and deter organizational success. Porter-O'Grady and Malloch (2007) suggested that *rational risk taking* is a leadership skill that can be learned and practiced. Rational risk taking requires shifting from the notion of risk taking as negative to developing the skills required to promote the success of a complex and rapidly changing organization. Decisions are made based on organizational values, the strategic plans of the organization, respect for others, the well-being of individuals, and availability of resources.

ASSESSING THE CONTEXT OF CARE FROM A FINANCIAL PERSPECTIVE

Effective projections and management of resources require some ability to understand history, including business history of the organization, history of the community or context of the business, and history of the services of the business within the business community as well as the general social geography. It is also necessary to connect with current affairs in business and in the community, and you must be able to predict the future to some degree. There are several mechanisms that can help you in such assessments, such as the environmental scan.

Environmental Scan

An environmental scan is a critical and intentional review of information available in order to make appropriate resource decisions related to the organization. Information is categorized and used to help guide planning, decision making, and use of resources. It is a critical step in financial management and necessary for strategic planning.

Cote, Lauzon, and Kyd-Strickland (2008) used critical browsing in an environmental scan to search, select, and summarize information found on the web related to interprofessional collaborative practice initiatives. Twenty-seven documents were selected for additional analysis and inclusion. The information was categorized using three main parameters: source, summary, and relevance to the practice model. Five broad themes were identified: promotion, networking, evidence, resources, and linkage between interprofessional education and care. The scan helped provide data for successful financial decisions.

Conducting a full-scale environmental scan to include national issues is time consuming and requires skill. Many organizations regularly conduct environmental scans. The information published from such studies is applicable in many health care settings. One example of this is the environmental scan conducted by the American Hospital Association (AHA). The 2015 AHA Environmental Scan:

> Identifies emerging trends to help hospital and health care leaders plan strategically. The annual Scan serves as the foundation of the AHA's rolling three-year strategic plan. Topics include consumers and patients; economy and finance; information technology and e-health; insurance and coverage; physicians; political issues; provider organizations; quality and patient safety; transforming care delivery; science and technology; and workforce. (AHA, 2014)

The AHA Environmental Scan is compiled from nationally recognized sources with recommendations from select AHA governance committees. Emerging or potential problems related to resources as well as opportunities can be recognized by a critical and systematic evaluation of information from an environmental scan. An example of a financial issue identified in the most recent AHA scan is an increase in the deductible amounts in insurance plans. The analysis cited this as the root cause of increased cost shifting (AHA, 2014). Cost shifting in health care occurs when organizations attempt to achieve a positive profit margin by enhancing revenues received from best payers, such as insurance companies, to make up shortfalls left by payers whose reimbursements are inadequate related to costs, such as Medicaid (Robinson, 2011).

External Trends in the Community

Changes in demographics of the local community can result in a shift in health care needs and affect potential revenue. For example, nearby construction of a high-rise residential building for the elderly may result in a greater demand for geriatric services. An increase in the number of manufacturing plants in the community may increase the need for services for young families with small children. Increased unemployment rates could mean that families no longer have health insurance and have fewer resources to pay for care. Changes in the economy on a local, regional or national level can result in decreased funding or changes in reimbursement levels.

Trends Within the Organization

An environmental scan of the internal environment, such as past experiences, present conditions, and expressions of future expectations, is important. The internal political climate should be assessed to place appropriate issues on the "front burner." Potential conflicts within multiple agendas may be identified, and alliances and areas of competition should also be defined.

Current terminology refers to this internal assessment as a microsystem analysis. A microsystem is a subsystem of a larger complex system that is the point of care and part of a larger infrasystem (Roussel, 2014). The present climate of dynamic change, requiring a merging of clinical and financial concerns, demands that leaders identify, analyze, and manage critical metrics related to both processes and outcomes. This is essential to improve care delivery, develop innovations, and meet expected benchmarks. The need to increase efficiency and effectiveness at the point of care is valued for its own sake, but also as a critical necessity for financial well-being. Barach and Johnson (2006) suggested that the conceptual perspective of a clinical microsystem also allows organizations to analyze such systems by process mapping of interactions between individuals and among microsystems. Clearly the importance of microsystem analysis is critical to the financial health of the organization, given links among payment methods and processes and outcomes.

The American Recovery and Reinvestment Act of 2009 (ARRA) supports the widespread use of electronic health records (EHRs) by the use of incentives. Whereas stage 1 focuses on the collection of clinical data and sharing this information with the individuals and other providers, stage 2 is designed to use capture data to improve quality (CMS, 2015a). Given the dependency of financial reimbursement upon quality measures (in addition to the financial incentive of participation in the EHR program), utilization of these data within a microsystem analysis will help identify and remedy conditions operating in less than desired capacities. In addition, information systems can be modified to collect data needed for more precise collection of metrics. For example, a recent graduate of a DNP program developed an information system add-on for her primary care practice that allows her to continually evaluate whether performance standards are met for diabetic patients. The systems vendor is interested in incorporating this and other applications into the information systems package for other practices (Shea, 2014). In addition to supporting compliance of practice standards—an actual requirement in some settings for maximum payment and a potential payment factor in others—this approach is also useful in verifying capture of charges, noting omissions, and providing adequate follow-up and continuity of care. The clinical and the financial aspects of care are no longer separate entities, but rather intertwined and interdependent.

Metrics obtained must be systematically organized before analysis and evaluation can take place. In addition to metrics on processes and outcomes, financial data can be integrated into the system. Some of these data can be linked to the clinical experience; for example, the amount of waiting time in the emergency department before being seen, the time before release or admission, or the patterns in utilization of services by demographics, payment methods or mix, or diagnosis, all in real time. Still other measures can be added to an integrated information system.

The 5 P Framework

The 5 Ps have been incorporated into a structured diagram providing a method to visually look into multiple aspects of a clinical microsystem and to make assessments. The concept originated at the Lucile Packard Children's Hospital at Sanford University Medical Center (Dartmouth Institute for Health Care Policy and Clinical Practice [DIHCPCP], n.d.-a; Godfrey, 2010).

The 5 Ps include the following: (1) "purpose," or desired outcomes; (2) "patients," referring to specific patient populations; (3) "professionals," or care providers; (4) "processes" of assessment, problem-solving, and treatment plans; and (5) "patterns," referring to patient outcomes related to styles and symbols of leadership, culture, and values of the microsystem (Godfrey, 2010, p. 8).

Workbooks, called *Greenbooks*, were developed for major practice areas, which include (a) inpatient, (b) emergency department, (c) long-term care, (d) outpatient primary care, (e) outpatient specialty care, and (f) neonatal intensive care. Each *Greenbook* can be downloaded and utilized in the appropriate clinical area, and clinicians are encouraged to do so (see Box 4.1).

Others have developed and utilized workbooks more closely aligned with a specific clinical practice, and these are available as well. As you will see in your reading, this organization encourages development, feedback, and contributions. Additional resources include descriptions of tools used in microsystem appraisal, problem identification, planning, and evaluation (DIHCPCP, n.d.-a, n.d.-b). Among the *Greenbooks* tools that you could apply are flowcharts, tracking cards, control charts, and Plan-Do-Study-Act (PDSA) templates. These tools cannot be explored here due to space concerns, but we invite you to review them.

BOX 4.1. GREENBOOKS

1. Access the Microsystem Academy supported by the Dartmouth Institute for Health Policy and Clinical Practice, at https://clinicalmicrosystem.org/workbooks/. Review the *Microsystems at a Glance* booklet.
2. Choose the *Greenbook* that most closely matches your clinical practice area.
3. Consider areas in your practice environment that could use improvement. For the purposes of this exercise, choose an area that would have an impact on financial well-being. *However, do recall the intertwining of quality measures and cost/finance.* For example, time delays in referrals, transfers, medication administration, laboratory results, and documentation—just to list a few—could affect quality scores as well as efficient use of resources and expanded liability.
4. After creating a clear statement of the area of concern, determine which section of the *Greenbook* you selected would be most helpful to you in understanding the problem. Give your rationale for this selection.
5. Determine the critical information you will need. Note that quantitative measures (referred to as metrics) may not be your only source. Many areas allow for qualitative data, such as interviews. Note the measures that you consider essential.
6. Develop your team. Such an undertaking can rarely be accomplished by an individual. Who in your work environment (or external, for that matter) could facilitate both the collection and analysis of your data? Whose support do you require?
7. To whom would your present your results? What means would you use to present the analysis? (charts, tables, software?)
8. Give some thought to strategies for change. What might be positive outcomes for change in terms of cost management or maximization of revenue?
9. Summarize your experience.

Business Models, Plans, and Budgets

Expert clinicians are not usually prepared as experts in business or finance. But in order to make a difference as a leader in any transformational manner, you must know the language, processes, and outcomes related to fiscal matters in health care. You must be able to clearly articulate the return on investment of the important work you do, and to interpret the work of promoting health and caring for the sick to professional colleagues whose world centers on providing, developing, or managing resources. Business models are depictions of the business, the theoretical picture, or the conceptual portrayal of the organization from a business or financial perspective. The business plan is the road map used to project the success and contingency plans of the enterprise. And the budget is the operational record of all financial resources and management of the endeavor.

Business Models. Formal and theoretical business models have been developed using a multitude of criteria. Models may be based on relationships with other businesses, type of product or service, physical location of infrastructure, corporate structure, and ownership, among other factors. Many models are complicated and seem to have little apparent application to health care delivery.

A business model is defined simply as "consisting of two elements: (a) what the business does, and (b) how the business makes money doing these things" (Weill, Malone, D'Urso, Herman, & Woermer, 2004, p. 6). Generally, health care is considered a service model. Using this definition, Weill and colleagues derived the four basic business model archetypes—creator, distributor, landlord, and broker—shown in Table 4.2. Under this model, provision of health care services would most often be classified as a landlord-type business. (It could additionally be subcategorized as "intellectual landlord.") Neither health care facilities nor providers are bought or sold by "customers," and "people are not 'assets' in an accounting sense"; however, "their time (and knowledge) may be 'rented out' for a fee" (Weill et al., p. 11).

TABLE 4.2 Characteristics of Archetypes for Business Models

MIT BUSINESS MODEL ARCHETYPES	CHARACTERISTICS OF ARCHETYPES
Creator	• Buys raw materials or components from suppliers and then transforms or assembles them to create a product sold to buyers • Designs products sold • Predominant business model in all manufacturing industries
Distributor	• Buys a product and resells essentially the same product to someone else • May provide additional value by, for example, transporting or repackaging the product, or by providing customer service • Ubiquitous in wholesale and retail trade
Landlord	• Sells right to use, but not own, an asset for a specified period of time • Also includes lenders who provide temporary use of financial assets (e.g., money), and contractors and consultants who provide services produced by temporary use of human assets • *Health care services would be classified as a landlord model*
Broker	• Facilitates sales by matching potential buyers and sellers

Adapted from Weill et al. (2004).

Weill and colleagues categorized the 1,000 largest public companies in the United States by archetype and evaluated them for financial performance by analysis of revenue stream. Results demonstrated that selling use of assets to customers (landlord archetype) was more profitable, and more highly valued by the market, than selling ownership of assets. In general, business models based on nonphysical assets were found to be more profitable than those based on physical assets (Weill et al., 2004). Clearly this is relevant to the skilled professional–based health care industry.

Not-for-Profit Status and Making a Profit. Nurses tend to dislike thinking about the probability of payment and making a profit for providing health care services. However, staff and rent must be paid, supplies purchased, and in many instances, investors repaid. The for-profit, or proprietary model, of conducting business has infused some variety and innovation into the delivery of health care in the United States. The number of health care facilities and providers who have moved to for-profit status continues to increase. A not-for-profit organization is an organization recognized by both the state and the federal government as not-for-profit and hence exempt from some specific taxes, based on documented return of income to the organization or to the community, or both. Actually, this does not mean that the organization does not wish, or need, to make a profit. However, any income after expenses is reinvested by the organization rather than being paid to owners or stockholders. Often, any overage of income beyond expenses is used to provide additional services, to subsidize those who cannot pay, or to fund charitable services.

Business Plans. A business plan is useful as it helps communicate the capital value of the health care professional and the services provided to those who may be the gatekeepers to funding. The willingness to support a particular type of venture is generally grounded in the perception that the business will be profitable, or at least an asset to the organization or community rather than a liability. Even charitable donors such as the United Way fund want to see evidence of sustainability. A significant gap in communication to the gatekeepers may be in creating the vision that the venture will be an asset; this can be articulated most authentically by the expert care providers.

A business plan functions as a developmental road map, integrating goals, resource needs, financial needs and planning, and projected outcomes to begin a business venture, clinical practice initiative, educational project, or some other innovation. It is a document most often prepared as a proposal in order to obtain funding (Baker & Baker, 2011, p. 271). The doctorally prepared nurse likely would develop a business plan before setting up a new practice, program, or service. This process could also be used to help choose among several competing service or business options or even when considering a new line of services or implementing a new program within the organization. Several factors should be considered before beginning such a venture. Bupert (2004) listed the following: need for the services in the community, community interest and willingness to use the services, number of potential clients or patients for the service, and reimbursement for services by third-party payers.

The business plan for a proposed innovation must include more than money matters. It should include analysis of "key assumptions, strategy, operating plan and tactics, resource requirements, financial plan/analysis, evaluation/measurement plan, and contingency plans" (Morjikian, Kimball, & Joynt, 2007, p. 400). It should also be based on the best available evidence (Brandt et al., 2009). As a leader, you need to know and articulately communicate whether your plan is budget neutral and why, or why your plan makes business sense. Your projections and subsequent evaluation should quantify cost savings while advancing the mission of the organization. Cost savings may be reflected in the actual budget by costs, charges, or new revenue, or indirectly by reduction in worker turnover or other employee costs such as workers' compensation. Thus, the business plan for a clinical practice initiative should reflect the best information available from those most knowledgeable on the project, good program design, evidence of practice expertise, evidence of expert economic and financial management, and strong evidence of effective leadership (Harris, 2010).

The business plan should be written, and should contain many of the following sections. Consider which element is most appropriate and will be most useful and persuasive to launch your enterprise:

- Always include an executive summary. If you cannot make your case clearly on one page, no one will want to hear your pitch.
- Your vision or mission statement as well as background information on the initiative that reflects the rationale and need for your initiative, and specific objectives. The background and rationale should reflect a clear definition of your market and analysis of the market, including input from stakeholders; analysis of competition, if appropriate; and a profile of the clients or community your project will serve. Objectives should flow from your rationale.
- Current products or services and needed research and development, as appropriate. Describe your management teams, your product or service strategies, key factors in delivering your service, and what your project will accomplish, including a timeline. Specifically describe capital requirements; business risks; financial plan, including repayment plans, if appropriate; and your plan to sustain the project.
- Outline a marketing plan for communication, dissemination, advertising, and promotion, and other publicity strategies (Bupert, 2004, pp. 341–342; Harris, 2010).

Two financial activities are critical components of the business plan: the break-even analysis and the projected payer mix. Simply stated, an organization's break-even point is that point after which revenues exceed costs. Both fixed costs, those costs that can be most easily predicted and tend to be stable, and variable costs, those that by their nature can fluctuate, are considered when projecting the break-even point. Estimation of the break-even point is especially critical in financial planning for new programs, services, and beginning organizations. Until that point is reached, operations can be thought of as being in the "red"; that is, operations expend more money than is received. Funds must be available to meet cost (expenses) until the revenue can at least equal expenses. Even then, it must not be assumed that revenue will continue to exceed expenses. However, accurate projection of the break-even point can assist in (a) estimating acceptable risk in beginning a new service, (b) approximating the amount of funds needed for "start up" (i.e., the amount of funding required to maintain operations until a profit is realized), and (c) communicating potential business success to potential funding sources.

Projection of the break-even point is also useful in determining charges for units of service, such as the charges for a clinic visit. However, the amount charge for unit of service is also influenced by market conditions, including competition; by participation in third-party payer programs; by conditions set forth by funding organizations or affiliated organizations; and by other factors.

Baker and Baker (2011, p. 69) illustrated the break-even point as cost–volume–profit (CVP) analysis. The break-even point is defined as the "point when the contribution margin (that is, net revenue less variable costs) equals fixed cost." Additionally, the break-even point can be expressed in two ways: as an amount per unit of service, or as a percentage of net revenues. CVP projections or portrayals are often displayed in graph form, with the horizontal axis being the volume (e.g., number of visits) and the vertical axis showing cost. Low-cost or free software can assist in plugging in various scenarios of volume, revenue, and fixed and variable costs. Adaptation of electronic spreadsheets can be used to generate graphs showing the intersection between revenue and cost. Changing the variables can illustrate how differences in projections might produce different potential outcomes. Contingency plans can then be made to help minimize risks.

Estimating the Volume. Estimating the projected volume of units, such as clinic visits, is an inexact science. To start, the intended recipients of the service need to be defined in terms of characteristics (e.g., emerging families, the elderly, migrant workers) and by geographical location. These recipients would be the target market. Need and demand for services then can be projected based on demographics of the community, services already in place or gaps in services, client loyalty to and satisfaction with these services, and comparison of charges to existing services. Another potential consideration may be market conditions. Is the service considered a necessity by potential target market? Is a comparable alternative available to clients? How competitive is the proposed service? Is the service consistent with expectations and community norms, and congruent with the culture of the target market?

The decreasing reliance on fee-for-service options changes the dynamic somewhat, shifting the focus away from the total reliance on unit volume (e.g., patient visits) for estimating revenue. However, this factor remains an important consideration and analyses must be conducted with a mind not only to payer mix, but also to probable payment programs within payer (e.g., Medicare) reimbursement models. Additionally, projection of volume is necessary to estimate needs such as facilities, supplies, and staff.

Estimating the Payer Mix. The payer mix is the variety of sources that pay, or reimburse, for health care services. Information about varied demographic groups, such as the percentage of the population eligible for Medicaid, those older than age 65 who would have Medicare coverage, unemployment rates, and age distribution of the population, help estimate the mix of third-party payers. The type of services provided may also provide insight into the payer mix. Services targeted toward the elderly, for example, would tend to have Medicare as the predominant third-party payer. Health care organizations located where poverty is prevalent likely would have a higher percentage of Medicaid recipients, and recipients who rely on other sources for subsidized care. These organizations might also have a higher percentage of patients who are not covered by third-party payers and cannot afford to self-pay.

Variations in the mix of payers can have a great impact on the revenue of an organization. Shifts in payer mix or failure to project a near approximation can severely alter income projections, as seen in Tables 4.3 and 4.4. Note

TABLE 4.3 Scenario 1 Payer Mix

SCENARIO 1 VOLUME × REIMBURSEMENT RATE = TOTAL REIMBURSEMENT			
THIRD-PARTY PAYER	VOLUME (NUMBER OF VISITS)	PER VISIT	TOTAL REIMBURSEMENT
Payer Uni	10 visits	$55.00	$550.00
Payer Medi	25 visits	$85.00	$2,125.00
Insurance A	30 visits	$95.00	$2,850.00
Insurance B	35 visits	$105.00	$3,675.00
Total	**100 visits**		**$9,200.00**

TABLE 4.4 Scenario 2 Payer Mix

SCENARIO 2 VOLUME × REIMBURSEMENT RATE = TOTAL REIMBURSEMENT			
THIRD-PARTY PAYER	VOLUME (NUMBER OF VISITS)	PER VISIT	TOTAL REIMBURSEMENT
Insurance B	10 visits	$105.00	$1,050.00
Insurance A	25 visits	$95.00	$2,375.00
Payer Medi	30 visits	$85.00	$2,550.00
Payer Uni	35 visits	$55.00	$1,925.00
Total	**100 visits**		**$7,900.00**

that scenario A and scenario B both show revenue for 100 visits. Reversing the number of visits per payer source in this payer mix results in a difference of revenue of $1,300 for the same number of visits.

Choosing to Participate. Some health care providers choose to not provide care to individuals whose services are billed to specific payers, due to the potential loss or liability incurred by decreased revenue. Others provide services, but limit the percentage of patients whose payment is from a particular source. An example is providers who refuse or limit the number of patients covered by Medicaid. In many states the amount allowed for payment of Medicaid services is lower than payment by other sources. It is not uncommon in a community to find few or no providers for services paid by Medicaid. Whether to accept all payers or restrict those accepted into care based on the payment sources is a decision that encompasses financial, legal, and ethical considerations and the ability to fulfill the mission of the organization.

Projecting Revenue. When calculating projected revenue, the difference between charges and reimbursement, or payment, must be recognized. Only the actual reimbursement amount can be projected as potential revenue. For example, Medicare and Medicaid only pay within specific dollar limits. Planning and targeting marketing of services should include defining all potential payers and estimating reimbursement levels. Contracts and agreements, such as care under preferred provider organizations (PPOs), rarely pay at the level of charges, but rather another amount agreed upon, or a contractual charge. Some payers use the "customary and usual" guidelines for payment. Customary and usual payments are those the payer determines by evaluating local or regional markets and assessing the usual charges for like services. Currently, this method is less prevalent than are negotiated contracts, such as those involving PPOs. Many contracts state a maximum amount per service that can be billed to the client. Whether or not the client can be billed for any difference between the charges and the designated reimbursement depends on the contract, and this can vary by service from the same provider of services. For example, a payer may not require a client

---

REFLECTION QUESTIONS

Among several issues in health care finance are cost shifting and "cherry-picking" (e.g., accepting into services those who have the best payers or demographics).

1. What ethical considerations come into play with these issues?
2. Are any ethical principles violated by limiting accepted payers?
3. How are the financial needs of the organization balanced with ethical concerns?

copayment for an annual physical examination but have a set copayment for an illness visit. Expressed deductibles can usually be billed to the client. In addition to set rates, other factors to consider when projecting revenues are discounts, contractual allowances, the likelihood of uncollectable bills, and client copayments.

The time intervals between provision of services and billing, and between billing and payment for services, are significant factors when minimal operating funds are available. Scrutiny of these time intervals will reveal the impact on the organization's ability to meet financial obligations and the level of operating funds needed to meet obligations. Using a device such as a control chart that indicates the lengths of time from discharges to filing of claims, processing, and to receipt of payment can help evaluate monetary flow of the organization. Any variances between expectations and actual time can be investigated. Lagging payments (i.e., increased time between receipt of claims and payments) are an ongoing concern.

In undertaking a business venture that requires funding, you must consider the level of *personal* financial liability that may be assumed. The structure and legal designation of the organization provides for specific "ownership" of liability. Consultation with legal experts on such issues is imperative. For example, liability, either personal or corporate, has to be defined in the event the organization does not generate enough revenue to meet payroll, utilities, rent, and repayment of loans or other obligations.

BUDGETS

Oversimplified, financial management is simply a matter of managing, balancing, and projecting resources. Most simply, a budget "is a plan with a timetable that guides an organization's activities" (Finkler & Kovner, 2000):

> A budget is based on *revenue* (income generated, owed, or [received] for services) and *expenses* (expenditures and costs of activities needed for the organization's operations). The difference between the projected cost and the actual cost of services is called a *variance*. The major types of budgets include the *operating budget* (the daily income and costs in one year for workload, personnel . . ., supplies, and overhead), the *capital* budget (buildings, land, long-term investments, or durable expensive equipment), the *cash* budget (actual/expected monthly income and cash disbursements), and the *long-range* budget (a strategic plan of goals over a 3- to 10-year period). (Greenberg, 2008, p. 74)

A simple traditional budgeting approach calculates annual incremental increases or decreases based on historical information about revenue and expenses. If it is "zero based," it is developed and justified anew (or from zero) each fiscal year. Creating a budget, or a financial road map, for an organization is an ongoing process. Possibly the biggest mistake made in budgeting is to assume that once a budget is constructed and implemented, the work is done until "next year."

Generally, budgets are created at the institutional or organizational level around designated cost centers. A cost center is a unit or department for which a budget is created and to which expenses are charged. A cost center may also be a designated source of revenue; however, depending on how the cost center is defined, revenue may be difficult to define. An example of this is a centralized cost center for nursing services in a hospital. The revenue for nursing services is often not detectable but rather embedded with other services or charges. Thus, expenses can be clearly defined but not the contribution to revenue.

Approaches to Budgeting

Budgets most often span a fiscal year. The fiscal year for a private organization is self-defined; for example, it could be from January 1 to December 31 or from July 1 to June 30. The choice of inclusive dates is influenced by the fiscal year of funding sources and reporting requirements of associated or governmental agencies. Public organizations would most often follow the appropriate government fiscal year.

There are two basic approaches to budgeting, as well as variations and combinations of the two. They are the historical or incremental approach and the zero-based budgeting or budgeting-by-objectives approach.

The Historical or Incremental Approach. The simplest and most commonly used approach is to base the following year's budget on budgets of the past, usually that of the previous year, assisted by data from the current year. A certain percentage is added or subtracted based on increases or decreases in projected expenses. Investigations are conducted on more or less predictable changes, such as employee salaries, benefits, and costs for energy, supplies, and equipment. Actual expenditures of the preceding year are also considered. This expected increment or decrease (the difference between last year's budget and the expected expenses for the coming year) is added to the current year's budget, producing the new proposed budget.

The historical approach to budgeting is attractive because it requires less time commitment and expertise for those preparing the budget. The assumption of this approach is that business will continue into the future relatively unchanged. Therefore, it is especially useful in an organization with intentionally enduring services or programs and in a stable economy.

The downside of historical or incremental budgeting is that it tends to sustain existing departments, programs, or activities for better or worse. While change is not incompatible with this approach to budgeting, neither is it fostered by this process. A tendency toward maintaining the status quo may make it difficult to align organizational objectives with the needs of the community or with changes in the economy, reimbursement practices, or health care delivery.

This could stem from a tendency to look within the organization rather than considering the external environment.

The Zero-Based or Budgeting-by-Objectives Approach. In contrast to the historical approach, the zero-based or budgeting-by-objectives approach makes no assumptions regarding the continuation of specific programs of the organization or of services provided. The budget is presented as a package that includes objectives, projected outcomes, and cost and revenue. Each budget unit must be justified and have definite objectives in line with the mission of the organization. Priorities are assigned to each of the unit budget proposals related to the mission and needs of the organization.

One of the strengths of zero-based budgeting is that a mechanism for discontinuing ineffective or inefficient departments or programs is inherent to the process, whereas historical budgeting tends to perpetuate the status quo. If the costs of a program or department cannot be justified in terms of intended outcomes or ratio of cost to benefits, then deletion has to be considered. The danger of this approach is that financial benefit to the organization may be the sole factor used for this determination. Care should be taken to ensure that intangible benefits are considered. Public expectations, goodwill, mission, and community needs must be considered.

An additional strength of zero-based budgeting is that new and creative programs have an equal footing in terms of possible funding as do established programs. The organization can be more responsive to changes in the social, economic, and health delivery environments. Rather than being grounded in established traditions, new creative and innovative approaches to health care delivery can be grounded in community needs, results of evidence-based practice, trials of community interventions, and opportunities for collaborative ventures.

Zero-based budgeting does have potential drawbacks. It is more time consuming than the historical approach and requires a higher level of budgetary expertise. Employees may feel threatened by a perceived lack of long-term stability and viability of their work environment, because continued funding will be questioned and may suffer in competition with other programs. In this same vein, a sense of negative competition may exist among departments and programs. A department or program's continued existence may be seen to depend on the manager's ability to develop unit objectives, assign cost to achieving defined outcomes, and analyze the impact on the overall organization. The leader has an obligation to assist the units in best presenting their budgetary package.

Several conditions may influence the manner in which budgets are framed. Budgets are framed within a specific time period in each organization, which may include a set fiscal year or a continual rolling process over time. Budgets may be relatively fixed or flexible.

Rolling Budget. A rolling budget is projected for a selected time frame in the future, for example, 3 or 6 months. While that budget is in effect, a new budget to follow that time period is developed. Thus, a budget is always in use and a new budget is always in development. Though this approach appears to be time consuming (and it is), it is not as great a variation from the yearly budget as it may appear. In actuality, organizations are engaged in developing future budgets on an ongoing basis, even when employing yearly budgets. The advantage of the rolling budget is that it allows for shifts in needs and proprieties that become apparent during the current budget span, allowing for adaptation to changes in priorities and needs without having to restructure a budget or miss an opportunity due to budget constraints.

Trended Budget. A trended budget is useful when there is a predictable unevenness in services over the budget year. If 20% more services are provided in September, October, and November than in June, July, and August, budget appropriation for those time periods differ by that same percentage difference. This prevents unnecessary budget variances in these months, as well as a surplus of funds in one period that might have been better utilized in a different period.

Fixed Versus Flexible Budget. A fixed budget assumes that both revenue and expenses will be essentially the same from month to month. The total amount allotted to an expense for the year is divided by 12 to determine the allotment for each month. A flexible budget, in contrast, is a budget that automatically adjusts variables to reflect changes such as volume, labor costs, and capital expenditures (Barr, 2005). The advantages of a flexible budget also apply to a trended budget but are enhanced. The ability to respond to changes in economics, patient care delivery, personnel needs, and emergencies is inherent in the flexible budgeting approach. What could be thought of as a disadvantage of flexible budgeting techniques—that is, the requirement for constant surveillance and synchronicity with both internal and external environments—is actually a business advantage. The biggest advantage of a flexible budget is the ability to make timely operational adjustments, if necessary (Sharpe, 2009). For example, a home health agency may recognize that the cost of gasoline has increased and that travel expenditures are running over budget. Using a flexible approach, alternatives could be identified immediately and set in place to mitigate the cost increases. Collaboration with those at the point of care might provide assistance in defining alternatives without diminishing quality of care. In the previous example, it might be possible to sequence home visits more efficiently without diminishing quality.

In the past, the ability to access the data needed for successful flexible budgeting would have been impossible. Today, electronic processes and sources of information make it relatively easy. The first challenge to implementing a flexible budget is to ensure that a system is in place to collect the needed data (Sharpe, 2009). Barr (2005, p. 26) explained:

> Patient volume can be plugged into a flex[ible] budget to make it more useful. The percentage of patients participating in Medicare, Medicaid and private insurance as well as the percentage of

uninsured will have varying effects on revenue and costs, and during the traditional budget preparation time those can only be estimated. A flex[ible] budget allows those numbers to be updated frequently over the year, creating new budgetary estimates of how the current year is unfolding and how the coming year looks financially based on those complicated interrelationships.

Components of the Budget

Organizations often have a format for creating the budget that includes several components. The most common components are outlined here. The operating budget, mentioned earlier in this discussion, is the expenditure plan for daily operating activities of the organization. It includes budgets for each cost center and all expense units in the organization, as well as a projection of revenue (Yoder-Wise, 2011). The personnel budget is usually the largest portion of an operating budget, accounting for about 85% of the projected expenditures (Liebler & McConnell, 2004). Personnel costs include wage and salary for each position and for each person, anticipated compensation raises, adjustments resulting in changes in personnel status, vacation relief, overtime pay, and temporary or seasonal help (Liebler & McConnell, 2004, p. 311). Consideration is also given to the cost of recruiting and orienting new personnel. Most organizations include a separate section on the cost of benefits, such as any health insurance and life insurance premiums that the employer pays or payments made into retirement benefits by the employer on behalf of the employee. Both time worked and time paid but not worked must be included in the budget. (See Table 4.5.)

TABLE 4.5 Components of an Organizational Operating Budget

MAJOR COMPONENTS OF THE OPERATING BUDGET
Personnel
Salary and Wages
Anticipated Compensation Adjustments
Benefits
Recruitment & Orientation
Capital Items
Facilities: land, buildings, lease agreements
High-cost Equipment
Appreciation/Depreciation
Supplies
Necessary Dispensable Items
Travel
Local Travel Costs for Personnel
Out-of-Town Travel Costs for Personnel

Personnel needs are usually calculated by full-time equivalents (FTEs), which, in turn, are calculated using projections of units of service or volume of services. Usually, an FTE is equated to working 40 hours per week for each week of a year, or 2080 hours yearly (Yoder-Wise, 2011). The unit of service is defined by the organization (though influenced strongly by payers' definitions) and may be the number of clinic visits, admissions to service, treatments, and so on. For a continuing budget, past volume and productivity can be used to estimate future needs. For new services, descriptions of expected services, examination of similar services, and expert opinion of providers are useful in projecting personnel needs. For added or new services, orientation time for employees is a special consideration, although there is an expense any time there is turnover in staff.

The capital budget items are facilities and other nondisposable or high-end purchases such as land and buildings, machinery, and equipment. Each organization has its own guidelines regarding what constitutes a capital expenditure. For example, criteria may dictate that to be included in the capital budget, equipment and machinery items must cost at least $1,000 and have a life expectancy of more than 5 years. Acquisition costs of equipment are calculated and prorated over the expected life of the equipment. Operating and depreciation costs are also calculated (Liebler & McConnell, 2004). Choices in equipment should be grounded in many factors, including the overall operating and maintenance expenses, human resource costs in educating staff to use the equipment, and clinical usefulness and ease of use.

Capital budget items may originate as a part of a cost center or work unit or be a part of the organization's strategic plan. In some instances, depending on the organization's policies, lease agreements may be subjected to the same type of budget proposals. A separate budget may be developed for future planned construction and may be referred to as the building or construction budget.

The supply budget ranges from disposable office materials such as pens and paper clips to clinical supplies, and is usually the most flexible component of the overall budget. Some materials may require requisition forms; others must be immediately available. Some supply charges are considered a part of "doing business"; others may be billable patient supplies. Some of the supplies are stable in price; others vary over time. All potential supply costs must be examined in order to adequately budget. Tracking systems must be able to capture and match the classification of supplies and their accounting to a unit budget.

The Budgeting Process

Regardless of the approach or technique used in budgeting, budget items or components must be justified. That is, it should be clear to decision makers why each proposed expenditure is necessary. All expenditures should be tied to the mission, goals, objectives, and strategic plan of the organization.

As participation of stakeholders in the budgeting process increases, commitment to the budget priorities and outcomes also increases. An inclusive approach is especially important when resources may be limited. The leader can bring into the process midlevel managers and providers of care across disciplines in a workshop environment. Working collaboratively to complete a budget is not only fruitful, but it also establishes a forum for educating staff about the budget process, discussing mission and goals of the organization, and addressing concerns. Bradley (2008, p. 57) described the vision of a budget workshop thus:

> The vision for the budget workshop included streamlining and simplifying the process as follows: 1) Providing access to tools and resources including finance, payroll, and decision support staff— in a single environment, 2) Scheduling a specific time for related departments to attend the workshop, and 3) Establishing a goal of "relevant completion" (substantial or 90 percent completion) at the beginning of the process.

Managing the Budget

Flexibility. The degree of flexibility of budget parameters is affected by the type of budget, the seat of power and decision making, and policies of the organization. Decisions can be swayed by perceived inflexibility of the budget, expressed as "The budget won't let us do it!" Rigid adherence to a budget may dampen creativity and squelch innovation, or even avert disaster, but choices about how to expend money are human choices. The budget is a management tool, it is not a management entity in and of itself. Although resources must always be considered when making choices, accountability and responsibility for making a particular choice do not lie with "the budget," they lie with leadership.

Oversight and Understanding Budget Variances. One of the most useful tools for determining if a budget is on course is the variance report. The "variance" in this context means that the funds expended on certain budgetary items (e.g., salaries or supplies) are over or under the amount allotted. At first glance, you may think that being over budget is inherently a negative, while being under is a desired occurrence. Although this is true, in general, it is critical to evaluate each occurrence. Being over budget on supply items may be detrimental to the organization if services provided are constant, but not if that overage is offset by an increase in revenue. Accordingly, revenue should also be monitored for consistency with budget expenditures. For example, an organization that provided services at the same level while revenue for units of services remains steady might still see total reimbursement decrease because supplies that could once be billed now must be absorbed into the organization. Due to efficient electronic data retrieval and management, reports can be generated in nearly "real time," providing an opportunity to correct any deficiencies.

Control charts can be useful tools in determining patterns of variances, both for financial performance and for the related quality indicators. Control charts are graphically displayed measurements, presented over time, that help in determining variations, possible causes, and meaning of changes in metrics. Often, benchmarks are used so that variances outside desired ranges can be immediately noted. Specialized computer programs allow for easy creation of such charts, but office-based software that is probably accessible to you can be adapted for this purpose. Most large organizations employ their own charts or contract with providers of such programs. An example of a commonly used, ubiquitous program is Microsoft Excel, which provides templates and many tutorials. However, these charts alone are not sufficient to perform the analysis. Connections must be made to real-world occurrences. For example, if overtime spiked over a period of time, it would be important to know whether patient visits were also higher due to seasonal illness as this might have caused staff members to become ill, leading to absences.

Finkleman (2006, pp. 455–456) presented a question guide for assessing patterns in variance management:

- What effect does the variance have?
- Why did the variance occur?
- What can be done to prevent its reoccurrence?
- What needs to be done to make the best of the situation?

Additionally, it may be asked: What needs to be done to make the *most* of the situation?

RESOURCE DEVELOPMENT

As you advance to higher levels in leadership, you will become more responsible for acquiring resources beyond existing budgets based on revenues and expenditures. Such fundraising is an art unto itself. To be successful, you must be committed to your organization from the heart. Donors invest where they see vision, energy, need, and the capacity to make a difference.

REFLECTION QUESTIONS

Recall your experiences with budgeting.

1. Have you been involved in creating a budget or in managing one?
2. What is your comfort level in budgeting?
3. What issues might concern you?
4. What approach to budgeting is used at your workplace (or former workplace)?
5. Is it a "good fit"? Why or why not?
6. What would you recommend as positive changes to improve the budgetary process?
7. What approach to budgeting do you find most attractive? Why?

Philanthropy

Most health care organizations have foundation or advancement staff members who are experts in philanthropy and develop relationships with potential donors. You may be asked to work with them if your area of responsibility is being considered by a donor for support. In other situations you may be part of a fundraising campaign in which certain priority areas are being highlighted. The essential tool for such fundraising is called the case statement. It is a formal document that reflects your vision statement from the perspective of those outside your organization. Its purpose is to inform potential donors, but the sheer activity of developing the case statement may help crystallize your vision and mission from within.

The case statement is told from the heart and should answer the following questions (Fritz, 2016; Panas, 2003):

- What is the need? This should be stated in the most urgent and compelling manner. It needs to be specific, and stated in such a way that potential donors can identify how they can personally make a difference.
- How is your organization uniquely positioned to resolve the need? The idea that your organization is the best or only means to resolve the need should become clear to the donor and should draw the donor to your enterprise.
- What are the benefits of your action to resolve the need? Again, a specific, urgent, heartfelt but authentic rationale needs to be articulated.
- How much will it cost? The donor should have a clear idea of the appropriate donation that would resolve the need. You must also articulate the consequences should you be unable to fulfill the need.

Grants

Funding sources for health care services, aside from the obvious reimbursement for services, may also be secured from local, regional, and national private and government grants. Monetary amounts of such grants, qualifications for grant recipients, and targeted programs vary widely. Some grants require an affiliation with a university or established health care organization. Some are dedicated to not-for-profit organizations only. Many require a research component; others require a community collaborative partner.

Grant sources include federal and state government agencies, private foundations and other philanthropic organizations, commercial businesses, local charities, and professional organizations. For example, advanced practice nurses who seek to improve patient outcomes may find good matches at the Agency for Healthcare Research and Quality (AHRQ, n.d.). Unlike many grants sources, such as the National Institutes of Health (NIH), where emphasis is targeted toward research, AHRQ focuses on the effectiveness of interventions in everyday practice (Edwardson, 2006).

Most grant applications require a justified budget, usually in a specified format. If you are new to the grant writing process, consider partnering with someone who has had success. But do not be deterred by inexperience. Funding sources provide considerable guidance and are usually available for telephone consultation. Also, many organizations offer grant writing courses for minimal or no cost, and some are available online.

Leaders are required to sustain the energy, keep the strategic plan fresh, and establish ongoing significant relationships with friends and stakeholders. Philanthropy and resource development is fast becoming a key element of leadership in health care. Engagement in philanthropic relationships stimulates creativity, opens the perspective of leadership, and can energize the leader. Grantors and donors give because they are drawn emotionally to your cause. It is a unique relationship between leader and donor, often profound because both believe in the vision.

Other potential funding sources, of course, are lending institutions. Again, personal liability must be considered. That said, banking institutions will examine any proposal as a potential business venture. Having a well-constructed business plan and projected budget is critical.

LEADERSHIP AND FINANCE

Health care leaders, providers, and members of our communities currently face many critical economic challenges, including reductions in funding, changes in budget allocations, and elimination of or reductions in programs and services. Nurses prepared at advanced levels are looking for alternative methods of care delivery and changes in practice environments. One nurse, dissatisfied with the philosophy, approach, and financial provisions of her employer's care environment, chose to begin her own practice (Muscari, 2004). The important role of her business plan—not only in establishing the practice but in sustaining her through the launching process—surprised her.

> Unexpectedly, the business plan provided me with emotional reassurance during slow referral times in the first year. The business plan allowed analysis of the number of referrals, timing of the referrals, and from whom they came. Gradual movement into self-employment, as opposed to complete cessation of a secure, income-providing job, decreases the stress on a businessperson because revenue still comes in while the new, self-employed position reaches the point of producing a steady and sufficient cash flow. A business plan can guide that process because it helps forecast when that time will occur and the amount of business that needs to come in before an individual can work solely for himself or herself. (Muscari, 2004, p. 177)

Attention to financial planning, careful mapping of strategy, marketing that is relevant and correctly targeted, accurate estimations of revenue and expenditures, and adherence to a vision can result not only in financial success, but in personal fulfillment as a leader. Further, it can be the beginning of your personal contribution toward transforming health care.

EMERGING MODELS OF CARE DELIVERY: A GLIMPSE INTO THE FUTURE OF FINANCING

One of the criticisms of health care reform legislation is that it seeks to create a free marketplace atmosphere for the procurement of health care commodities in much the same fashion that other consumer goods are marketed and sold (Nix, 2013). Most might agree that the purchase of health care often carries with it emotional aspects and, not infrequently, emergent needs. Still, terms such as *value-based purchasing* and *reward value*—reimbursements linked to quality indicators—have invaded the literature and are our current reality. Finance and quality *are* linked. *Fee for service* is becoming an obsolete term. While these changes may be fast moving, confusing, and consumptive of energy and resources, they also present an excellent atmosphere for innovative change. This is the perfect time to be a DNP student!

Many of the obvious and most often discussed changes in finance have been present in the models of hospital payment by Medicare, and we know that other payers often follow suit. Aetna Insurance Company paid more than one-quarter of reimbursements for health care in 2014 through value-based contracts and plans to increase this figure to three-quarters by 2020. Blue Cross/Blue Shield paid 20% of claims in 2012 as value-based care, an amount that exceeded $65 billion. In addition, the insurer reported saving $500 million in 2012 as a result of fewer emergency visits and admissions, and improved access to preventive care, attributed to value-based contracts (Bryant, 2015).

Changes in payment models continue in the provision of primary care. In a survey of 1,624 primary care physicians and 525 nurse practitioners and physician assistants, more than half reported receiving financial incentives based on quality or efficiency. Only one-third of the physicians were being paid exclusively on a fee-for-service basis, and the percentage of nurse practitioners and physician assistants was even lower (13%). One-third of the physicians acknowledged that their practice qualified as a patient-centered medical home (PCMH; Ryan et al., 2015).

Presently, Medicare has a multipronged effort under way to enact value-based payment, comprising PCMHs, the Transitions programs, and emerging chronic care management programs and population-focused initiatives. A PCMH is a primary care model that provides accessible, comprehensive care to patients using a team approach. Patients and families are key members of the team. Other approaches to care are being tested through demonstration projects under the Comprehensive Primary Care Initiatives (CMS, 2015b). Details about this program and others are beyond the scope of this chapter, but they illustrate the opportunity to create new approaches to practice in your care environment.

It is worth saying again that opportunities abound. The current health care environment is in acute need of the skills of the DNP. Clinical redesign is a financial imperative that must be accomplished by a partnering of financial and clinical experts. Collaboration and valuing of each team member's contributions is necessary to achieve the difficult balance of cost containment and revenue maximization; of sustainability/stability and responses to change; and of the continuing need of "traditional" care and the movement toward population-focused and preventive care. The dynamics of care must be explored by the expert clinician (that is, you) to ensure not only the best in care to individuals, but also the restructuring of care delivery from an improved systems perspective.

REFERENCES

Agency for Healthcare Research and Quality. (n.d.). *Defining the PCMH*. Retrieved from https://pcmh.ahrq.gov/page/defining-pcmh

American Hospital Association. (2014, September 8). Take a look at how market forces will impact health care: The AHA Environmental Scan pinpoints changes in costs, economy, aging generations, and more as factors affecting health care. *Hospitals & Health Networks*. Retrieved from http://www.hhnmag.com/articles/4012-take-a-look-at-how-market-forces-will-impact-healthcare?dcrPath=/templatedata/HF_Common/NewsArticle/data/HHN/Magazine/2014/Sep/gate-aha-environment-scan-2015

Baker, J. J., & Baker, R. W. (2011). *Healthcare finance: Basic tools for nonfinancial managers* (3rd ed.). Sudbury, MA: Jones & Bartlett.

Barach, P., & Johnson, J. K. (2006). Understanding the complexity of redesigning care around the clinical microsystem. *Quality and Safety in Health Care, 15*(Suppl. I), i10–i16.

Barr, P. (2005). Flexing your budget: Experts urge hospitals, systems to trade in their traditional budgeting process for a more dynamic and versatile model. *Modern Health Care, 35*(37), 24, 26.

Bradley, L. S. (2008, March). Budgeting—or refusing to budge? How budget workshops can reduce the pain. *Health Care Financial Management*, 56–59.

Brandt, J. A., Reed Edwards, D., Cos Sullivan, S., Zehler, J. K., Grinder, S., Scott, K. J., . . . Maddox, K. L. (2009). An evidence-based business planning process. *Journal of Nursing Administration, 39*(12), 511–513.

Bryant, K. (2015, December). Shift toward population health hampered by lack of coordination. *Law & Health*. Retrieved from http://health.wolterskluwerlb.com/2015/12/shift-toward-population-health-hampered-by-lack-of-coordination/

Bupert, C. (2004). *Nurse practitioner's business practice and legal guide* (2nd ed.). Sudbury, MA: Jones & Bartlett.

Carlson, J. (2009). A retiring bunch. *Modern Health Care, 39*(26), 6.

Carlson, J., Evans, M., Lubell, J., Rhea, S., & Zigmond, J. (2009). The exodus continues: More executives leaving top health care jobs. *Modern Health Care, 39*(28), 4.

Centers for Medicare and Medicaid Services. (2013, January). *Inpatient measures.* Retrieved from https://www.cms.gov/Medicare/Quality-Initiatives-Patient-Assessment-Instruments/HospitalQualityInits/InpatientMeasures.html

Centers for Medicare and Medicaid Services. (2014, August). *Acute inpatient PPS.* Retrieved from https://www.cms.gov/Medicare/Medicare-Fee-for-Service-Payment/AcuteInpatientPPS/index.html

Centers for Medicare and Medicaid Services. (2015, September). *Outcome measures.* Retrieved from https://www.cms.gov/Medicare/Quality-Initiatives-Patient-Assessment-Instruments/HospitalQualityInits/OutcomeMeasures.html

Centers for Medicare and Medicaid Services. (2015a). *Electronic health records (EHR) incentive programs.* Retrieved from https://www.cms.gov/Regulations-and-Guidance/Legislation/EHRIncentivePrograms/index.html

Centers for Medicare and Medicaid Services. (2015b). *Comprehensive primary care initiative.* Retrieved from https://innovation.cms.gov/initiatives/Comprehensive-Primary-Care-Initiative/index.html

Cote, G., Lauzon, C., & Kyd-Strickland, B. (2008). Environmental scan of interprofessional collaborative practice initiatives. *Journal of Interprofessional Care, 22*(5), 449–460.

Dartmouth Institute for Health Care Policy and Clinical Practice. (n.d.-a). Workbooks/Greenbooks. *The Microsystem Academy.* Retrieved from https://clinicalmicrosystem.org/workbooks/

Dartmouth Institute for Health Care Policy and Clinical Practice. (n.d.-b). Transforming microsystems in health care. *The Microsystem Academy.* Retrieved from https://clinicalmicrosystem.org/

Edwards, S. T., & Landon, B. E. (2014). Medicare's chronic care management payment reform for primary care. *New England Journal of Medicine, 371*(22), 2049–2051.

Edwardson, S. R. (2006). Securing successful funding for nursing research through the Agency for Healthcare Research and Quality. *Nursing Economics, 24*(3), 160–161.

Finkleman, A. W. (2006). *Leadership and management in nursing.* Upper Saddle River, NJ: Pearson, Prentice Hall.

Finkler, S. A., & Kovner, C. T. (2000). *Financial management for nurse managers and executives* (2nd ed.). Philadelphia, PA: Saunders.

Fritz, J. (2016). *Writing a great case statement.* Retrieved from http://nonprofit.about.com/od/fundraisingbasics/a/casestatement.htm

Godfrey, M. M. (Ed.). (2010). *Microsystems at a glance.* Lebanon, NH: Dartmouth Institute for Health Policy & Clinical Practice. Retrieved from http://tdi.dartmouth.edu/about/facts-figures

Greenberg, M. J. (2008). Budget management. In H. R. Feldman, M. Jaffe-Ruiz, M. L. McClure, M. J. Greenberg, & T. D. Smith (Eds.), *Nursing leadership: A concise encyclopedia* (pp. 74–75). New York, NY: Springer Publishing Company.

Halloran, E. J. (2008). Financing health care. In H. R. Feldman, M. Jaffe-Ruiz, M. L. McClure, M. J. Greenberg, & T. D. Smith (Eds.), *Nursing leadership: A concise encyclopedia* (pp. 229–234). New York, NY: Springer Publishing Company.

Harris, J., Holm, C. E., & Inninger, M. (2015, March). Financial leadership imperatives in clinical redesign. *Healthcare Financial Management*, 66–72.

Harris, J. L. (2010, January). *Improving healthcare outcomes: Building the business case.* Paper presented at the meetings of the American Association of Colleges of Nursing Doctoral Education Conference, Captiva Island, FL.

Issac, T., Zaslavsky, A. M., Clearly, P. D., & Landon, B. E. (2010). The relationship between patients' perceptions of care and measures of hospital quality and safety. *Health Services Research, 45,* 1024–1040.

Jha, A. K., Orav, E. J., Zheng, J., & Epstein, A. M. (2008). Patients' perceptions of hospital care in the United States. *New England Journal of Medicine, 359,* 1921–1931.

Kibort, P. M. (2005, November/December). I drank the Kool-Aid—and learned 24 key management lessons. *Physician Executive,* 52–55.

Liebler, J. G., & McConnell, C. R. (2004). *Management principles for health professionals* (4th ed.). Sudbury, MA: Jones & Bartlett.

Morjikian, R. L., Kimball, B., & Joynt, J. (2007). Leading change: The nurse executive's role in implementing new care delivery models. *Journal of Nursing Administration, 37*(9), 399–404.

Moseley, G. B., III (2009). *Managing healthcare business strategy.* Sudbury, MA: Jones & Bartlett.

Muscari, E. (2004). Establishing a small business in nursing. *Oncology Nursing Forum, 31*(2), 177–179.

Nix, K. (2013, November). What Obamacare's pay-for-performance programs mean for health care quality. *Heritage Foundation: Backgrounder.* Retrieved from http://report.heritage.org/bg2856

Panas, J. (2003). *Making the case: The no-nonsense guide to writing the perfect case statement.* New York, NY: Institutions Press.

Porter-O'Grady, T., & Malloch, K. (2007). *Quantum leadership: A resource for healthcare innovation* (2nd ed.). Sudbury, MA: Jones & Bartlett.

Robinson, J. (2011). Hospitals respond to Medicare payment shortfalls by both shifting costs and cutting them, based on market concentration. *Health Affairs, 30*(7), 1265–1271.

Roussel, L. A. (2014). The nature of the evidence: Microsystems, macrosystems, and mesosystems. In H. A. Hall & L. A. Roussel (Eds.), *Evidence-based practice: An integrative approach to research, administration, and practice* (pp. 171–184). Burlington, MA: Jones & Bartlett.

Ryan, J., Doty, M. M., Hamel, L., Norton, M., Abrams, M. K., & Brodie, M. (2015, August). Primary care providers' views of recent trends in health care delivery and payment. *Commonwealth Fund and The Kaiser Family Foundation.* Retrieved from http://www.commonwealthfund.org/publications/issue-briefs/2015/aug/primary-care-providers-views-delivery-payment

Sharpe, M. (2009, June). New approach to budgeting can improve bottom line: Flexible budget gives a true picture. *Hospice Management Advisor,* 67–68.

Shea, J. L. (2014). *Prevention of coronary artery disease in patients with type 2 diabetes mellitus: Development of a checklist.* Unpublished DNP project. University of Alabama–Huntsville, College of Nursing, Huntsville, AL.

U.S. Small Business Administration. (2016). *Accounting glossary.* Retrieved from http://www.sba.gov/smallbusinessplanner/plan/getready/serv_sbplanner_gready_glossory.html

Weill, P., Malone, T. W., D'Urso, V. T., Herman, G., & Woermer, S. (2004). *Do some business models perform better than others? A study of the 1000 largest U.S. firms.* MIT Sloan

School of Management working paper. Boston, MA: Sloan School of Management, Massachusetts Institute of Technology. Retrieved from http://seeit.mit.edu/Publications/BusinessModels6May2004.pdf

Wilson, L. (2011, September 12). Pursuing value: Providers aim for rewards by emphasizing quality metrics used in the new CMS' new purchasing system. *Modern Healthcare*, 14–23. Retrieved from http://www.modernhealthcare.com/article/20110912/SUPPLEMENT/309129999

Yoder-Wise, P. S. (2011). *Leading and managing in nursing* (5th ed.). St. Louis, MO: Mosby Elsevier.

CHAPTER 5

Collaborative Leadership Contexts: Networks, Communication, Decision Making, and Motivation

Marion E. Broome and Elaine Sorensen Marshall

Never doubt that a small group of thoughtful, committed citizens can change the world. Indeed, it is the only thing that ever has
—Margaret Mead

OBJECTIVES

- *To understand the changing nature of roles in response to change in health care*
- *To describe how emerging leaders build networks with other leaders within and across organizations to effect change that will support growth*
- *To describe the core values needed to enable effective intra- and interprofessional collaboration*
- *To identify key interprofessional collaboration competencies to ensure successful organizational impact*
- *To describe facilitative infrastructures that support intra- and interprofessional collaboration models*
- *To describe how a leader utilizes expert opinion and others to make the best decisions possible*

As you advance in clinical preparation, formal education, and leadership development, you have a responsibility to expand your influence. You become a citizen of the larger discipline of health care leadership and a leader among leaders. The world awaits your ideas, skills, and the unique contributions you will make. If you have the courage to use your voice, experience, and expertise you will claim membership among thoughtful, committed people who can make a difference. Doors will open and opportunities appear for you to make transformational change in ways you could not imagine before you entered this society of leaders. The challenges in health care of patients, their families, and those who seek to live healthier lives are too complex to be overcome by a sole creative person or even by a collection of representatives from a single discipline. Transformational change happens only through the collaborative choreography of groups and teams of leaders.

Other emerging leaders struggle with similar issues in their work. They may share your concerns but have different perspectives, complementary skills, and new ideas that can amplify your abilities. Leaders in other disciplines offer so much that nurses can use to transform our vision of practice to improve lives. Just as this book and your program focus on the talents and skills for leadership among nurses, the need for effective leadership across health care is recognized and promoted among various professions, each of which offers ideas, advice, and rationales for why members of that discipline are best poised to be the leaders of the future. For example, some have proclaimed that "most physicians possess the traits essential for leadership" (Falcone & Satiani, 2008, p. 87), which is likely an accurate statement but ignores the need for health care leaders who have different skills, expertise, and perspectives. In fact, it will "take a village" of health care disciplines to address the complex problems we face (Dietz et al., 2015). Others claim that this is the time for nurses to take the helm as leaders to transform health care (Mason, Jones, Roy, Sullivan, & Wood, 2015), and studies have shown that nurses can and do in fact evolve their leadership to address new challenges (Pittman & Forrest, 2015). Box 5.1 describes one example.

BOX 5.1 EVOLVING ROLES FOR NURSES IN THE HEALTH SYSTEMS OF TODAY AND TOMORROW

Pittman, P., & Forrest, E. (2015). The changing roles of registered nurses in pioneer accountable care organizations, *Nursing Outlook*, 3(5), 554–565.
The purpose of this study was to explore how leaders of pioneer accountable care organizations (ACOs) proposed that the roles of registered nurses must evolve to bring about decreased health care costs. The findings of this study, gleaned from interviews with nurse leaders in 18 of the original 32 pioneer ACOs, reported eight types of changes in roles of the registered nurse:

- Enhancement of the role
- Substitution
- Delegation
- Relocation of services
- Transfer of nurses across settings
- Use of liaison nurses across settings
- Partnerships of nurses coordinating patients' care in acute care and primary care settings

These findings suggest the need for broad-based changes in health care that require the ongoing attention and focus of nursing leaders to support the growth of registered nurses who provide direct and indirect care within their evolving organizations.

Still others propose that the best leadership can come only from a business model. The truth is that we are all in this together. Success in the next century can come only from a community of leaders who understand each other's values, theories, and approaches so as to finally invent true interprofessional leadership. You will be a leader among those leaders!

FORMAL AND INFORMAL NETWORKS

The commonly assumed context of leadership is the formal organization, with divisions, departments, positions, job descriptions, and tasks. Entry and advancement are usually validated by credentials, qualifications, merit, or seniority. Leaders and other workers are employees with designated titles, and the higher the position, the greater is the *presumed* authority to lead. Decisions that have organization-wide impact are usually made by those in authoritative positions, and it is presumed that each leader is representing his or her constituency when such decisions are made.

But every organization also has an informal network that provides the real context for how any decision makes (or doesn't make) an impact. The informal structure is an extension of the social structures that develop within the formal context. It includes individuals with personal qualifications, goals, and motivations, as well as the spontaneous emergence of smaller groups and organized units with their own activities and goals. Leaders often emerge from the informal context by their charisma, personal qualities, and the ability to influence others. Formal leaders are wise to be sensitive and supportive of informal leadership contexts, to recognize and emulate influence and interest in others, and to care for individuals and their goals and means of communication. Informal leaders do what they do through strong communication channels with powerful relationships in which they help others.

In a context of complex adaptive systems, or simply within any community, most people are willing to notice, risk, help, and lead. Indeed, many great movements worldwide can be attributed to one person noticing a need, persistently working on the problem, enlisting the help of others, and not giving up. That is precisely how Lillian Wald founded public health nursing, how Loretta Ford invented nurse practitioners, and how you will make a difference. It is not easy, but it does work: One person picks up the cause and wears his or her heart out; others take note and join. And thus a movement is formed and changes the world. But it is not only the individual who makes the difference. The individual champion provides the leadership to move forward, but the difference is made with a local network, then a community or perhaps a community of practice, then communities that become systems of influence (Wheatley & Frieze, 2006).

Wheatley and Frieze (2006) described the power of networks as the most effective way of organizing for change. They pointed out that networks are formed only by living systems, are born of self-organization, and have always existed but are just now being observed through a new lens. Networks self-organize where individuals of a species "recognize their interdependence and organize in ways that support the diversity and viability of all" (Wheatley & Frieze, 2006). Consider migrating birds in fight, citizens for ecological sustainability, surgeons working on a new technique, or nurse leaders dealing with practice design. All are networks that make a difference from the synergy of the natural confluence of talented individuals. Wheatley and Frieze (2006) further pointed out that networks provide the conditions for and become the first step toward emergence, "which is how life changes."

Academic–Practice Partnerships: Intraprofessional Networks

One specific and important collaboration model in health care is the academic–practice partnership (Beal et al., 2012; Broome, Everett, & Wocial, 2014). Although such partnerships are often discussed, there is a broad range of types and degrees of success. The most common academic–practice partnership is between a school of nursing and a clinical agency. Such partnerships may include innovative initiatives such as dedicated teaching units (Jeffries et al., 2013; Warner & Burton, 2009), expanding educational enrollment capacity (Clark & Allison-Jones, 2011), improving clinical education (Mulready-Shick, Kafel, Banister, & Mylott, 2009), or clinical staff recruitment (Clark & Allison-Jones, 2011). However, such successful partnerships seem to fall at one end of the continuum; many schools of nursing exist separately, lacking strong networks with clinical departments of nursing in health systems.

Effective nursing partnerships incorporate a variety of different models. They may include joint appointments (Broome et al., 2014), implementation science and evidence-based practice projects (Stetler, Ritchie, Rycroft-Malone, Schultz, & Charns, 2009), or original research collaborations (Granger et al., 2012).

Beal et al. (2012, p. 333) proposed the following guiding principles for academic–practice partnerships:

- Collaborative relationships between academia and practice are established and sustained
- Mutual respect and trust are the cornerstones of the academic–practice partnership
- Knowledge is shared among partners through a variety of mechanisms
- A commitment is shared by the partners to maximize the potential for [nurses] to reach the highest level within their individual scope of practice
- A commitment is shared by the partners to work together to determine an evidence-based transition program for students and new graduates that is both cost-effective and sustainable

MacPhee (2009) proposed a logic model for such partnerships. The model outlined inputs that include partnership champions, compatible philosophies of partners, a shared vision, key stakeholder commitment, formalized agreements, shared goals and accountabilities, and dedicated time and resources. Activities include open, ongoing communications; shared decision making; and shared professional development. Outputs include shared or compatible action and strategic planning, and outcomes include productive short-term, action-plan, or tactical goals and successful completion of long-term strategic goals.

Successful academic–clinical partnerships bring together key stakeholders, create a common vision to enhance the mission and culture of each organization, and commit to effective collaborative communication and shared decision making. This requires uncommon mutual leadership and exemplary collaboration and shared vision among staff, students, and all other constituents. In addition, it requires sustained human and fiscal resources from each partner and commitment to track outcomes that support the work of both the clinical and academic endeavors.

In the long run, results and outcomes become secondary to effective personal relationships. That is, the individuals involved continue the important work and projects with their partners as a result of energizing and satisfying relationships (Broome et al., 2014). Some examples of specific outcomes reported by some successful partnerships have been reported. These include increases in the number of evidence-based and research projects that involved direct care nurses, increase in the number of baccalaureate-prepared nurses; and increases in the number of clinicians involved in teaching students in areas of their expertise (Broome et al., 2014; Granger et al., 2012; Jefferies et al., 2013; Stetler et al., 2009).

REFLECTION QUESTIONS

If you are in a class or a work setting, team up with another individual. Review and discuss the guiding principles outlined by Beal et al. (2012), the conceptual model and outcomes in the Indiana University Nurse Learning Partnership (Broome et al., 2014), and the Academic–Practice Partnerships tool (2015) found on the Association of Colleges of Nursing website (http://www.aacn.nche.edu/leading-initiatives/academic-practice-partnerships/tool-kit).

1. If you created a partnership team, who would be members of that team from each setting? What critical logistical steps would you take to develop those commitments?
2. What barriers do you think you would face, and how would you begin to address those?
3. What are some common outcomes on which your partnership might focus?
4. What resources would you need to develop and sustain the partnership?
5. What criteria would you use to evaluate the effectiveness of the partnership?
6. How would such a partnership help you as a leader to develop a professional network? How could that work inform the formal leadership structures and networks in the two settings?

Informal Networks

As a leader, you will have many opportunities for a variety of different kinds of informal networks. Some will provide support and enrichment to your work, some will allow you to solve problems or develop new initiatives, and some will launch you to new heights of creative endeavors.

One effective and supportive informal network most emerging leaders find useful is the "community of practice" model. Such self-organized communities, often supported with technology by a larger organization, are networks of people who come together because of shared interest in a specific domain. Often, such communities form through distance media. They share stories, resources, skills, and information to solve a problem, enhance information, share experience, collaborate, and map knowledge in the domain. A community of practice may reflect interdisciplinary practitioners, government groups, educational groups, and members of social groups.

Informal networking is also an important benefit of participating in professional and community organizations. As a leader, your role can be greater than simply paying dues and going to meetings. Opportunities to serve on committees, or simply taking the time to get to know and collaborate with colleagues, can add so much to your outlook and your accomplishments.

Seldom discussed in the context of networking is the cost to enter and sustain networks. Sometimes efforts at networking are random and haphazard, based on the assumption that the more participants, the merrier, and the more involvement per individual, the better. Engagement in networks requires time and energy of members—for communication, meetings, and other personal contributions—which can sometimes detract from performance or quality. Cross, Grey, Cunningham, Showers, and Thomas (2010) explained how one can use network analyses (e.g., determining what individuals connect with others and how many they influence) to take a strategic outlook and determine specific goals from networking, what patterns and levels of connectivity would best meet the goals, and how to develop initiatives that secure effective networks.

The formal concept of networking probably emerged 30 to 40 years ago. New technologies and perspectives on emergent creation of communities will continue to change the traditional view of networking. Tomorrow's leader will have a whole new world of choices, relationships, and new means to sustain networking across disciplines, culture, and geography. It will require new ways of thinking and connecting and will change leadership as we know it.

Engaging in a variety of networks will enrich your work and be important in leading others through the dynamics of change. As you collaborate and simply share among colleagues within networks, the entire professional community will become better prepared to negotiate the challenges of change.

INTERPROFESSIONAL COLLABORATION

Most professionals, particularly those in health care, are educated and socialized into discipline-specific bodies of knowledge built on strong discipline-specific theories and frameworks. They are licensed and regulated into rigid professional practice jurisdictions. It is an impressive challenge for such highly trained professionals to move out of the comfort and habit of their specific occupations to work together. Such work requires sensitivity to other theoretical foundations and ways of knowing and thinking. It requires learning new languages and skills. Interprofessional collaboration requires applying a major change in professional logic, adopting new paradigms, and working in new social environments (D'Amour, Ferrada-Videla, Rodriguez, & Beaulieu, 2005).

D'Amour et al. (2005) reviewed concepts and theoretical frameworks among empirical reports of interprofessional collaboration. Such collaboration was described as a dynamic, interactive, and evolving process. Process steps might include negotiation and compromise in decision making or shared planning and intervention, transcending professional or disciplinary boundaries. They identified five major overarching concepts of collaboration, partnership, interdependency, power, and team. They found the following concepts most often mentioned in definitions of collaboration: sharing, partnership, interdependency, and power. Furthermore, they identified several uses of the concept of sharing as a construct of collaboration, including shared responsibilities, decision making, health care philosophy, values, data, and planning and intervention.

Partnership was characterized by a collegial relationship that is authentic and constructive, open, and honest, and noted by awareness of and value of the contributions and perspectives of others, common goals, and specific outcomes. Interdependency implies mutual dependence. The concept of power was conceived of as shared and symmetrical in power relationships, and characterized by empowerment of all parties. D'Amour et al. (2005) also identified a variety of terms in the context of team environments. This model was examined for clinical utility with health care providers in practice related to shared decision making in clinical care (Legare et al., 2011). Stakeholders suggested that the patient should be placed at the center of the model, and that it would be important to clarify expected outcomes and to recognize how environment and emotions of those on the team influence the utility of the model.

Barriers to successful interprofessional collaboration include poor communication, lack of knowledge of other professional roles, minimal understanding of when and to whom to refer specific patient problems, the need for training in successful team function, and the need for evidence of improved patient outcomes (Moaveni, Nasmith, & Oandasan, 2008). Additional challenges include differential power between team members, the time it takes to collaborate, and insufficient resources to support collaboration (Legare et al., 2011).

More recently the concepts of interprofessional education (IPE), interprofessional practice, and interprofessional collaboration have been emphasized in documents, standards, and competency white papers in the health professions. In 2011, five professional associations in nursing, allopathic medicine, pharmacy, osteopathic medicine, public health, and dentistry published *Core Competencies for Interprofessional Collaborative Practice* (Interprofessional Education Collaborative Expert Panel [IPEC], 2011) in which they described four domains of competency: (a) values and ethics for interprofessional practice, (b) roles and responsibilities, (c) interprofessional communication, and (d) teams and teamwork.

Each of these domains contains 8 to 11 subcompetencies that illustrate how critically important core values of respect, accountability, communication, and teamwork are to successful collaborations that shape quality care for patients and families (see Table 5.1).

Although calls for interprofessional approaches to solve the many crises of American health care are heard above the sound of nearly every other cry, reaction has been slow. Numerous national organizations and commissions have

TABLE 5.1 Interprofessional Collaborative Practice Competency Domains

COMPETENCY	DOMAIN	SUBCOMPETENCIES
1	Values/ethics for interprofessional practice	**VE1**: Place the interests of patients and populations at the center of interprofessional health care deliver. **VE3**: Embrace the cultural diversity and individual differences that characterize patients, populations, and the health care team. **VE9**: Act with honesty and integrity in relationships with patients, families, and other team members.
2	Roles/ responsibilities	**RR3**: Engage diverse health care professionals who complement one's own professional expertise, as well as associated resources, to develop strategies to meet specific patient care needs. **RR6**: Communicate with team members to clarify each member's responsibility in executing components of a treatment plan or public health intervention. **RR8**: Engage in continuous professional and interprofessional development to enhance team performance.
3	Interprofessional communication	**CC2**: Organize and communicate information with patients, families, and health care team members in a form that is understandable, avoiding discipline-specific terminology when possible. **CC4**: Listen actively, and encourage ideas and opinions of other team members. **CC6**: Use respectful language appropriate for a given difficult situation, crucial conversation, or interprofessional conflict.

(continued)

TABLE 5.1 Interprofessional Collaborative Practice Competency Domains (*continued*)

COMPETENCY	DOMAIN	SUBCOMPETENCIES
4	Teams and teamwork	**TT4**: Integrate the knowledge and experience of other professions—appropriate to the specific care situation—to inform care decisions, while respecting patient and community values and priorities/ preferences for care.
		TT7: Share accountability with other professions, patients, and communities for outcomes relevant to prevention and health care.
		TT8: Reflect on individual and team performance for individual, as well as team, performance improvement.

Source: IPEC (2011). Used with permission.

officially mandated interdisciplinary collaboration as one of the primary hopes for improved health care of the future. Richardson, Haber, and Fulmer (2008) pointed out the efforts of several other major organizations toward encouraging interprofessional collaboration. Richardson and colleagues further reminded that nearly every major professional document on preparation, practice, and research includes some element of interdisciplinary collaboration. Health care has become far too complex for any single organization to rely on its own dedicated employees without collaboration either across the organization or across disciplines (IPEC, 2011).

Porter-O'Grady and Malloch (2008, p. 177) suggested, "What is needed is less emphasis on individual role specificity or clarity and more emphasis on role complement and contribution to patient outcomes." Although each discipline must be able to distinguish the specific scope of its contribution to patient care, as an individual each member of the group must understand his or her own unique contributions as well as respect the unique knowledge and skills of the other members. No single individual is viewed as the consistent leader; rather, depending on the context of the patient or organizational situation, team leaders will change. Few can argue that interprofessional collaboration in health care would best be facilitated at the foundation of educational preparation of the various professions. This is where individual understandings are formed and the respect and value for all health professions is learned. Although valiant attempts are ongoing, actual formalized, integrated collaboration is not yet widespread. Thibault (2010) outlined the following barriers to generalized IPE:

- *Cultural:* Strongly held value systems of each profession
- *Structural:* Different schedules and locations (in educational preparation)
- *Faculty:* Not comfortable and not rewarded (for interprofessional collaborative endeavors)
- *Temporal:* Establishing the ideal developmental times for (interprofessional) interaction. (E.g., are first-year medical students and first-year nursing students [at parallel developmental points] in their preparation?)

- *Noncore:* Elective experiences at off-hours. (Many groups who have tried interprofessional collaboration in education provided such opportunities only as elective experiences requiring additional time beyond the requisite program.)
- *Nonsustaining:* Series of "cameos." (Most programs have been short-term demonstration projects dependent on limited or temporary resources.)
- *Lack of leadership from the top:* Usually driven by passion of one or two faculty members
- *Asymmetry:* [Have not been] equally supported by all participating professions

Despite the barriers to interprofessional preparation, there are some hopeful initiatives to support such collaboration between medicine and nursing. Two examples of promising models of IPE those at the University of Colorado and at Arizona State University. At the University of Colorado, all health professions students are oriented together and then share, across their education years, educational experiences related to bioethics, quality and patient safety, and simulated patient care scenarios. At Arizona State University, the Schools of Nursing and Social Work, along with the University of Arizona–Phoenix Schools of Medicine and Pharmacy, have developed a primary care curriculum and team-based care clinical practicum for students from those disciplines who work as teams in clinics across the city and surrounding areas (Josiah Macy Jr. Foundation, 2016).

Furthermore, many doctor of nursing practice (DNP) programs promote interprofessional collaboration as a core component of preparation. Such programs offer promise for a brighter future of collaboration in the daily work of health care among a variety of professions. Effective collaboration not only is personally and professionally satisfying to those involved, but also contributes to a unified and holistic approach to patients and clients, facilitates faster internal decision making, reduces cost through shared resources, and promotes innovation (National Center for Interprofessional Practice and Education, 2015).

Successful partnerships are particularly enriching to the leaders involved, who are able to work with new friends, new perspectives, and new supporters outside the daily work environment. We are just beginning to understand the real-world value of interprofessional collaboration on actual patient outcomes (Zwarenstein, Goldman, & Reeves, 2009). It will be the responsibility of leaders of the future to develop working models for collaboration and shared decision making (Stacey, Légaré, Pouliot, Kryworuchko, & Dunn, 2010) but initial findings on the positive effects of interprofessional practice models for patient outcomes in diabetes, emergency department patient satisfaction, and the reduction of clinical error rates have been documented (Zwarenstein et al., 2009).

As you enter a new leadership role, regardless of the setting, efforts to connect and secure collaborative projects with leaders outside your organization are likely to produce lasting professional friendships and collegial relationships, creative contributions, and renewed energy and insights. Such personal benefits spill into effective service to patients and to the community.

COMMUNICATION

Effective networking cannot happen without effective communication and decision making. Communication and making decisions are skills discussed in every leadership class and described in every leadership book. Theories on these issues abound across business management and health care leadership. But do not be fooled: no teacher, no guru, no book has the answers. They will offer great advice, helpful insights from experts, and abundant evidence from research, but they will not be able to tell you exactly what will work best for you, for your style, or in your situation. A commonly heard principle of organizational leadership is, "It's all about the people"—and we would add, "It's all about communicating, communicating, and communicating with those people." Throughout your career, you will learn your own lessons about communication, how to handle conflict, and how to make better decisions, so you must share your own learning along the way. Here you learn what has worked for others.

Communication to Build Relationships and Facilitate Productivity

Human communication is among the few things absolutely essential to life. Human beings must connect physically, emotionally, intellectually, and spiritually. It is as necessary as breathing, but much more complex (Yoder-Wise & Kowalski, 2006). We all know that there is the message sender and the message receiver, but myriad factors affect actual communication. When two people interact, each brings filters that include attitude, assumptions, intentions, beliefs, emotional state, physical conditions, history, culture, and experience. All affect the nature or the quality of the communication.

Verbal and written communication is a deal maker and breaker for the aspiring leader. Mastery of all forms of communication, including nonverbal, makes all the difference in how you present yourself. You are the package that people will notice before they take in your message. Keys to effective communication are self-knowledge and sensitivity to what others want and need to know. The well-known Johari Window (Oestreich, 2008; Yen, 1999) helps to illustrate interpersonal processes and facilitate personal refection on skills in interpersonal relationships. It includes four rooms or panes (think of window panes). The first is called the "open arena," which includes what others know about you and what you know about yourself. The second is called "blind" or the "blind spot"; this is what others know about you, but what you do not know about yourself. The third pane is the "hidden" or "façade," or what others do not know about you, but what you know about yourself. And finally, the last pane is the "unknown," or what others do not know about you and what you do not know about yourself. All rooms affect a person's communication. The panes of the window help to understand nuances and complexities of human communication.

Communication is about dissemination of your ideas, thoughts, feelings and experiences (McBride, 2011). Leaders communicate in speech, writing, actions, body language, and even in silence. Effective communication begins with an

BOX 5.2 VERBAL COMMUNICATION SELF-ASSESSMENT

- Do you overuse jargon? Acronyms are often used as shortcuts for entities or practices it is assumed everyone understands—but, in fact, may not—such as "IPE (interprofessional education)" or "JCAHO (Joint Commission on Accreditation of Healthcare Organizations)"?
- Do you use colloquial phrases such as "my docs" or "the folks in housekeeping"?
- Do you have a soft voice or an accent that makes people strain to understand you?
- Is your style either too informal or too pedantic?
- Is your voice harsh, whiny, or intimidating?
- Do you speak too fast?
- Are you comfortable expressing yourself?

awareness of your own style, of how others respond to you. For example, when considering speech communication, recognize that others respond to your tone, volume, word choices, and ethnic or regional accent—and that does not even take into account your body language or facial expressions. As you aspire to leadership at the highest levels, it is most important to examine your own style of verbal communication (see Box 5.2).

Among the most effective tools for successful communication is active listening. Indeed, listening is often more important and effective than speaking. Many problems are solved simply by listening. Successful listening simply requires that people feel "heard." In today's world of handheld distractions, it is a treasured gift to give full focused attention and listen to another human being. Active listening is especially important. Yoder-Wise and Kowalski (2006) outlined the characteristics of active listening. They noted that the purpose is to assure the speaker that he or she has been heard, that the intensity of tone or emotion is heard and understood, and that it is safe to continue. As an active listener, paraphrase both the content and the tone of the message and reflect them back to the speaker in a genuine, empathetic manner. Sometimes, it is simply helpful to reflect the person's own words, but you must be truly interested. If you are just practicing a technique, it will not be helpful and will come off as near mockery.

Meeting Management

After listening, speaking is the most important signature of your leadership style. One of the most common means of communication for leaders is the "meeting." When I (Marshall) moved from a faculty position to an administrative role, the first, biggest, and most distressing shock was the sheer number of meetings. Then I began to note the length of the meetings. I found that if you set a meeting for 2 hours, it will take 2 hours and 5 minutes. Furthermore, if you set a meeting for 1 hour, it will take 1 hour and 5 minutes. The tradition was for our meetings to be scheduled in 2-hour blocks. I found that every meeting of every group, committee, and task force required the full 2 hours and 5 minutes. I changed the meeting schedule to 1½ hours. Guess what? The work still got done and we cut 2½ hours off each meeting day.

Now, that is not to say that the work might have been done in 1-hour or 15-minute meetings. But not knowing the threshold of time needed, we simply filled the time space allotted. It is important to hold face-to-face meetings in many situations, and it is often preferred. But think about the purpose of the meeting and what is to be accomplished. Communication must be clear, must be fair, and must facilitate the views of all. The following strategies for meeting management help you to accomplish your goals (and everyone else's) in the most efficient manner.

- Think about not only your agenda but also the agenda on the mind of every member of the group. Meetings should be for group process or for very important messages from the leader that can only be delivered personally.
- Place times next to each agenda item (e.g., 3:00–3:15). Initially, it will be difficult to gauge which items will take more time and which less, but after a few meetings of the group this will become easier.
- Meetings are also important to promote *esprit de corps* and a sense of belonging. It therefore is good to check in with each member, welcome new members, celebrate those leaving related to their accomplishments while a member, and so on. This will be an important investment of a few minutes of time at the beginning of the meeting.

After the meeting, other means of communication, such as e-mail, should be used appropriately to facilitate sharing the meeting results. Using a stream-lined three-column format to summarize the takeaway notes from each meeting (column 1 = topic discussed; column 2 = large areas of the discussion; column 3 = responsibility for follow-up) will increase the likelihood of busy people reading them and provide items for the next agenda. If any item with a complex background is scheduled to come before the group for a decision, it is most helpful if the individual bringing the issue or challenge prepares in advance a one-page document that outlines (a) the scope and background of the issue; (b) two or three proposed solutions; (c) resources (i.e., suggested reallocations or new resources), including people, time, talent, funding, or a combination of these; and (d) how the success of the strategy implementation will be evaluated, and (e) when the evaluation will be done. This approach allows group members to prepare to give their best advice, even if the document is received the day before the meeting. In my (Broome) experience it is also not uncommon for those preparing the document to decide not to bring a challenge forward after completing a description of the issue in writing. Simply preparing to bring up the issue helps them realize they have the authority to implement one of the proposed strategies without involving everyone in the group.

Presentation as Persuasion

Presenting a talk to a large (and often powerful group) is often intimidating. Several experts provide helpful strategies to consider whenever you make a presentation to a group:

- Know your purpose. Ask both yourself and your audience why you are there. Do your homework. One tip is to send e-mails to 8 or 10 people in the group before the meeting and ask them about their issues, desires, and challenges (Sue, 2001).
- Know your subject and be prepared to help the audience understand it using terms they can identify with (Bradlow, 2012; McBride, 2011).
- Make sure your opening is powerful. Capture attention and create interest. You might begin with some startling attention-getting information specifically about your topic. Keep it grounded in the audience's experiences or potential experiences (Sue, 2001).
- State your case and support it with evidence, facts, and examples. The importance of data cannot be overstated, but their inclusion must make the case for the compelling premise you want the audience to leave with (e.g., "we must increase the number of advance practice nurses in this subpopulation of patients to manage their care" (McBride, 2011).
- Use visual information, but only if it is powerful. Do not rely on your PowerPoint to *be* your presentation. Remember, it is only a blue screen with a few words or bullet points. *You* must convey the message (Bradlow, 2012; Sue, 2001).
- Reengage your audience every 6 to 8 minutes. Tell a relevant story, share a surprising statistic, have the group do something, but keep them with you.
- Use notes, but never memorize or read your presentation (Bradlow, 2012; Sue, 2001).
- Set the rules early for how questions and answers will be handled. Is this an open discussion? Is it an information session during which you expect to be peppered with questions? Will you take questions only at the end (Sue, 2001)?
- If this is not a formal presentation, rehearse what you are going to say at least four times without interruption, especially when the information is a surprise or bad news. Make an outline, keep it to only the number of points you can remember (for us, that is only three to five items), and know them (Bradlow, 2012; Sue, 2001).
- Check the environment before you present. Be sure you have set the stage by considering as many environmental factors as possible. Arrange the room, the chairs, the temperature, the clutter, the equipment, water, and food. Take away distractions and remove all barriers to your message (Sue, 2001).

Written Communication

After listening and speaking, written communication is your most important tool as a leader (McBride, 2011). Leaders are required to write every day. First, you must decide which form of written communication is most appropriate for the situation: e-mail, formal memo, letter, or public announcement. Even before that decision, you must decide to be a good writer. That means you must practice. Get help. Nothing will defeat your leadership more quickly than poor writing. Consult models and collect "templates" to use as models for documents such as letters of recommendation, executive summaries, proposals, or other communications that you write regularly.

Decide the purpose of your writing. Do you need to persuade, get information, clarify, motivate, solve a problem, make a recommendation, or defuse a crisis? Regardless of what you write, *always* make an outline. It helps to clarify your purpose and gives a structure for your message.

Even after you have become an expert in all aspects of communication, some challenge will erupt that tests all of your best skills. It helps in those times to step aside from yourself and examine your communication skills. You may need to edit your style. Take care not to be drawn into a style that is unbecoming or ineffective.

Preparing to Present Bad News

The skills discussed for use in both developing written communications and presenting information to members of the organization are essential competencies to develop. This is especially true when the organization is experiencing stress as a result of financial concerns, community disasters, tragedy within its walls, or any other sudden, unexpected event that threatens the well-being of the organization and its members. No matter how well prepared the leader, how earnest the followers, or how successful the organization appears, in today's complex health care environment it is inevitable that at some moment, things will go bad. Whether it is an unconscionable error, an economic crash, a disappointing employee, or a painful lawsuit, one day, suddenly, the leader will wish that she or he had aspired to be anything but to be "in charge."

Such situations may include any of the following and range from the micro to the macro environment, such as when you must deliver a negative performance review; when you must confront unfair treatment, deception, breaches of confidentiality, or lack of commitment; when you must deal with a person who is abusive, needy, or irresponsible; when you must deliver bad news or share the results of a difficult decision; when a safety breach occurred and patients or employees were at risk; when you must say "no"; or when you must surmount enormous barriers (e.g., mixed messages, sabotage) to effective communication. At times you may wonder, "How will I survive this?" It may be a painfully public issue or one that is born in a quiet, hurting heart. Its source may be a circumstance or a person.

It is very important for all leaders of the organization to be engaged in conveying the same message to employees, outside constituencies, and others. This is commonly referred to as being "on the same page." To accomplish this requires a level of transparency between executive leadership and mid-level managers who are most responsible for communicating with employees closest to care delivery. Key message points should be developed jointly and discussed daily during any crisis, and every leader should be comfortable with the messaging. If not, when pointed questions are asked by employees, those conveying the message will not be able to provide genuine answers, even if the answer is, "We don't have any more information than what I have shared about the situation at the current time."

Sharing the Good News: Your Story and the Organization

On the other hand, when you are doing something great from which others might learn or benefit, do not assume that your good work will be automatically valued and recognized. Indeed, unless you tell your story in an effective manner, it may be barely noticed. Regardless of your initiative, build relationships with others who may help you tell your story. Remember to include your network colleagues. Think about including the public relations or public communications officer of your organization, if one exists, or invite a local journalist to be part of your team. Invite key policy makers, such as local or state public officials, who might influence resources to translate your work to the larger community. And do not forget to go beyond traditional means of communication by using social media tools such as Twitter, Facebook, and blogging to tell your story.

As you advance in leadership roles, the clinical background that has connected you with real patients will be invaluable in marketing discussions of your organization. Your stories are grounded in authentic clinical experience. As a DNP-prepared leader in an organization, you have a unique set of skills to contribute to the message about today's health care system—especially in conveying how the profession of nursing contributes to increased access, decreased costs, and improved quality of care (see Box 5.3).

Heinrichs (2009) described the changing face of nursing, the increasing acceptance of nurse practitioners, and the future of the DNP. He offered specific

---

BOX 5.3 PREPARE YOUR STORY

Ultimately as a leader, you must know the story of your organization so well that you are able and eager to tell it at any moment with passion. Purposely prepare a story moment.

- Prepare your "elevator moment," a 30-second version of your story. When someone asks what you do, you have already chosen the story and set each word as a jewel in a setting to share your clear and compelling message.
- Prepare your 5-minute moment for any opportunity when you are called to a podium or around a table to introduce yourself.

Take advantage of opportunities to be in the right meetings where you will be invited to tell your story, then stand up prepared to share. Do not confuse the 30-second moment with the longer one. Never overstay your welcome with your message. And above all, remember that your story is not about you; it is about the great organization that you have the opportunity to lead.

suggestions for marketing approaches to invite the public to see the nurse beyond the culture of subservient roles and gender-specific stereotypes without losing the positive attributes that endear nurses to the public trust. The mission was to portray the nurse as a healer educated at the highest level. He asserted that appropriate marketing might follow the success of nurses expanding their scope of practice and influence to become recognized and valued players in health care reform. He proposed that such a marketing approach would saturate the markets with positive images of nurses in such advanced roles. Nurse leaders have a unique and valuable story to tell.

DECISION MAKING: THE ART AND SCIENCE OF ORGANIZATIONAL LEADERSHIP

Regardless of the message, the nature of decisions and the manner in which they are made in the organization are of highest priority. Effective or ineffective decision making can "make or break" the message, even with the best communication. Decision making is one of the most studied topics in the social sciences, yet we continue to wonder how good decisions get made. Campbell, Whitehead, and Finkelstein (2009) studied faulty decisions made by otherwise capable leaders from a neuroscience perspective. They confirmed that when faced with a situation calling for a decision, we make assumptions and take a perspective based on previous experiences, judgments, and emotional patterns. Thus, we may think we understand a pattern based on past history or emotional experience when, in fact, we do not *really understand* the new situation. Campbell et al. (2009) identified three "red-flag conditions" of distorted patterns or "emotional tagging."

1. First was inappropriate self-interest or conflict of interest that can bias judgment and decisions even unintentionally. An example of this would be a leader who served on the board of a local nonprofit agency that developed a proposal for a health care system to consider in funding a new care model though which patients from the emergency department would be cared for at home. If the health care system was also where the leader worked, it would be best to recuse, or remove, herself from any final decision making about the choice of proposals and sharing with others the conflict of interest.
2. The second red flag is distorted attachments to people, places, or things. An example would be the reluctance of a leader to cut a program in which he had been directly involved. In this case it would be important for the leader to be exceptionally open to other leaders' assessments, while providing information about the history and performance of the unit. When sharing that information, the leader should work to present information as objectively as possible.
3. The third red flag is misleading (or selective) memories that take our thinking in an inappropriate direction, or to a place where we might overlook or overvalue some important factor in a situation. One example might be the

leader who, relying on prior successes in managing conflict with a group of nurses, then assumes that the same strategies can be used successfully with a group of emergency department physicians who are negotiating with the health system to increase compensation. To counteract such potential flaws, it is helpful to involve another person in the decision. Look to add a fresh mind, a different experience. Invite debate and challenge.

Another systems-level approach to these potential influences on decision making is to institute governance safeguards, such as a process for ratification of decisions. This can range from board-level decisions to those within units of the organization. On the other hand, Hayashi and Ewert (2006) pointed out the value of instinct and the intuitive skills of wise leaders to make critical decisions. We have all known leaders whose experience, native wisdom, and emotional sensitivity contribute to sound decisions. Some emotional context and business instinct is essential, especially at the highest levels of leadership. Higher levels of emotional intelligence have, in fact, been found to be associated with more effective leadership decisions (Hess & Bacigalupo, 2011; Yip & Côté, 2013).

Many routine, daily tactical decisions can be delegated. In strategic decision making, however, the stakes are high. There may be novelty or ambiguity, or the decision may represent substantial change or commitment of financial or human resources. Thankfully, most leaders make relatively few life-or-death strategic decisions, but it *is* the leader who makes the strategic decisions. Further, leadership does not end with making the decision, however difficult that decision may be. After the decision is made, the leader must mobilize people and resources, sustain motivation of the entire organization, and navigate the sometimes troubled waters of disagreements, doubters, resisters, and those who simply do not know how to respond.

Regardless of the strategic or tactical value of a decision, the wise leader is always painfully aware of impact on real people's daily lives. Regardless of the organization, people are the greatest asset, to be treasured and highly regarded. Wise decision making does not grow from leadership style or personality; instead, leadership style should be adapted to circumstance. Ken Chenault explained:

> In some situations you have to be highly directive, because people are looking for clear direction from the leader. You always want to understand different perspectives, but in certain situations, you cannot manage by consensus. However, in being directive, you want to make sure that you're taking time to consider the consequences of your actions. Even in a crisis, you want to demonstrate to people that you understand what they're going through. You need to be empathetic and compassionate, but you must remain decisive, because the objective is to navigate the choppy waters and get people through it. (Feinberg, 2005, p. 9)

Remember, the easy things have been done by the time the challenge arrives on your doorstep. Although it is a big responsibility to make the final decision, with adequate outreach and inclusion of others in decision making along the way, the final decision will be easier for you. Doing nothing and not making decisions when one is in a position of responsibility is simply unconscionable. Lack of action frustrates others who are looking to you to decide so that they can move on and implement plans aligned with that decision. That is your job as the leader. Know your personality preferences and style. Learn to bracket your personal viewpoints. Learn to consult counsel and cultivate a network of sages and mentors. Educate yourself on the issues. Try on the alternatives. Rehearse the potential outcomes. Then be brave. Trust your wisest instinct. Plan, decide, and then move forward!

MOTIVATION: LEADING BY INSPIRATION AND MODELING

Motivation is so much more than providing incentive for productivity. It is about inspiring and giving hope to colleagues and followers within the organization. And marketing is so much more than selling. It is also about inspiring and giving hope to colleagues and the public outside the organization. To motivate others is to listen to their aspirations for themselves and their careers, as well their aspirations for the organization they work for. It is also the responsibility of the leader to listen for the signs of others' fears and to show the way to hope.

For years, motivation experts have argued over whether intrinsic or extrinsic motivators are most effective. But motivation is larger than a polarized paradigm between external and internal rewards. The truth is that everyone responds to *both* extrinsic and intrinsic sources of motivation. Extrinsic factors include such things as power, money, and status; and intrinsic factors include finding meaning, growing, and learning. We all respond to both. Of course many workers whose basic needs have been satisfied are best motivated by higher needs of achievement, emotional fulfillment through relationships, flexibility, and personal growth (Bal, De Jong, Jansen, & Bakker, 2012; Yoder-Wise & Kowalski, 2006).

Intrinsic or internal motivation is personal passion. Behind it is energy to engage in the work, to set and pursue personal and organizational goals, to overcome obstacles, and to press forward. External incentives, such as money or status, are secondary to the satisfaction of engagement and achievement (Porter-O'Grady & Malloch, 2007). The transformational leader in a healthy organization believes that others respond to both internal motivators and external motivators (Broome, 2013). Thus, the assumption is that people who are valued, encouraged, supported, and provided with the environment and resources to succeed will take initiative and perform creatively and effectively. From such groups will emerge collective wisdom, creativity, and some degree of self-governance.

REFLECTION QUESTIONS

1. What motivates you the most related to your professional career? Identify both intrinsic and extrinsic motivators.
2. How would you respond (think, feel, behave) if one of the extrinsic motivators (decrease in pay but more flexibility in role) changed?
3. If one of your colleagues was upset about a change in some factor that clearly motivated him or her (position title, scope of responsibility) and came to talk with you about leaving the organization, what would you say?

Motivation is a powerful internal and external force that influences behavior. Motivation is neither manipulative nor coercive. Yoder-Wise and Kowalski (2006, p. 135) refer to the following ideas of Kim (1996) in seeking to understand motivation in leadership:

- Motivation is a force, positive or negative, that creates action.
- Understanding the underlying motive that leads to taking action is the key to motivating people, including ourselves.
- Every motive for taking action comes from a need and a desire to satisfy it.
- Motives come in many forms and change throughout life.
- Motives can change rapidly, even during a specific activity.

Wise leaders stay in touch with the people with whom they work. The leader can do this in a variety of ways, including making rounds throughout the organization to be visible and to talk with employees and other leaders. Other strategies include sending personal congratulatory notes when an individual does something of note and calling when something (e.g., a death, an illness) occurs to share condolences or concern. Leaders are individually more or less comfortable with each of these strategies and must find the strategies that, individually, best enable them to stay in touch with colleagues and staff. There is no magic theory, strategy, or practice for motivation that works universally every time. Motivation requires authentic passion about the work, genuine interest in the workers, and vigilance to human needs for encouragement, support, autonomy, and meaning.

REFERENCES

Bal, P., De Jong, S., Jansen, P., & Bakker, A. (2012). Motivating employees to work beyond retirement: A multilevel study of the role of I-deals and unit climate. *Journal of Management Studies, 49*(2), 303–331.

Beal, J. A., Alt-White, A., Erickson, J., Everett, L. Q., Fleshner, I., Karshmer, J., . . . Gale, S. (2012). Academic partnerships: A national dialogue. *Journal of Professional Nursing, 28*(6), 327–332.

Bradlow, J. (2012). *6 easy to apply tips to giving an effective presentation.* Retrieved from http://www.workhappynow.com/2012/05/6-easy-to-apply-tips-to-giving-an-effective-presentation/

Broome, M. E. (2013). Self-reported leadership styles of deans of baccalaureate and higher degree programs in the United States. *Journal of Professional Nursing, 29*(3), 323–329.

Broome, M. E., Everett, L. Q., & Wocial, L. (2014). Innovation through partnership: Building leadership capacity in academe and practice. *Nurse Leader, 12*(6), 91–94.

Campbell, A., Whitehead, J., & Finkelstein, S. (2009). Why good leaders make bad decisions. *Harvard Business Review, 878*(2), 60–66, 100.

Clark, R., & Allison-Jones, L. (2011). Investing in human capital: An academic-service partnership to address the nursing shortage. *Nursing Education Perspectives, 32*(1), 18–21.

Cross, R., Grey, P., Cunningham, S., Showers, M., & Thomas, R. (2010, Fall). How to make employees networks really work. *MIT Sloan Management Review*, 83–90. Retrieved from http://sloanreview.mit.edu/article/the-collaborative-organization-how-to-make-employee-networks-really-work/

D'Amour, D., Ferrada-Videla, M., Rodriguez, L. S. M., & Beaulieu, M. (2005). The conceptual basis for interprofessional collaboration: Core concepts and theoretical frameworks. *Journal of Interprofessional Care, 19*(Suppl. 1), 116–131.

Dietz, W. H., Solomon, L. S., Pronk, N., Ziegenhorn, S. K., Standish, M., Longjohn, M. M., . . . Bradley, D. W. (2015). An integrated framework for the prevention and treatment of obesity and its related chronic diseases. *Health Affairs, 34*(9), 1456–1463.

Falcone, R. E., & Satiani, B. (2008). Physician as hospital chief executive officer. *Vascular and Endovascular Surgery, 42*(1), 88–94.

Feinberg, P. (2005, Fall). Q and Anderson: Kenneth Chenault on leadership. *Assets: UCLA Anderson School of Management*, 8–9.

Granger, B., Prvu-Bettger, J., Aucoin, J., Fuchs, M. A., Mitchell, P. H., Holditch-Davis, D., . . . Gilliss, C. L. (2012, March). An academic-health service partnership in nursing: Lessons from the field. *Journal of Nursing Scholarship, 44*(1), 71–79.

Hayashi, A., & Ewert, A. (2006). Outdoor leaders' emotional intelligence and transformational leadership. *Journal of Experiential Education, 28*(3), 222–242.

Heinrichs, J. (2009, October). Re-brand nurse. *Southwest Airlines Spirit*, 44–50.

Hess, U. J. D., & Bacigalupo, A. C. (2011). Enhancing decisions and decision-making processes through the application of emotional intelligence skills. *Management Decision, 49*(5), 710–721.

Interprofessional Education Collaborative Expert Panel. (2011). *Core competencies for interprofessional collaborative practice: Report of an expert panel.* Washington, DC: Interprofessional Education Collaborative.

Jeffries, P., Rose, L., Belcher, A., Dang, D., Hochuli, J., Fleischmann, D., . . . Walrath, J. (2013). A clinical academic practice partnership: A clinical education redesign. *Journal of Professional Nursing, 29*(3), 128–136.

Josiah Macy Jr. Foundation. (2016). *Interprofessional education and teamwork.* Retrieved from http://macyfoundation.org/priorities/c/interprofessional-education-and-teamwork

Kim, S. H. (1996). *1001 ways to motivate yourself and others.* Hartford, CT: Turtle Press.

Legare, F., Stacey, D., Gagnon, S., Dunn, S., Pluye, P., Frosch, D., . . . Graham, I. (2011). Validating a conceptual model for an inter-professional approach to shared decision-making: A mixed methods study. *Journal of Evaluation in Clinical Practice, 17*(4), 554–564.

MacPhee, M. (2009). Developing a practice-academic partnership logic model. *Nursing Outlook, 57*(3), 143–147.

Mason, D. J., Jones, D. A., Roy, C., Sullivan, C. G., & Wood, L. J. (2015). Commonalities of nurse-designed models of health care. *Nursing Outlook, 63*(5), 540–553.

McBride, A. (2011). *The growth and development of nurse leaders.* New York, NY: Springer Publishing Company.

Moaveni, A., Nasmith, L., & Oandasan, I. (2008). Building best practice in faculty development for interprofessional collaboration in primary care. *Journal of Interprofessional Care, 22,* 80–82.

Mulready-Shick, J., Kafel, K. W., Banister, G., & Mylott, L. (2009). Enhancing quality and safety competency development at the unit level: An initial evaluation of student learning and clinical teaching on dedicated education units. *Journal of Nursing Education, 48*(12), 716–719.

National Center for Interprofessional Practice and Education. (2015). *Informing, connecting, engaging, advancing.* Retrieved from https://nexusipe.org/home

Oestreich, D. (2008). *What is reflective leadership?* Retrieved from http://www.unfoldingleadership.com/blog/?p=171

Pittman, P., & Forrest, E. (2015). The changing roles of registered nurses in Pioneer Accountable Care Organizations. *Nursing Outlook, 63*(5), 554–565.

Porter-O'Grady, T., & Malloch, K. (2007). *Quantum leadership: A resource for health care innovation* (2nd ed.). Sudbury, MA: Jones & Bartlett.

Porter-O'Grady, T., & Malloch, K. (2008). Beyond myth and magic: The future of evidence-based leadership. *Nursing Administration Quarterly, 32*(3), 176–187.

Richardson, H., Haber, J., & Fulmer, T. (2008). Interdisciplinary leadership in nursing. In H. R. Feldman, M. Jaffe-Ruiz, M. L. McClure, M. J. Greenberg, & T. D. Smith (Eds.), *Nursing leadership: A concise encyclopedia* (pp. 310–314). New York, NY: Springer Publishing Company.

Stacey, D., Légaré, F., Pouliot, S., Kryworuchko, J., & Dunn, S. (2010). Shared decision-making models to inform an interprofessional perspective on decision-making: A theory analysis. *Patient Education and Counseling, 80*(2), 164–172.

Stetler, C. B., Ritchie, J. A., Rycroft-Malone, J., Schultz, A. A., & Charns, M. P. (2009, November). Institutionalizing evidence-based practice: An organizational case study using a model of strategic change. *Implementation Science, 4,* 78–96.

Sue, M. P. (2001). *Sparkle when you speak: 10 presentation tips for communicating results.* Retrieved from http://www.presentation-pointers.com/showarticle/articleid/463/

Thibault, G. E. (2010, January). *Interprofessional healthcare education and teamwork: Making it happen.* Paper presented at the meetings of the American Association of Colleges of Nursing Doctoral Education Conference, Captiva Island, FL.

Warner, J., & Burton, D. (2009). The policy and politics of emerging academic-service partnerships. *Journal of Professional Nursing, 25*(6), 329–334.

Wheatley, M., & Frieze, D. (2006). *Using emergence to take social innovation to scale.* Provo, UT: The Berkana Institute.

Yen, D. H. (1999). *Johari window.* Retrieved from http://www.noogenesis.com/game_theory/johari/johari_window.html

Yip, J. A., & Côté, S. (2013). The emotionally intelligent decision maker. *Psychological Science, 24*(1), 48–55.

Yoder-Wise, P. S., & Kowalski, K. E. (2006). *Beyond leading and managing: Nursing administration for the future.* Philadelphia, PA: Mosby Elsevier.

Zwarenstein, M., Goldman, J., & Reeves, S. (2009). Interprofessional collaboration: Effects of practice-based interventions on professional practice and healthcare outcomes. *Cochrane Database of Systematic Reviews, 8*(3), CD000072.

PART II

BECOMING A TRANSFORMATIONAL LEADER

CHAPTER 6

Frameworks for Becoming a Transformational Leader

Marion E. Broome and Elaine Sorensen Marshall

While many people believe that transforming organizations . . . is the most difficult, the truth is that transforming ourselves is the hardest job. And if we transform ourselves, we transform our world.

—Dag Hammarskjold

OBJECTIVES

- *To deepen appreciation for two current models: authentic leadership and the leadership challenge model*
- *To identify and explore competencies and/or habits for leadership*
- *To develop a vision in leadership*
- *To recognize the importance of the use of evidence to support vision*
- *To define and understand the significance of power as a leader*
- *To consider the role of a leader as an entrepreneur*
- *To understand servant leadership*
- *To recognize the responsibility of a leader for generativity*

Stephen Covey devoted a career to convincing us that there are seven or eight habits of a successful leader (Covey, 1989, 2004). Hamric, Spross, and Hanson (2009, p. 254) reviewed current leadership models and concluded that only three habits are most important to the transformational leader in clinical practice: (a) empowerment of colleagues and followers, (b) engagement of stakeholders within and outside nursing in the change process, and (c) provision of individual and system support during change initiatives. But we all know there are many more essential habits for the effective transformational leader. Consequential leadership requires the cultivation of a lifetime of habits that build others and strengthen self.

In Chapter 1, we reviewed various dimensions of transformational leadership—the focus of this book. At the beginning of this chapter, we introduce two complementary leadership frameworks that you may find useful in thinking about your own personal leadership philosophy, style, and behaviors: Authentic Leadership (Avolio & Gardner, 2005) and Leadership Challenge (Kouzes & Posner, 2010). Consideration of these models provides a foundation for examining and developing personal leadership styles. A discussion of how competencies of leadership have evolved over time expands the conversation. We then show how leaders can take these frameworks to build their own leadership skills and competencies.

TWO MODELS TO USE IN BUILDING A FOUNDATION TO BECOME A TRANSFORMATIONAL LEADER

Authentic Leadership Model

Authentic leadership is one of the frameworks that emphasizes relationships between leaders and followers and focuses on the self-development potential of the leader. At the same time, the model reflects a recognition that this potential and subsequent interactions are in service of the larger organization and context, as well as the individuals within the organization. Authentic leaders are perceived as hopeful and optimistic, exhibiting behaviors reflective of a moral compass they can articulate. Such individuals speak with a clear voice for the needs of those in their organization (Avolio & Gardner, 2005). Key characteristics of these leaders include self-awareness, relational transparency, internalized moral perspective, and balanced information processing (Bamford, Wong, & Laschinger, 2013).

Nurse leaders who are authentic are able to be honest and open in their relationships with individuals to whom they report, as well as those who work for them. Their sense of integrity also facilitates, actually mandates, their need to seek diverse perspectives from others and use multiple sources of evidence when making an important decision. Bamford et al. (2013) conducted a secondary analysis of data from 280 nurses who worked with nurse managers. Those nurses who worked for nurse leaders who exhibited higher levels of authentic leadership were more fully engaged in the workplace and reported a greater sense of alignment in multiple areas of their work life.

Leadership Challenge Model

Kouzes and Posner (2007, 2010) developed a model of leadership by analyzing practices of leaders to provide emerging leaders with a description of behaviors and practices that develop strengths. The model consists of five practices: (a) model the way, (b) inspire a vision, (c) challenge the process, (d) enable others to act, and (e) encourage the heart.

The nurse leader who *models the way* understands his or her own beliefs and is able to articulate how the mission of the organization is an important responsibility of all. Such leaders are visible and committed to the organization and those who work with them. They are experts in their field. It is through their efforts to connect with others and set an example of how to maximize their own and others' strengths that they are able to *inspire a vision* for the organization. Their assessment of the group's potential based on listening to the hopes and aspirations of others and enthusiasm about where the organization is capable of going enlists others in working toward a common goal. However, as the leader begins to set the stage it becomes clear that traditional ways of being and doing will need to be challenged in order to develop new thinking and ways of behavior to achieve the goals. The leader will then engage in questioning and *challenging existing processes*. Experimenting with new ways of doing things and challenging others to develop their skills and take risks will enable them to act. *Enabling others to act* will require the leader to set a challenge and provide resources for them to draw on to meet the challenge. As they achieve success others will grow and develop leadership skills themselves. From the collaborations they form while working to solve the challenge, they will learn the value of working with others with complementary knowledge and skills. The final exemplary practice, to *encourage the heart*, is one threaded throughout the leadership journey although clearly more important to stress at times when the challenges are more difficult. Individuals working with the leader rely on coaching, celebrating small victories, and the presence of the leader when stress runs high in the organization. Kouzes and Posner developed the *Leadership Practices Inventory*® series (2016) which allows individuals to assess their own leadership strengths in each of the five exemplary practices and provides tools and activities to use to grow their leadership skills.

These two leadership frameworks reflect a clear emphasis on authentic and meaningful relationships between the leader and others. Leaders in each framework articulate their beliefs that serve as a foundation for their vision for the organization and for how the potential of others can be developed and leveraged for success of all. Leaders who are relationship based have a clear moral compass, are secure in their belief system, and are open to and seek out diverse perspectives in order to shape how they think about challenges and solutions. These models are broader and more philosophical, and frankly more inspiring from our perspective, than some other approaches that include lists of competencies for leadership performance.

LEADERSHIP COMPETENCIES: HABITS FOR PERFORMANCE

There is growing agreement on the need for better leadership in health care but little consensus or evidence regarding which specific areas of knowledge, skills, attitudes, habits, or competencies are best suited to the leaders of the next century (Baker, 2003) or how they are best acquired. Thus, it seems that every leadership guru creates a list. We have lists of competencies from experts and expert panels, from authorities in business and health care, from government agencies, from the Institute of Medicine, and from every practice discipline.

Much of the literature on leadership in health care actually refers to specific management skills with a focus on performance. And performance is usually defined by competencies. Although the idea of *competency* carries an intuitive, implied definition, there is little agreement on a generally accepted operational definition. There are numerous examples of competency lists for health care managers and many definitions of the concept. One author mused, "Definitions and terminology surrounding the concept of competency are replete with imprecise and inconsistent meanings, resulting in [a] certain level of bewilderment among those seeking to identify the concept" (Shewchuk, O'Connor, & Fine, 2005, p. 33). A commonly accepted definition of competency is the following: "a cluster of related knowledge, skills, and attitudes that: (1) affect a major part of one's job, role, or responsibility, (2) correlate with performance on the job, (3) can be measured against well accepted standards, and (4) can be improved by training and development" (Lucia & Lepsinger, 1999, in Shewchuk et al., 2005, p. 33). Five underlying characteristics of competencies are motives, traits, self-concept, knowledge, and skills that optimize job performance (Shewchuk et al., 2005; Spencer & Spencer, 1993).

Competency models originate from private and public sector business and industry as well as academe, each one with its own list of dimensions. The dimensions usually include items related to productivity, personal characteristics, and personnel relationships (Simonet & Tett, 2013). Such models have now found their way into health care organizations.

Many of the competency models rely on some sort of 360-degree evaluation model, which refers to regular, formal, and direct leader feedback related to performance on specific goals based on stated organizational values. This model begins with self-evaluation and then integrates formal evaluation from superiors, peers, and subordinates. The critiques are reviewed with an immediate supervisor, and a plan for improvement is developed. This evaluation model is commonly used in business and increasingly incorporated into health care environments (Burkhart, Solari-Twadell, & Haas, 2008; Day, Fleenor, Atwater, Sturm, & McKee, 2014).

As in the business literature, it seems that every health care writer has a list of the most important, or core, competencies for the health care manager. Many come from the personal experience and thoughts of the author, with little reliable empirical data to adequately distinguish, predict, or even to teach the most important competencies. For example, one study sought the most important competencies for physicians to become health care leaders. Most highly ranked were interpersonal communication skills, professional ethics, and social responsibility. Other desired competencies were influencing peers to adopt new approaches in medicine and administrative responsibility in a health care organization (McKenna, Gartland, & Pugno, 2004).

There is increasing interest in the empirical discovery and measurement of competencies for successful leaders (Day et al., 2014). Guo and Anderson (2005) and Guo (2009) promoted a paradigm that identified four essential dimensions: conceptual, participation, interpersonal, and leadership. They subsequently identified the following core competencies: health care system and environment competencies, organization competencies, and interpersonal competencies (Guo, 2009). Stoller (2008) outlined six more specific key leadership competency domains: (a) technical skills and knowledge (operational, financial, information systems, human resources, and strategic planning), (b) industry knowledge (clinical processes, regulation, and health care trends), (c) problem-solving skills, (d) emotional intelligence, (e) communication, and (f) commitment to lifelong learning.

Another list includes planning, organizing, leading, and controlling (Anderson & Pulich, 2002). Still another cluster includes teamwork, negotiation, interpersonal skills, communication, vision, customer service, and business operations (Finstuen & Mangelsdorff, 2006). And yet another model outlines 52 competencies in four domains: (a) technical skills (operations, finance, information resources, human resources, and strategic planning/external affairs), (b) industry knowledge (clinical process and health care institutions), (c) analytical and conceptual reasoning, and (d) interpersonal and emotional intelligence (Robbins, Bradley, & Spicer, 2001). Intuitively, the list seems to be comprehensive and useful. Each of the competencies has been defined theoretically and operationally. Nevertheless, it is daunting to the aspiring leader who might ask, "Where do I begin?"

One group of competencies that has been extensively researched originates from the National Center for Healthcare Leadership (NCHL) in Chicago, Illinois. Its *Health Leadership Competency Model* (NCHL, 2015) was developed from extensive academic and clinical study. The model comprises three domains of transformation, execution, and people. Under each domain is a list of the following competencies:

1. *Transformation competencies:* achievement orientation, analytical thinking, community orientation, financial skills, information seeking, innovative thinking, and strategic orientation
2. *Execution competencies:* accountability, change leadership, collaboration, communication skills, impact and influence, information technology management, initiative, organizational awareness, performance measurement, process management/organizational design, and project management
3. *People competencies:* human resources management, interpersonal understanding, professionalism, relationship building, self-confidence, self-development, talent development, and team leadership (Calhoun et al., 2004; NCHL, 2015)

The *Healthcare Leadership Alliance Competency Directory* (Evans, 2005; Healthcare Leadership Alliance [HLA], 2013; Stefl, 2008) lists 300 competences under the five domains of leadership, communications and relationship management, professionalism, business knowledge and skills, and knowledge of the health care environment. If leadership performance could be learned from a dictionary, this would be the one of choice. It is a large classification system of knowledge and skill areas searchable by an elaborate system of key words. Sponsored by the American College of Healthcare Executives, the American College of Physician Executives, the American Organization of Nurse Executives (AONE), the Healthcare Financial Management Association, the Healthcare Information and Management Systems Society, and the Medical Group Management Association, it provides an impressive inventory of leadership concepts that can enable managers and leaders to meet the challenges of navigating and leading through the complexities of today's current health care environment (HLA, 2013). Unfortunately, it does not provide mentorship, role models, personal experience, or inspiration for the soul of the aspiring leader. For nurse leaders, these supports must be found through the many available leadership academies, conferences, short intensive courses, and other similar options.

Each new list or model (which may or may not be grounded in evidence) announces something along these lines: "The model of leadership competencies presented . . . [here] will become an essential tool for organizations in their pursuit of leaders to implement and drive successful change. This leadership competency model … will ensure that essential steps of change are followed and provide organizations with a blueprint for success" (Hall, 2004). If nothing else, current experts appear to be confident in their competency paradigms.

Nursing leaders also have their own lists of competencies. These include competencies specific to areas of practice, such as professionalism, network and team building, communication, problem solving and prioritizing, vision, awareness of nurse subordinates, and knowledge of policies and procedures of the unit and larger organization (Grossman, 2007). Most lists developed by nurses are not uniquely distinct from those of the management disciplines. A study using focus groups of nurses produced the following "essential nursing leadership competencies": skills in listening and conflict resolution; the ability to communicate a vision, motivate, and inspire; and "technological adroitness, fiscal dexterity, and the courage to be proactive during rapid change" (Eddy et al., 2009, p. 1). Stichler (2006, pp. 256–257) asserted that creating and fostering a vision were most important, followed by 15 positive personal attributes, leadership skills that "ignite passion in others and influence them to make things happen," clinical knowledge and skills, and business competencies. Sherman, Bishop, Eggenberger, and Karden (2007) developed a competency model from a list of six competency categories. The categories were systems thinking, personal mastery, financial management, human resource management, interpersonal effectiveness, and caring.

Huston (2008, p. 906) outlined eight "essential" leadership competencies for the nurse leader of 2020:

1. A global perspective of health care and professional nursing issues
2. Technology skills that facilitate mobility and portability of relationships, interactions, and operational processes
3. Expert decision-making skills rooted in empirical science
4. The ability to create organization cultures that permeate quality health care and patient/worker safety
5. Understanding and appropriately intervening in political processes
6. Collaborative and team-building skills
7. The ability to balance authenticity and performance expectations
8. Being able to envision and proactively adapt to a health care system characterized by rapid change and chaos

Whew! The list is as daunting as the health care system itself.

In health care organizations, one of the frequently referenced models of competencies is that produced by the AONE (2016). They provide an assessment tool that emerging leaders can use to examine their own competencies and where they are in their leadership journey. Nurse educators can also use the tool to help guide curricular development. The AONE noted the need to delineate differences in leadership competencies among leaders of health care systems, leaders working outside of traditional hospital or inpatient settings, and those who are nurse managers.

The current emphasis on competencies and competency measurement appears to be in direct response to economic and social pressures of health care organizations for performance as well as the fact that "rapid change in the organization, financing, and provision of health care services … demand greater efficiencies and better clinical and organizational performance" (Shewchuk et al., 2005, p. 33). With the proliferation of competency-based leadership evaluation that targets efficiencies and safety, caution seems prudent regarding the potential return to traditional mechanistic, industrial efficiency models of providing health care.

Despite our tongue-in-cheek journey through the world of competencies, it may be helpful to know the specific competencies on which nurse leaders might focus. Some observers say that there is a need for greater business acumen (Kleinman, 2003); others promote the need for more "caring competencies" (O'Connor, 2008). The Center for Nursing Leadership outlined nine dimensions of leadership that reflect unique caring competencies: holding the truth, intellectual and emotional self, discovery of potential, quest for the adventure toward knowing, diversity as a vehicle to wholeness, appreciation of ambiguity, knowing something of life, holding multiple perspectives without judgment, and keeping commitments to one's self (O'Connor, 2008). Again, there is little evidence of empirical testing. Some models from nursing include specific characteristics of transformational leadership, but most fall short of identifying clinical applications, and many borrow from models in business and health care management.

Competencies are necessary, of course, to provide a framework to document and assure performance, especially in areas of productivity, accuracy, and efficiency, but it is difficult to inspire workers or even endear clients or patients with catalogs of expectations. Without vision, competencies are only chore lists for managers. Porter-O'Grady and Malloch (2007, p. 421) reminded that "Leadership is not simply as set of skills [and competencies], but a whole discipline." Wear (2008, p. 625) warned that while competencies are important, turning every measure of practice into a competency "is an ill-advised leap that transforms a complex educational [clinical, and leadership] mission into a bottom-line venture." It is important that we broaden the focus to include "ongoing reflective processes and humility that mark the lifelong development of skilled, empathic" clinicians and leaders (Wear, 2008, p. 625).

As you consider new roles or simply a new perspective for an existing clinical leadership role with advanced preparation at the highest level of clinical practice, it would be most unfortunate if you were to attempt to reinvent the entire concept of competency. This review confirms the abundance of work on health care leadership competencies It is the responsibility of the next generation

REFLECTION QUESTIONS

1. What habits, skills, and competencies must the next generation of leaders in nursing in practice and academe possess?
2. Is health care leadership only about competencies or skills?
3. What are common assumptions and expectations related to leadership style and competencies? What needs might be uniquely met by a leader rooted in clinical practice?
4. If you are a leader with responsibilities across both academe and practice, what leadership skills must you possess?
5. Who and where are your role models for leadership? What knowledge, skills, and competencies do you see in them that you admire and would seek to emulate? What are the gaps in skill you see?
6. If you interview one of your role models what three questions would you ask them to help you understand how they developed their leadership skills?

of leaders to sort, identify, test, and apply most effective competencies that will support the vision of the transformational leader.

VISION: PERSPECTIVE AND CRITICAL ANALYSIS

Vision is probably one of the most discussed and commonly accepted attributes of leaders. Vision is their habit. Visionary leaders do not stop at simply holding workers accountable to competencies. They make it their habit to look up and beyond, foreseeing next steps and future challenges, opportunities, and accountabilities. Their own personal vision enlivens formal vision statements and integrates the meaning of the statements into their very beings. Vision releases forces that attract commitment and energize people to create meaning in the lives of others, to establish standards of excellence, and to bridge the present and the future (Kouzes & Posner, 2010; Nanus, 1992). If you have no vision of where you are going, why should anyone follow you? Followers expect leaders to know where they are going and to strike the path toward a vision. Kouzes and Posner (2007, 2010) are credited with the well-known statement, "There's nothing more demoralizing than a leader who can't clearly articulate why we're doing what we're doing." By the same token, to spare themselves their own personal demoralizing sense of daily drudgery and burden, visionary leaders take the larger perspective, beyond day-to-day tasks and operations.

What is vision and how do you cultivate the habit of sustaining your vision? Vision is the image of the future you want to create. It is your picture of what is possible. Vision requires a dream and a perspective that set a direction that others want to follow. Heathfield (2015) proposed the following fundamental requirements for vision to actually make a difference: The vision must clearly set a direction and purpose for the entire organization. It must inspire a commitment, loyalty, caring, and genuine interest in personal involvement in the enterprise. The vision should reflect the unique culture, values, beliefs, strengths, and the direction of the organization. It must "fit." The vision always promotes the feeling among followers that they are part of something greater than themselves, that their daily work is more than operational, but part of some greater future. Such a vision challenges others to stretch, to reach, and to produce beyond their own expectations.

The leader who sets such a vision will have the larger perspective not only of the official vision statement or strategic plan but also beyond. Nevertheless, the effective visionary leader does not only see the big picture of the vision, but also is able to sensitively support others in the daily work of all members of the organization. To the perceptive leader, the vision is more than a rallying cheer. It represents a substantive direction for action and achievement. The vision is only one aspect of a strategic plan for action, but it is the vital life force of that plan. Inspiring leaders have the courage and the drive to dream. In times of near despair, confusion, chaos, or even routine and boredom, we need dreams. As a leader, you must believe in your dream; you must believe that it can happen. Kouzes and Posner (2007, p. 17) observed:

> Every organization, every social movement, begins with a dream. The dream of vision is the force that invents the future…. Leaders gaze across the horizon of time, imagining the attractive opportunities that are in store…. They envision exciting and ennobling possibilities. Leaders have a desire to make something happen, to change the way things are, to create something that no one else has ever created before.

Dreams that actually become fulfilled are shared among members of a critical mass. A leader must have followers. Solitary vision that is not shared is only daydreaming. Transformational leaders must be vigilant that they do not follow their own light so far into the distance that followers are left in the dark. Shared dreams "fit," and they grow in the hearts of those committed to the organization. Stichler (2006, pp. 255–256) stated:

> The nurse leader is responsible for creating a vision for the organization and clearly articulating that vision to others. The vision must be so compelling that others can feel passionately enough about it to direct their efforts toward achieving the vision. The vision must be viewed as being for the "common good," and the [leader] must foster that sense of common commitment so that others are willing to follow on the quest toward the vision …
>
> Along with the vision, the [leader] is responsible for defining the philosophy of care and translating that philosophy with others into care delivery models…. [The leader] directs the care delivery process and accomplishes the mission and goals of the organization through others in a manner that empowers nurses and other professional providers to achieve autonomy in their practice.

BOX 6.1. VISION EXERCISE

Think of a team you are working with on a specific project. Even projects have a vision- that is a desired end state-a common goal—a place where the group wants to end up. It is a helpful exercise to engage people in creating a vision statement. This activity should take no longer than 1 hour of a meeting.

- When brainstorming to develop the vision statement, be bold to use metaphor, poetry, images, stories, and emotion. People need to truly experience the image. Ask each member of the group to draw a picture, image or a word that describes where they want to project look like when completed.
- Now ask each participant to take 1 minute and vividly describe it, discuss it, and encourage all to share in that person's their view of it.
- As the last person is done, ask the group to write down a clear, succinct statement that captures what the common theme was across everyone's "vision" or preferred end state.
- At the end there will be two to three different themes if 10 to 12 people are in the group. So next step is to come to one understanding that is so clear that the only response is, "Yes! That's who we are. That's what we want to be. That's where we are going!"

A vision statement is a helpful way to articulate the dream. The most effective vision statements are short (two to three sentences), reflect the values of the organization, and provide a picture of what the organization is about to become (see Box 6.1).

A shared vision for any project or organization gives perspective. It allows everyone to look up from many lists of competencies and the daily grind that hovers over nearly every team or organization at one time or another. As a leader with a vision in your heart, you are the guardian of perspective. You are able to critically appraise what is important and what simply appears to be urgent at the time. You help people cut through the daily lists of "stuff" that must be done to see what really might be done for a better future. Sometimes, it involves just a moment of reflection, a reminder; sometimes, a change of schedule or procedure; sometimes, a different use of language. Language is important, particularly in the vision statement. It must be beautiful so that it clearly reflects the image of where you are going, the picture of the desired future.

The leader who believes and constantly carries the vision is able to critically analyze decisions, solve problems, and effectively predict next steps. The vision is not about you, your career goals, or your personal desires. It is about the organization as a living organism, as a community, perhaps even as a family. You are the steward of the vision of the organization. For your vision to be authentic, you must love the place, the people, and the work you are doing.

Because the vision is integrated into your being as the leader, many plans and decisions will seem to automatically flow in the direction of the vision. Opportunities will appear, or you will suddenly see opportunities in a new way to allow you to move toward the vision. The vision becomes your habit. It will not be easy, but a clear vision allows purposeful critical analysis and helps to winnow away issues that cloud direction. It allows you to better trust your decisions because you know where you are going, and your actions are more likely to be trusted because you have the creditability of a clear direction. Critical analysis becomes easier, almost second nature, because you have set your own benchmark. You know where you are going.

USING EVIDENCE TO MAKE A DIFFERENCE

Vision is only dreaming without the use of evidence to make decisions that make it happen. The use of evidence in health care is no longer an option (Malloch & Melnyk, 2013). It must become the intellectual and practice habit of all leaders and clinicians. If use of evidence, or empirical research data, is truly to make a difference, it must be embraced at all levels, from point of contact to the broadest systems perspective. Furthermore, evidence must be implemented and evaluated from the perspective of all aspects of leader, clinician, and patient experiences. The effects or outcomes of evidence cannot be evaluated from any sole viewpoint. Evidence must be integrated and synthesized into the practice experience, into the patient response, into the entire caregiving or healing event. "Evidence of making a difference is … evidence of collaboration, integration, and systemization of all the related contribution" (Porter-O'Grady & Malloch, 2007, p. 54).

The recent sweeping movement toward evidence-based practice has been largely promoted by academics and targeted to clinicians in direct patient care. Nurse leaders have long been accustomed to the challenges of promoting research utilization within health care organizations. Current care settings are often laden with practices of habit, tradition, and routine. Nevertheless, Porter-O'Grady and Malloch (2008, pp. 185–186) warned against joining "the evidence-based practice fad," that the current surge toward use of evidence should "not exclude other non-quantitative sources of evidence," and cautioned not to oversimplify clinical nursing knowledge. It is important as we embrace evidence-based practice that we not lose, but rather empirically document, other significant ways of knowing and practice such as clinical intuition, attention to individual differences, the art of practice based on clinical expertise, and professional autonomy (Tracy, Dantas, & Upshur, 2003). Indeed, Råholm (2009, p. 168) "challenged the wisdom of basing the practice of leadership on a narrow, reductionist understanding" of evidence and defended the meaning of context in the definition of evidence. With the emerging focus on implications of genetic testing and genomics, health care practice is poised to move from the application of evidence-based protocols to a focus on individualized or customized care.

Although the development, discovery, and use of evidence for clinical practice continue to mount, there is a continuing need to close the gap between evidence and practice (Hay et al., 2008). In most clinical settings, truly integrated evidence-based practice is still not second nature. In the past several years much emphasis has been placed on the role of leadership for implementation of evidence-based practice. Aarons, Farahnak, Ehrhart, and Sklar (2014) discussed the critical importance of the leader in shaping a culture in which all clinicians value evidence versus tradition-based practices in their work. The leader's mandate is to expect, support, and reward those who demonstrate that value through their work. Examples of clinicians who demonstrate these behaviors include:

- The nurse who consults the pharmacist on the unit after a patient mentions that his wife brought his antinausea drug from home, and a check of the medication triggers an alert when entered into the electronic health record
- The new graduate who questions the use of 48-hour dressing changes in the manager's staff meeting after reading a related research study in a journal on the unit
- An experienced nurse who suggests a new procedure for communicating physician messages to nurses who are administering medications after reading new evidence on the relationship between information overload and medication errors

A movement is under way to emphasize the role of the nurse manager and leader in executing the appropriate use of evidence into practice. Unfortunately, we are only just beginning to compile adequate evidence for how this is best accomplished. Gifford, Davies, Edwards, Griffin, and Lybanon (2007) reviewed the literature on what may constitute effective nursing leadership in leading the charge toward evidence-based practice. They found the following leadership activities that influenced nurses' use of research: managerial support, policy revisions, and auditing. They also found that, often, organizational practice structures impose barriers to both leaders' and nurses' access to, promotion of, and ultimate use of evidence. They concluded that "both facilitative and regulatory" measures for leaders are necessary and recognized the need for research to confirm the role of leadership in promoting evidence-based practice to improve patient outcomes. DeSmedt, Buyl, and Nyssen (2006) found that implementation of evidence-based practice is best facilitated by clear communication, summaries of evidence, easily understood protocols, and web-based databases accessible within the work environment, as well as by leaders whose practice is grounded more thoroughly in evidence and less by personal experience.

It is the role of the leader to remove barriers and provide resources for clinicians to access the best research evidence. Such practice often represents a change of culture and total integration of use of evidence in clinical communications (Aarons et al., 2014). And all leaders throughout the nursing department, from nurse manager to nurse executive, must be aligned in their expectations about implementation of innovative approaches (O'Reilly, Caldwell, Chatman, Lapiz, & Self, 2010). If they are not engaged and aligned, nurses at the bedside may revert to become tradition and trial-and-error bound in their practices caring for patients.

It continues to be largely the responsibility of the leader to break the path, to facilitate the culture for evidence-based practice to be comprehensive throughout all systems. Use of evidence must simply become a way of doing and being in clinical practice. Indeed, leadership and operational structures must align to "place clinical practice at the center of the organization's purpose and build the structures and processes necessary to support it" (Goad, 2002; Porter-O'Grady & Malloch, 2008, p. 177). The entire organizational culture, especially its leadership, must support the ongoing practice of evidence-based decision making, actions, and evaluation of outcomes.

Holloway, Nesbit, Bordley, and Noyes (2004) and Quinlan (2006) pointed out that although the literature may offer methods to teach evidence-based practice, traditional teaching methods for integrating such practice do not lead to sustained, integrated change. This can be accomplished only by setting standards, clearly outlining role expectations, and supporting practices that instill and promote the wise use of evidence. Leaders must incorporate the language and concepts of evidence-based practice into the organizational mission and strategic plans, establish clear performance expectations related to the use of evidence, integrate the work of evidence-based practice into the governance structures of the system, and recognize and reward performance and outcomes based on the use of evidence (Titler, Cullen, & Ardery, 2002). The transformational leader coaches and promotes collaboration among clinicians, patients, and researchers to create a "professional culture and transformed environment of care in which decisions are made on the basis of best evidence, patient preferences and needs, and expert clinical judgment" (Worral, 2006, p. 339).

Thus, it is well established that evidence-based practice will not thrive without leadership support (Aarons et al, 2014; Berwick, 2003; Everett & Titler, 2006; Stetler, 2003). Leaders must provide access to evidence, authority to change practice, an environment of collaboration, and policies that support evidence-based practice (Everett & Titler, 2006; Malloch & Melnyk, 2013; Titler, 2004).

Although we have become more careful to seek and use research for aspects of patient care, with all of our attention on the trend of the past decade toward evidence-based practice we have largely neglected the need to generate and use evidence specifically related to leadership practices. A growing body of clinical guidelines are in use internationally (Hutchinson, McIntosh, Anderson, Gilbert, & Field, 2003; Mäkelä & Kunnamo, 2001), but we are just beginning to assemble an empirically tested knowledge base for best practices in leadership. Vance and Larson (2002) reviewed nearly 20 years of research on leadership outcomes in health care. Of 6,628 articles, only 4% were data based, and 41% were purely descriptive of the demographic characteristics or traits of leaders. Thus, we know little about either what actually works for leaders or what or how to teach effective leadership (Welton, 2004). Day et al. (2014) recently reviewed 25 years of research on leadership development and called for a continuing focus on gathering data that support the effectiveness of certain leadership strategies and education/training programs.

In health care we are just beginning to document and promote models for evidence-based decision making in leadership (Aarons et al., 2014; Nicklin & Stipich, 2005). Effective leaders pay attention to the need to recruit nurses who enjoy innovative approaches to old challenges, support those nurses who can influence others using positive evidence-based strategies for change in policies and procedures, and provide vision and time to teams who invest in the work culture. The next generation of transformational leaders must continue the task of discovering and utilizing best evidence for successful leadership. Valid use of evidence for leadership will define and strengthen the entire concept of power to leaders of the future.

USING POWER EFFECTIVELY

Leadership, authority, and power are often confused. *Leadership* may be formal or informal and is always characterized by the ability to influence others toward the attainment of some task or goal. We have already described transformational leadership as value driven and grounded from an ethical foundation. It includes the personal qualities and behaviors of the leader. *Authority* is a formally designated or organizationally endowed ability, accountability, or right to act and make decisions. *Power* is the ability to exert influence, but may or may not be rooted in an ethical value system. It may also be formal or informal. Gardner is said to have defined power as "the basic energy needed to initiate and sustain action or … the capacity to translate intention into reality and sustain it" (National Defense University [NDU], n.d., p. 2). Positional power "confers the ability to influence decisions about who gets what resources, what goals are pursued, what philosophy the organization adopts, what actions are taken, who succeeds and who fails" (NDU, n.d., p. 4). The source and use of power by world leaders has been a fascination throughout the centuries.

Power is key to leadership. It is its underlying energy. To become an effective leader, you must become comfortable with power. It takes many forms. There is power of position, power of personality, power in presence or of charisma, power of informal authority, and power by relationships with others of greater power. Power is the ability to move others, to move causes forward, and to extend both energy and assurance or confidence. No matter what the external source of authority, power is eventually ineffective if some sense of personal power does not burn from within. It emanates from conviction, drive, and confidence in self; from a greater self; and from the direction of the organization.

The use of power can be subtle and positive or cunning and ruthless. History has long shown that seeking or using power for its own sake or for personal satisfaction reflects an unfortunate level of professional immaturity that undermines ethics and effectiveness and can do damage to the organization in the long run.

To lead with power, you must build a power base. The power base is both a process and a structure of connecting to personal attributes, skills, organizations, and people to contribute to the creation and control of strategic goals, direction, and resources. A power base is built by engaging in communication, information, and personal networks; reaching out to influential others for mentorship; acquiring your own reputation as powerful; and reflecting the influence and reputation of your own organization (NDU, n.d.).

Pfeffer (1992) outlined the following attributes of a leader to acquire and sustain a strategic power base:

- High energy and physical endurance, including the ability and motivation to personally contribute long and sometimes grueling hours to the work of the organization
- Directing energy to focus on clear strategic objectives, with attention to logistical details embedded with the objectives
- Successfully reading the behavior of others to understand key players, including the ability to assess willingness and resistance to following the leader's direction
- Adaptability and flexibility to redirect energy, abandon a course of action that is not working, and manage emotional responses to such situations
- Motivation to confront conflict, willingness to face difficult issues, and the ability to challenge difficult people to execute a successful strategic decision
- Subordinating the personal ego to the collective good of the organization, by exercising discipline, restraint, and humility

Authentic, transforming power emanates from values and principles. Such principles carry their own form of power to be expanded by the person who carries them forward. Principle-based power is not self-aggrandizement or self-advancement. Rather, the more one empowers others, the more power is generated.

Power is not control; indeed, it is often enhanced by letting go of control. In new paradigms of self-organization and transformational leadership, power is generated from sharing, enhanced by a shared vision, and becomes the amplified energy for change when understood and used as the secret treasure of the leader who shares it strategically within the organization. In fact, the judicious and other-centered use of power and influence are often defined as empowerment of others (MacPhee, Skelton-Green, Bouthillette, & Suryaprakash, 2012). Giving the gift of power actually expands the power of the giver. When people feel that power is being taken from them, they engage in actions to "hoard" power: sabotage, passive resistance, withdrawal, or outright rebellion. But a sense of having power frees energy and promotes a sense of self-efficacy, positive influence, commitment, and greater willingness to give. Conflict is reduced as influence becomes more positive and shared. This discussion makes the process sound reasonable and easy. It is not easy. But it is worth the effort to cultivate skills in sharing power and influence, and empowering others.

THINKING AS AN ENTREPRENEUR

Appropriate use of power releases freedom to innovate and tap into your entrepreneurial leanings. Yet, preparation as a health care professional is not rooted in entrepreneurial thinking. Entrepreneurship is largely absent in American professional clinical curricula. Indeed, a review of entrepreneurial activities of nurses and other health care workers revealed that most of the studies have been done in Scandinavia and the United Kingdom (Austin, Luker, & Roland, 2006; Exton, 2008; Mackintosh, 2006; Sankelo & Akerblad, 2008, 2009; Traynor et al., 2008). Marshall remembers when a creative, non-conformist nurse asked, while they were at work years ago, "Do you ever think of your entrepreneurial self?"

> I did not have a clue what she was talking about. I have often wondered what happened to her. I always imagined that she started her own care business or consulting firm. I have always assumed that entrepreneurs either had patrons to support their inventive habits or put their family fortunes at risks on whimsical new business ideas. I was wrong. Entrepreneurial habits are ways of thinking, creating, and solving problems.

Never have there been more opportunities for entrepreneurial thinking in health care. The U.S. system cries out for innovative answers to difficult, complex problems. It may be a new kind of independent practice; it may be a consultation service to solve unique problems (Shirey, 2006; Tumolo, 2006; Zaccagnini, 2012); it may be a new kind of business relationship between the practitioner and the agency. But we need more independent, creative approaches to solve problems. Some outstanding examples of entrepreneurial nurses who developed businesses to improve health are highlighted by the American Academy of Nursing (AAN, 2016).

You can be a system employee and still be an entrepreneur. Synonyms for entrepreneur include adventurer, promoter, producer, explorer, hero, opportunist, voyager, and risk taker. Our health care systems need entrepreneurial thinkers. We need those willing to risk a new idea, to provide evidence for its value, to take the responsibility for its implementation and evaluation, and to nurture teams to risk innovative practices for positive outcomes. An entrepreneurial thinker resists habits of "stuck" thinking and forms new habits of looking at old problems in new ways. If such approaches are done within the system effectively, the entrepreneur may become even more valued by the system. When you see a problem, before lamenting its existence, reflect on the problem, let it simmer, then brainstorm at least three ways to solve it. Search for evidence on the problem. Think some more. Create a plan to address the problem, marshal the team to commit, implement the new idea, and then test the outcomes. The process is as old and familiar as practice, but it is the reframing of problems and search for ideas and solutions that calls for some adventure.

Given the pioneering roots of professional nursing, in general, and of advanced practice nursing, in particular, it is ironic that the entrepreneurial spirit seems so foreign to current daily practice. Lillian Wald dared to envision, champion, and create public health nursing. Following the loss of her own two children and the heartache of observing the lack of health care in rural America, Mary Breckinridge did not hesitate to nearly single-handedly bring the independent practice of nurse-midwifery to the United States. And Loretta Ford legitimized the primary care practice of public health nurses by establishing the first nurse practitioner program. Why, then, is entrepreneurial nursing not evident in the everyday practice of every nurse leader today? Several authors have pointed out that worldwide, although expertise among nurses is increasingly recognized, traditional organizational bureaucratic and hierarchical mechanisms, ingrained cultures, and ambivalence and ambiguity among practitioners in shaping "new" identities and practices continue to restrain entrepreneurial activities that might improve health care (Aranda & Jones, 2008; Austin et al., 2006; Exton, 2008).

Entrepreneurial habits need to be fed. Ideas are not born of nothing. They come from watching, listening, and reading widely. Begin today with the habit of reading within and outside the health care literature. Read business magazines and newspapers. Notice how chiefs of other industries are solving problems. Drucker (2004, p. 59) chided:

> Ask what needs to be done. Note that the question is not, "What do I want to do?" Asking what has to be done, and taking the question seriously, is crucial for managerial success. Failure to ask this question will render even the ablest executive ineffectual.

Is there a policy that must be changed? What is your idea to change it? Are you willing to give the time and commitment to see it through (Traynor et al., 2008; Whitehead, 2003)?

Once you are committed to a new idea, passion alone is not enough for success. Nurses are generally not prepared to face the challenges of an entrepreneurial practice. You must commit to becoming an expert in securing resources and relationships to help with legal issues, financial management, marketing strategies, payment plans, defining your role and niche, time management (Caffrey, 2005), and outcomes measurement. It takes courage and the willingness to risk, but the world needs more nurses willing to break new paths in health care leadership in entrepreneurial ways.

CARING FOR OTHERS: WHAT SERVANT LEADERSHIP REALLY MEANS

Unlike some entrepreneurs in the general marketplace who creatively feed self-interest, effective entrepreneurial leaders in health care foster some aspect of altruism. At the root of health care leadership is caring for and about others. No industry is more appropriate for servant leadership.

"Leadership is giving. Leadership is an ethic, a gift of oneself to a common cause, a higher calling" (Bolman & Deal, 2001, p. 106). The unique power and prerogative of a leader is the freedom to share yourself, your style, your values, and your influence for a better future. Bolman and Deal (2001, p. 106) stated:

> The essence of leadership is not giving things or even providing visions. It is offering oneself and one's spirit. Material gifts are not unimportant. We need both bread and roses. Soul and spirit are no substitute for wages and working conditions. But … the most important thing about a gift is the spirit behind it…. The gifts of authorship, love, power, and significance work only when they are freely given and freely received. Leaders cannot give what they do not have…. When they try, they breed disappointment and cynicism. When their gifts are genuine and the spirit is right, their giving transforms an organization from a mere place of work to a shared way of life.

The concept of servant leadership was introduced by Robert Greenleaf in the 1970s (1977, 1998) and has been further developed by Spears (1995). Servant leadership releases powerful energy and proposes skills that are particularly effective in health care disciplines, at the heart of which is some degree of altruism. It resonates in special ways within the discipline of nursing (Howatson-Jones, 2004; Swearingen & Liberman, 2004). It encourages the professional growth of the leader and clinician and promotes positive health outcomes. It facilitates collaboration, teamwork, shared decision making, values, and ethical behavior (Barbuto & Wheeler, 2007).

Eleven characteristics of servant leadership include having a sense of calling, listening, empathy, healing, awareness, persuasion, conceptualization, foresight, stewardship, growth, and building community. Senge (1990, 2006) suggested the following five elements of the servant-leader: (a) personal mastery, or "continually clarifying and deepening personal vision … focusing energies, developing patience, and seeing reality objectively" (1990, p. 7); (b) mental models, or deep assumptions, generalizations, or images "that influence how we understand the world and how we take action" (1990, p. 8); (c) building shared vision, or sharing the image we create of the future; (d) team learning, or fundamental learning as a team unit rather than as individuals; and (e) systems thinking.

Some people are natural servant-leaders. You know who they are in your own life. But more important, one can learn to become a servant-leader. It begins with commitment to and practice of lifelong personal and professional learning. Personal mastery is the first step. It means to commit to continual engagement in redefining and clarifying your own personal mission. It means that you cultivate exquisite self-knowledge and personal growth, that you set personal goals related more to the advancement of others than to self-aggrandizement, and that you take time for reflection and feeding your inner self. You come to see your work with a sense of calling.

To be aware of mental models means that you are sensitive to your own personal biases, viewpoints, history, and style and that you strive to use your best self to promote the effective work of others to achieve organizational goals. You examine your own thinking and strive to create a clear vision that you can valiantly communicate and defend. You cultivate exquisite sensitivity in listening, awareness, and empathy. You approach your work and relationships from a perspective of healing.

The shared vision is the common and persuasive image of the future. As the leader, you conceptualize and facilitate that picture with foresight and empower others to share the dream and focus energies to make the changes and do the work to achieve shared goals.

Team learning reflects your ability to suspend your personal assumptions and pace in order to bring the team together to listen to each other and to work in synchrony or harmony. It means that your focus is on the needs and strengths of the team and that you create ways to develop the team to foster collaboration and effectiveness. You lead the team with a sense of stewardship and interest in the growth of its members and help them build a community together. Systems thinking allows you to see the whole as a synergistic concept rather than simply as parts put together. It allows you to see the influence of your own actions and the work of the team on the entire system.

Secretan (2016a) identified the following five "shifts" in servant leadership: (a) from self to other, (b) from things to people, (c) from breakthrough to "kaizen" (celebration of doing things differently rather than simply doing things better), (d) from weakness to strength, (e) and from competition and fear to love. He reminded leaders to ask how we use our gifts to serve. He further outlined six values or principles for Higher Ground Leadership®:

1. *Courage:* Being brave enough to reach beyond the boundaries created by our existing, often deeply held, limitations, fears, and beliefs. Initiating change in our lives—of any kind—happens only when we are courageous enough to take the necessary action.
2. *Authenticity:* Committing oneself to show up and be fully present in all aspects of life, removing the mask and becoming a real, vulnerable, and intimate human being, a person without self-absorption who is genuine and emotionally and spiritually connected to others.
3. *Service:* Focusing on the needs of others by listening to them, identifying their needs, and meeting them. Being inspiring, rather than following a self-focused, competitive, fear-based approach.
4. *Truthfulness:* Listening openly to the truth of others and refusing to compromise integrity or to deny universal truths—even when avoiding the truth might, on the face of it, especially in testing times, seem easier.

5. *Love:* Embracing the underlying oneness with others and life. Relating to, and inspiring, others and touching their hearts in ways that add to who you both are as persons.
6. *Effectiveness:* Being capable of, and successful in, achieving the physical, material, intellectual, emotional, and spiritual goals we set in life. (Secretan, 2016b)

When a leader adopts the transformational stance, along with efforts to transform the organization is a tacit promise to transform others. This is an unspoken covenant to promote and model integrity, respect, and good works of others. This can be achieved in myriad ways. Create traditions replete with ceremonies and rituals that provide a sense of community and belonging, and reinforce the message that significant things are happening and that the people involved are important. Celebrate successes, and rejoice in the achievements of others. Find ways to distinguish good work and reward it. Create an environment of high standards to which people are drawn with assurance that their work is appreciated. Servant leadership is based on the assumption that people are more important than the task and that authentic service to people gets the task done.

GENERATIVITY: PREPARING THE NEXT GENERATION

The transformational leader in health care has an eye on and a heart for the next generation of leaders. Leadership development, coaching, and mentoring are integrated into the very life of the transformational leader. This is the only hope of society for a better future. It is how you leave a living legacy. As the number of experienced managers and leaders in health care continues to diminish at the same time that demand for competent and visionary leaders is increasing, entire organizations are now beginning to integrate leadership development into the everyday life of clinical practice (Spallina, 2002). Unfortunately, too many disciplines in professional health care have histories of a kind of professional hazing (as in, "If I did it, so should you"), including long hours with assigned shift work; sink-or-swim approaches to practice; see-one, teach-one, do-one; "probie" approaches to learning; or even condescending bullying. Such traditions simply will not work in a more competitive environment that must focus on quality improvement, patient outcomes, cost containment, and professional recruitment and retention. A study in Belgium attempted to identify the impact of a specific clinical leadership development program on the clinical nursing leader, the nursing team, and the caregiving process. Although the study uncovered insights related to the leader's progress toward a transformational style and its effects on nursing staff, effects on care processes were more challenging (Dierckx de Casterlé, Willemse, Verschueren, & Milisen, 2008). Another exploration in England demonstrated the value of structured planning and programs in professional development and coaching for future leaders (Alleyne & Jumaa, 2007). There is certainly room for more study in this area. Drucker (2000) proposed four ways to motivate and develop future leaders: (a) know people's strengths, (b) place them where they can make the greatest contributions, (c) treat them as associates, and (d) expose them to challenges. Wells and Hijna (2009) proposed five key elements to develop new talent for leadership in health care: (a) identification of leader competencies; (b) effective job design; (c) a strong focus on leadership recruitment, development, and retention; (d) leadership training and development throughout all levels of the organization; and (e) ongoing leadership assessment and performance management. Of course, this is common-sense jargon, but how do we do it in a way that inspires the dreams and hopes of new leadership?

One way to inspire the next generation for leadership is to tell your own story. Some research has demonstrated that storytelling, especially directly related to the aspiring leader, is effective in developing managers with high potential for success (Ready, 2002). Stories need to be related to the context of current situations and at the level understood by the potential leader. Effective stories are told by respected role models. Share the passion and drama of your experiences, how you failed and learned from the failure, what your successes were, and how you learned to survive. And listen to the stories of aspiring leaders. What is their context and where are they going? How can you help them get there?

Stichler (2006, p. 256) advised that the leader "must consider a logical succession plan in developing tomorrow's nurse leaders and demonstrate competencies and skills as a mentor, coach, role model, and preceptor. The [leader] teaches by example and fosters continual growth" and extends increasing responsibilities to those to assume future leadership. One nurse leader suggested specific steps to approach succession management as a professional obligation, calling it a "migration risk assessment" (Ponti, 2009). First, assess potential attrition and emerging leaders within the organization, establish core competencies for leadership positions, and develop individual plans while identifying critical success factors for upcoming leaders. Then prioritize, coach, and mentor aspiring leaders.

The transformational leader with a constant eye on developing others for leadership is investing in the future. Generativity is a characteristic of leaders with passion for what they do, a vision for a better future, and a genuine interest in helping others to grow. By enabling the next generation, you extend a living legacy of your own efforts, you enliven our own experiences, and you contribute to a positive human investment in making the world a better place.

REFERENCES

Aarons, G. A., Farahnak, L. R., Ehrhart, M. G., & Sklar, M. (2014). Aligning leadership across systems and organizations to develop a strategic climate for evidence-based practice implementation. *Annual Review of Public Health, 35,* 255–274.

Alleyne, J., & Jumaa, M. Q. (2007). Building the capacity for evidence-based clinical nursing leadership: The role of executive co-coaching and group clinical supervision for quality patient services. *Journal of Nursing Management, 15*(2), 230–243.

American Academy of Nursing. (2016). *Raise the voice: Edge runner.* Retrieved from http://www.aannet.org/edgerunners

American Organization of Nurse Executives. (2016). *Resource library*. Retrieved from http://www.aone.org/resources/?search=competencies

Anderson, P., & Pulich, M. (2002). Managerial competencies necessary in today's dynamic health care environment. *Health Care Management, 21*(2), 1–11.

Aranda, K., & Jones, A. (2008). Exploring new advanced practice roles in community nursing: A critique. *Nursing Inquiry, 15*(1), 3–10.

Austin, L., Luker, K., & Roland, M. (2006). Clinical nurse specialists as entrepreneurs: Constrained or liberated. *Journal of Clinical Nursing, 15*(12), 1540–1549.

Avolio, B. J., & Gardner, W. L. (2005). Authentic leadership development: Getting to the root of positive forms of leadership. *Leadership Quarterly, 16*, 315–338. Retrieved from http://marklight.com/Resources-Presentations/MPS594%20Ethical%20 Leadership/Authentic%20leadership%20development,%20Avolio.pdf

Baker, G. R. (2003). Identifying and assessing competencies: A strategy to improve healthcare leadership. *Healthcare Papers, 4*(1), 49–58.

Bamford, M., Wong, C. A., & Laschinger, H. (2013). The influence of authentic leadership and areas of worklife on work engagement of registered nurses. *Journal of Nursing Management, 21*(3), 529–540.

Barbuto, J. E., & Wheeler, D. W. (2007). Becoming a servant leader: Do you have what it takes? In *NebGuide*. Lincoln, NE: University of Nebraska–Lincoln Extension. Retrieved from https://aspireonline.org/aspire2015/wp-content/uploads/sites/ 9/2015/10/BECOMING-A-SERVANT-LEADER-OVERVIEW.pdf

Berwick, D. M. (2003). Disseminating innovations in health care. *Journal of the American Medical Association, 289*(15), 1969–1975.

Bolman, L. G., & Deal, T. E. (2001). *Reframing organizations: Artistry, choice, and leadership*. Hoboken, NJ: John Wiley & Sons.

Burkhart, L., Solari-Twadell, P. A., & Haas, S. (2008). Addressing spiritual leadership: An organizational model. *Journal of Nursing Administration, 38*(1), 33–39.

Caffrey, R. A. (2005). Independent community care gerontological nursing: Becoming an entrepreneur. *Journal of Gerontological Nursing, 31*(8), 12–17.

Calhoun, J. G., Vincent, E. T., Baker, G. R., Butler, P. W., Sinioris, M. E., & Chen, S. L. (2004). Competency identification and modeling in healthcare leadership. *Journal of Health Administration Education, 21*(4), 419–440.

Covey, S. R. (1989). *The seven habits of highly effective people*. New York, NY: Simon & Schuster.

Covey, S. R. (2004). *The 8th habit: From effectiveness to greatness*. New York, NY: Free Press.

Day, D. V., Fleenor, J. W., Atwater, L. E., Sturm, R. E., & McKee, R. A. (2014). Advances in leader and leadership development: A review of 25 years of research and theory. *Leadership Quarterly, 25*(1), 63–82.

DeSmedt, A., Buyl, R., & Nyssen, M. (2006). Evidence-based practice in primary health care. *Student Health & Technology Information, 124*, 651–656.

Dierckx de Casterlé, B., Willemse, A., Verschueren, M., & Milisen, K. (2008). Impact of clinical leadership development on the clinical leader, nursing team, and caregiving process: A case study. *Journal of Nursing Management, 16*(6), 753–763.

Drucker, P. (2000). Managing knowledge means managing oneself. *Leader to Leader, 16*. Retrieved from http://rlaexp.com/studio/biz/conceptual_resources/authors/ peter_drucker/mkmmo_org.pdf

Drucker, P. (2004, June). What makes an effective executive? *Harvard Business Review, 82*(6), 58–63.

Eddy, L. L., Doutrich, D., Higgs, Z. R., Spuck, J., Olson, M., & Weinberg, S. (2009). Relevant nursing leadership: An evidence-based programmatic response. *International Journal of Nursing Education Scholarship, 6*(1 Art. 22), 1–17.

Evans, M. (2005). Textbook executive: The skills and knowledge that all healthcare execs need to master can now be found in one big directory. *Modern Healthcare, 35*(37), 6–16.

Everett, L. Q., & Titler, M. G. (2006). Making EBP part of clinical practice: The Iowa model. In R. F. Levin & H. R. Feldman (Eds.), *Teaching evidence-based practice in nursing* (pp. 295–324). New York, NY: Springer Publishing Company.

Exton, R. (2008). The entrepreneur: A new breed of health service leader? *Journal of Health Organization Management, 22*(3), 208–222.

Finstuen, K., & Mangelsdorff, A. D. (2006). Executive competencies in healthcare administration: Preceptors of the Army-Baylor University graduate program. *Journal of Health Administration Education, 23*(2), 199–215.

Gifford, W., Davies, B., Edwards, N., Griffin, P., & Lybanon, V. (2007). Managerial leadership for nurses' use of research evidence: An integrative review of the literature. *Worldviews on Evidence Based Nursing, 4*(3), 126–145.

Goad, T. W. (2002). *Information literacy and workplace performance.* Westport, CT: Quorum Books.

Greenleaf, R. K. (1977). *Servant leadership: A journey into the nature of legitimate power and greatness.* New York, NY: Paulist Press.

Greenleaf, R. K. (1998). *Power of servant leadership.* San Francisco, CA: Bennett-Koehler.

Grossman, S. (2007). Assisting critical care nurses in acquiring leadership skills: Development of a leadership and management competency checklist. *Dimensions of Critical Care Nursing, 26*(2), 57–65.

Guo, K. L. (2009). Core competencies of the entrepreneurial leader in health care organizations. *Health Care Management, 28*(1), 19–29.

Guo, K. L., & Anderson, D. (2005). The new health care paradigm: Roles and competencies of leaders in the service line management. *International Journal of Health Care Quality Assurance Including Leadership in Health Services, 18*(6–7), suppl. xii–xx.

Hall, L. (2004). A palette of desired leadership competencies: Painting the picture for successful regionalization. *Healthcare Management Forum, 17*(3), 18–22.

Hamric, A. B., Spross, J. A., & Hanson, C. M. (2009). *Advanced practice nursing: An integrative approach* (4th ed.). St. Louis, MO: Saunders Elsevier.

Hay, M. C., Weisner, T. S., Subramanian, S., Duan, N., Niedzinski, E. J., & Kravitz, R. L. (2008). Harnessing experience: Exploring the gap between evidence-based medicine and clinical practice. *Journal of Evaluation in Clinical Practice, 14*(5), 707–713.

Healthcare Leadership Alliance. (2013). *HLA competency directory.* Retrieved from http://www.healthcareleadershipalliance.org/directory.htm

Heathfield, S. M. (2015). *Secrets of leadership success: Choose to lead.* Retrieved from http://humanresources.about.com/od/leadership/a/leader_success.htm

Holloway, R., Nesbit, K., Bordley, D., & Noyes, K. (2004). Teaching and evaluating first and second year medical students' practice of evidence-based medicine. *Medical Education, 38*(8), 869–878.

Howatson-Jones, I. (2004). The servant leader. *Nursing Management, 11*(3), 20–24.

Huston, C. (2008). Preparing nurse leaders for 2020. *Journal of Nursing Management, 16*, 905–911.

Hutchinson, A., McIntosh, A., Anderson, J., Gilbert, C., & Field, R. (2003). Developing primary care review criteria from evidence-based guidelines: Coronary heart disease as a model. *British Journal of General Practice, 53*(494), 690–696.

Kleinman, C. S. (2003). Leadership roles, competencies, and education: How prepared are our nurse managers? *Journal of Nursing Administration, 33*(9), 451–455.

Kouzes, J. M., & Posner, B. Z. (2007). *The leadership challenge* (4th ed.). San Francisco, CA: Jossey-Bass.

Kouzes, J., & Posner, B. Z. (2010). *The five practices of exemplary leadership* (2nd ed.). Hoboken, NJ: John Wiley & Sons.

Kouzes, J., & Posner, B. Z. (2016). *LPI: Leadership Practices Inventory®*. Retrieved from http://www.leadershipchallenge.com/professionals-section-lpi.aspx

Lucia, A. D., & Lepsinger, R. (1999). *The art and science of competency models: Pinpointing critical success factors in organizations*. San Francisco, CA: Jossey-Bass.

Mackintosh, M. (2006). Transporting critically ill patients: New opportunities for nurses. *Nursing Standard, 20*(36), 46–48.

MacPhee, M., Skelton-Green, J., Bouthillette, F., & Suryaprakash, N. (2012). An empowerment framework for nursing leadership development: Supporting evidence. *Journal of Advanced Nursing, 68*(1), 159–169.

Mäkelä, M., & Kunnamo, L. (2001). Implementing evidence in Finnish primary care: Use of electronic guidelines in daily practice. *Scandinavian Journal of Primary Health Care, 19*(4), 214–217.

Malloch, K., & Melnyk, B. M. (2013). Developing high-level change and innovation agents: Competencies and challenges for executive leadership. *Nursing Administration Quarterly, 37*(1), 60–66.

McKenna, M. K., Gartland, M. P., & Pugno, P. A. (2004). Development of physician leadership competencies: Perceptions of physician leaders, physician educators and medical students. *Journal of Healthcare Administration Education, 21*(3), 343–354.

Nanus, B. (1992). *Visionary leadership*. San Francisco, CA: Jossey-Bass.

National Center for Health Care Leadership. (2015). *NCHL health leadership competency model*. Recruited from http://www.nchl.org/static.asp?path=2852,3238

National Defense University. (n.d.). Leveraging power and politics. *Strategic leadership and decision-making*. Retrieved from http://www.au.af.mil/au/awc/awcgate/ndu/strat-ldr-dm/pt4ch17.html

Nicklin, W., & Stipich, N. (2005). Enhancing skills for evidence-based health care leadership: The executive training for research application (EXTRA) program. *Nursing Leadership, 18*(3), 35–44.

O'Connor, M. (2008). The dimensions of leadership: A foundation for caring competency. *Nursing Administration Quarterly, 21*(1), 21–26.

O'Reilly, C. A., Caldwell, D. F., Chatman, J. A., Lapiz, M., & Self, W. (2010). How leadership matters: The effects of leaders' alignment on strategy implementation. *The Leadership Quarterly, 21*(1), 104–113.

Pfeffer, J. (1992). *Managing with power: Power and influence in organizations*. Boston, MA: Harvard Business School Press.

Ponti, M. A. (2009). Transition from leadership development to succession management. *Nursing Administration Quarterly, 33*(2), 125–141.

Porter-O'Grady, T., & Malloch, K. (2007). *Quantum leadership: A resource for health care innovation* (2nd ed.). Sudbury, MA: Jones & Bartlett.

Porter-O'Grady, T., & Malloch, K. (2008). Beyond myth and magic: The future of evidence-based leadership. *Nursing Administration Quarterly, 32*(3), 176–187.

Quinlan, P. (2006). Teaching evidence-based practice in a hospital setting: Bringing it to the bedside. In R. F. Levin & H. R. Feldman (Eds.), *Teaching evidence-based practice in nursing* (pp. 279–293). New York, NY: Springer Publishing Company.

Råholm, M. B. (2009). Evidence and leadership. *Nursing Administration Quarterly, 33*(2), 168–173.

Ready, D. A. (2002, Summer). How storytelling builds next-generation leaders. *MIT Sloan Management Review, 43*(4), 63–69.

Robbins, C. J., Bradley, F. H., & Spicer, M. (2001). Developing leadership in healthcare administration: A competency assessment tool. *Journal of Healthcare Management, 46*(3), 188–202.

Sankelo, M., & Akerblad, L. (2008). Nurse entrepreneurs' attitudes to management, their adaptation of the manager's role, and managerial assertiveness. *Journal of Nursing Management, 16*(7), 829–836.

Sankelo, M., & Akerblad, L. (2009). Nurse entrepreneurs' well-being at work and associated factors. *Journal of Clinical Nursing, 18*(22), 3190–3199.

Secretan, L. (2016a). *The Secretan Center*. Retrieved from http://www.secretan.com/about-us/higher-ground-leadership/

Secretan, L. (2016b). *The higher ground leadership challenge*. Retrieved from http://www.secretan.com/tools/media-and-learning-tools/higher-ground-leadership-challenge/challenge/

Senge, P. (1990). *The fifth discipline: The art and practice of the learning organization*. New York, NY: Doubleday.

Senge, P. (2006). *The fifth discipline: The art and practice of the learning organization* (rev. ed.). New York, NY: Doubleday.

Sherman, R. O., Bishop, M., Eggenberger, T., & Karden, R. (2007). Development of a leadership competency model. *Journal of Nursing Administration, 37*(2), 85–94.

Shewchuk, R. M., O'Connor, S. J., & Fine, D. J. (2005). Building an understanding of the competencies needing for health administration practice. *Journal of Healthcare Management, 50*(1), 32–47.

Shirey, M. R. (2006). Building authentic leadership and enhancing entrepreneurial performance. *Clinical Nurse Specialist, 20*(6), 280–282.

Simonet, D. V., & Tett, R. P. (2013). Five perspectives on the leadership-management relationship: A competency-based evaluation and integration. *Journal of Leadership & Organizational Studies, 20*(2), 199–213.

Spallina, J. M. (2002). Clinical program leadership: Skill requirements for contemporary leaders. *Journal of Oncology Management, 11*(3), 24–26.

Spears, L. C. (1995). *Reflections on leadership: How Robert K. Greenleaf's servant leadership influenced today's top management thinkers*. New York, NY: John Wiley & Sons.

Spencer, L. M., & Spencer, S. M. (1993). *Competence at work: Models for superior performance*. New York, NY: John Wiley & Sons.

Stefl, M. E. (2008). Common competencies for all healthcare managers: The Healthcare Leadership Alliance model. *Journal of Health Care Management, 53*(6), 360–373. Retrieved from http://healthcareleadershipalliance.org/Common%20Competencies%20for%20All%20Healthcare%20Managers.pdf

Stetler, C. B. (2003). Role of the organization in translating research into evidence-based practice. *Outcomes Management, 7*(3), 97–105.

Stichler, J. F. (2006). Skills and competencies for today's nurse executive. *AWHONN Lifelines, 10*(3), 255–257.

Stoller, J. K. (2008). Developing physician-leaders: Key competencies and available programs. *Journal of Health Administration Education, 25*(4), 307–328.

Swearingen, S., & Liberman, A. (2004). Nursing leadership: Serving those who serve others. *Health Care Manager, 23*(2), 100–109.

Titler, M. G. (2004). Methods in translation science. *Worldviews on Evidence-Based Nursing, 1,* 38–48.

Titler, M. G., Cullen, L., & Ardery, G. (2002). Evidence-based practice: An administrative perspective. *Reflections of Nursing Leadership, 28*(2), 26–27.

Tracy, C. S., Dantas, G. C., & Upshur, R. E. (2003). Evidence-based medicine in primary care: Qualitative study of family physicians. *BMC Family Practice, 9*(4), 6.

Traynor, M., Drennan, V., Goodman, C., Mark, A., Davis, K., Peacock, R., & Banning. (2008). "Nurse entrepreneurs": A case of government rhetoric? *Journal of Health Services Research & Policy, 13*(1), 13–18.

Tumolo, J. (2006). Thinking outside the box: How nontraditional practice is paying off for some NP entrepreneurs. *Advanced Nurse Practitioner, 14*(4), 37–39, 40.

Vance, D., & Larson, E. (2002). Leadership research in business and health care. *Journal of Nursing Scholarship, 34*(2), 165–171.

Wear, D. (2008). On outcomes and humility. *Academic Medicine, 83*(7), 625–626.

Wells, W., & Hijna, W. (2009). Developing leadership talent in healthcare organizations. *Healthcare Financial Management, 63*(1), 66–69.

Welton, W. E. (2004). Managing today's complex healthcare business enterprise: Reflections on distinctive requirements of healthcare management education. *Journal of Health Administration Education, 21*(4), 391–418.

Whitehead, K. (2003). The health-promoting nurse as a health policy career expert and entrepreneur. *Nurse Educator Today, 23*(8), 584–592.

Worral, P. S. (2006). Traveling posters: Communicating on the frontlines. In R. F. Levin & H. R. Feldman (Eds.), *Teaching evidence-based practice in nursing* (pp. 337–346). New York, NY: Springer Publishing Company.

Zaccagnini, M. (2012). Emerging roles for the DNP: Nurse educator, nurse administrator, nurse leader, nurse entrepreneur and community health. In S. DeNisio & A. Barker (Eds.), *Advanced practice nursing.* Boston, MA: Jones & Bartlett.

CHAPTER 7

Becoming a Leader: It's All About You

Marion E. Broome and Elaine Sorensen Marshall

Through imagination we can envision the worlds within us.
—Stephen Covey

OBJECTIVES

- *To identify the typical career journey of leaders in nursing*
- *To describe and use self-assessment tools to build leadership capacity*
- *To describe the challenges, such as fear and failure, that leaders may face, and identify strategies to manage them*
- *To apply the importance of caring for self, mindfulness techniques, and spirituality in a leader's journey*
- *To learn how to cultivate peer networks and consider career coaches to develop skills*
- *To describe key elements to enhance influence*
- *To explore a sense of spiritual self in leadership*

Few successful leaders began their careers thinking they would one day make a major impact in their profession. Most, on reflection, simply say they took advantage of opportunities as they came along, worked hard, and enjoyed what they were doing at the time. Yet they will also share that somewhere, someone believed in them and saw things in them that they often did not see in themselves. Emerging leaders are often heard to share that they were "just lucky," or "in the right place at the right time." Although there may be some truth in these statements, many people are in the right place at the right time to take advantage of an opportunity but do not. In this book, we have explored what transformational leadership is and what a transformational leader does. In this chapter we focus on how the transformational leader develops, how selected tools can be useful in developing leadership strengths and competencies, and the challenges any leader faces. We also discuss critically important ways a leader can sustain hope and optimism during her career (McBride, 2011).

CAREER JOURNEY OF NURSE LEADERS

Most nurses do not, as they begin their careers, intend to become a leader. Rather they talk about wanting to be good at what they do, learning how to apply the knowledge and skills they learned in their first nursing program to become an expert—usually in direct care for patients. As they return for advanced degrees they specialize in areas of practice, such as caring for patients with cardiovascular problems, informatics, nursing administration, and so on. Even at that point many rarely own the notion that, as a result of obtaining further education, they now are indeed leaders in the profession. Hence, there is often a discrepancy in how their patients, students, clients, and other system leaders view them and how they view themselves. The reality is that leaders in a field do not always hold a formal position, but others may look to them for direction, a way forward, and problem solving (Stanley et al., 2011). It is important that nurses think reflectively about their career, their own skills, strengths and weaknesses, and potential for leadership.

HAVING INFLUENCE

"Influence is more important than authority" (Sullivan, 2004, p. 3). Being influential is a characteristic that leaders must work to develop. Influence requires high levels of credibility, strong interpersonal skills, and a genuine interest in others. Making the decision to become influential is the first and most important criterion required to actually have influence. You must first decide to have influence.

Securing a New Position

Once you decide that you want to make a difference, that you want to have influence as a leader in health care, you may decide that it is time to aspire to the next step in an official leadership position. When that decision is made, the first step in gaining influence is "to assess the way you present yourself" (Sullivan, 2004, p. 8). Never underestimate the power of the image you portray to enhance your influence and success, especially in a first impression. Image will not sustain leadership effectiveness in the absence of other substantive knowledge and skills, but it can open or close doors, support or undermine whether you are taken seriously, and amplify or diminish the energy you must bring to exert and sustain your personal position of influence or leadership.

Career coaches Martin and Bloom (2003) outlined principles to avoid derailment and to facilitate success at the outset of your career in leadership. Personal presentation tops the list. Whether you like it or not, people evaluate your abilities within 8 to 30 seconds of the first meeting (Martin & Bloom, 2003). First impressions are important. People expect to see an open, interesting, positive, and hardworking general attitude. Walk tall, smile generously, make eye contact, and give a firm handshake. Dress appropriately. The old adage to dress for the position to which you aspire instead of the one you currently hold is true. When interviewing, and even after you secure the position, set the standard for dress and appearance. To be well groomed, neat, and clean goes without saying. For interviews, standards for men include neutral colors of navy, gray, and black jacket; conservative shirt color; and an interesting but not flamboyant tie. Women generally still find people less forgiving about informal attire upon presentation than men.

Attention to detail is critical. Avoid anything that calls attention away from you as a leader and instead directs eyes and comments toward your appearance. That means to avoid too many accessories, strange hair colors, bright nail polish, too-short skirts, or clunky shoes. Martin and Bloom (2003) shared their own experience, noting that they have rarely observed women candidates ascend to the highest levels of executive positions who wore pantsuits to first interviews, but be assured that you must be true to yourself and to your own style. Make sure the fit is right for you. Nevertheless, at the same time, part of your skill as a leader is sensitivity to the culture where you aspire to a position of leadership.

Many interviewees make the mistake of thinking that trendy, expensive attire is crucial. Others believe that women must dress conservatively in order to make an impression. Neither statement is true. Instead, be honest with yourself and look at the clothing you do have. What styles flatter your physique, what colors make you look bright and comfortable with yourself? Ask friends for their advice if you are not comfortable with your own assessment. You do not want your attire to detract from your presence; rather, you want to use it to help others take you seriously as a professional.

A second critical aspect of the interview is to be prepared. Know the job for which you are applying and the system in which it "sits"—the vision, mission, and expectations. As you prepare for the interview, look at each item on the job description and jot down notes about experiences you have had that related to the competency or skill. Recall examples of times when you used that skill in a previous job. Invariably you will be asked to share a story that illustrates a situation in which you were effective in achieving a goal and one in which you failed to achieve your objective. Be prepared to talk about what you might do differently the next time. Be prepared with some ideas about what your ideal job would be, and what supports you would need to be successful. Ask good questions of your interviewer, such as:

• How will I know I am successful after 6 months—what do you expect me to accomplish?
• How do you want me to keep you informed, and about what kinds of issues?
• I read about the new clinic the service. What are some areas of intersection that I (as the new manager of a related unit) would need to think about?

Interviewers are asked to evaluate several individuals for each job. Give them something to remember you by thorough illustrative examples of how you think and what your experiences have been to meet the specific needs of the organization.

Making the Difference

Once you secure the job, it is important to learn and practice some basic principles of influence to make the difference. The same team well known for creating *Crucial Conversations* (Patterson, Grenny, McMillan, & Switzler, 2002) have created an entire enterprise focused on leadership development directed toward positive influence (Grenny, Patterson, Maxfield, McMillan, & Switzler, 2013; Switzler, 2016; VitalSmarts, 2016). Here we will explore some of their fundamental ideas. One of their principles is to "change the way you change minds" (see Switzler, 2016). As a leader, you must decide for yourself and be willing to help others believe that a change of outlook, action, or behavior can be done and will be worth the effort. Grenny et al. (2013) and Switzler (2016) suggested creating personal experiences and sharing stories rather than just trying to persuade. In other words, help others to experience the change. Use field trips to other organizations where the values or environments you want to emulate exist. Develop friendships with colleagues at these organizations and secure invitations to send your staff to observe workers at these sites. This requires visibility with those you are trying to influence.

A second principle is to "find vital behaviors" (Grenny et al., 2013, pp. 35–64), meaning to identify what specific, essential *actions* are most necessary to lead to change toward the desired outcome. Identification of the actions needed must be informed by evidence of what works to make the difference. Especially in health care, we are sometimes lured by current trends in thinking and practice. Instead of sticking to the usual modes, the influential leader studies the evidence inside and out of the usual practices to discover what really works. The leader must also present the evidence to others in such a way that they understand it and can be persuaded.

A third principle is to "make the undesirable desirable" or "help them love what they hate" (Grenny et al., 2013, pp. 77–112). Sometimes, basic requirements to get the job done are "noxious, painful, boring, or simply less desirable than other tasks." Find ways to make such tasks palatable. Perhaps, that means changing the task itself, reframing it, or seeing that it is clearly tied to some reward or desirable outcome. In any case, such tasks need to be faced head-on and accomplished.

Another idea is to "surpass your limits" or "help them do what they can't" (Grenny et al., 2013, pp. 113–144). Do what it takes and help others to exceed expectations. This usually means acquiring superior abilities by practice. In the bestselling book *Outliers: The Story of Success,* Gladwell (2008) explained the "ten-thousand-hour rule"—that behind every great achiever is 10,000 hours devoted to practice, practice, and practice. You cannot expect to surpass your limits without committed practice to your art and skill. This holds true for others, too.

As a leader, you set the example and use your influence to encourage others to devote the time and energy needed to be the best. This will require getting to know others, which implies presence and visibility with those you lead.

The idea to "harness peer pressure . . . or the power of social influence" (Grenny et al., 2013, pp. 145–184) is a basic principle of making things work. To influence others, help them influence each other. Identify respected opinion leaders within your organization. Invite them as mentors or peers and involve them in change processes. Plant seeds of ideas among working groups, during informal gatherings, and in hall conversations, then let them grow. From such actions, you can create strength and support from the very people who can make things happen. Meanwhile, support yourself with positive peers who share your goals. Avoid or reduce the effects of potentially toxic individuals and find ways to mutually support people who nurture each other and the values of the organization.

Beyond the social environment, many leaders fail to extend sufficient attention to the actual physical environment where people spend most of their day working. Look at the physical, social, and intellectual environment with new eyes (Grenny et al., 2013, pp. 247–286): What needs to happen to influence others for success?

Meanwhile, reward early successes, punish only when necessary, and do not rely on incentives as the first line of motivation (Grenny et al., 2013, pp. 217–246). Reward positive, innovative, and healthy behaviors. Measure progress and reward success. Ensure that rewards are meaningful to the individual. A meaningful reward may not always be money, but perhaps time, flexible work hours, or just a show of genuine appreciation. The reward needs to meet the perspective of the recipient more than the giver. One person may love a framed "award" at the next public meeting, while another may prefer a 4-hour holiday away.

What needs to happen to influence others for success? Encourage honesty and candid feedback; give clear signals; manage fairness in worker input, being sure to include those most distant; and continually review processes. Attend to the environment, and join your workers in practice of pursuits to exceed expectations.

SELF-ASSESSMENT FOR GROWTH

Successful influence is always a product of continuing self-assessment. There are various approaches in such assessment. The support of another, more seasoned, leader can help. Despite the strong emphasis in nursing on the need for mentors during one's career, relatively few nurses can identify such individuals in their workplaces. Many claim that mentors are scarce, despite the demographics, which would suggest there are many seasoned nurses who might help others negotiate career challenges and advancement. In our experience, nurses often find it difficult to ask for help, and engaging with a mentor can appear to be doing just that (Broome & Gilbert, 2014a). In contrast, some nurses think they do not need help and can master any knowledge or competencies required, preferring to ask for help if they need it. Either of these stances is likely to shortchange the individual and preclude him or her from developing into a strong, influential leader who can make a difference in the lives of others. All of us who are labeled as strong leaders can, in fact, identify mentors and colleagues who helped us see things we could not see—about both ourselves and our situations. Sometimes those mentors chose us and sometimes we sought them out for their guidance and help. In each case we were willing to share, listen, and reflect.

Many of us also took formal courses or short-term intensive workshops that provided self-learning opportunities and often a project to work on to hone our skills as leaders (see Table 7.1 for a few examples). What does one learn and do in these courses? As much as one chooses. Most of these courses provide content about leadership frameworks, communication, vision setting, goal setting, leading teams, and so on. Most also ask participants to engage in some form of self-assessment using structured tools that provide the individual with information about leadership strengths and areas for improvement. Two of the most common and valuable components of these opportunities are small group work and a leadership project.

Small Group Work

Small group work, as a component of leadership training, involves three to five individuals assigned as a group to work as a unit throughout the experience. This setup allows the individuals to get to know each person's professional challenges, aspirations, and the skills he or she seeks or needs to develop. The value of this group is the shared space in which trust can grow and in which participants can

TABLE 7.1 Examples of Selected Leadership Training Opportunities

LEADERSHIP DEVELOPMENT OPPORTUNITY	DESCRIPTION OF COURSE	TIME FRAME AND COST	CONTACT INFORMATION
Sigma Theta Tau International	Maternal–Child Health Academy; Maternal–Child Health Africa; Geriatric Nursing Leadership; Nurse Faculty Leadership; Board Leadership Institute	Most of these are a 12- to 18-month commitment with some face-to-face intensive training, use a mentor–mentee model, use expert faculty leaders, and involve a project. Costs are defrayed for several by grants but range from $0 to $500 for participation fee and travel to intensives (usually 2) and to the convention, to present.	www.nursingsociety.org

(continued)

TABLE 7.1 Examples Of Selected Leadership Training Opportunities (*continued*)

LEADERSHIP DEVELOPMENT OPPORTUNITY	DESCRIPTION OF COURSE	TIME FRAME AND COST	CONTACT INFORMATION
Center for Creative Leadership	Offers five core programs, including Leadership at the Peak, Leading for Organizational Impact, and Leadership Development Program; and six specialized programs, including Navigating Change, and Women's Leadership Experience	These 2- to 5-day programs are offered throughout the year, require assessment prework, focused goal setting, etc. Tuition covers most meals and instruction, preassessment, and several post-coaching sessions. You are responsible for travel and lodging. Tuition costs are listed on the website and range from $2,500 to $7,500.	www.ccl.org
Amy V. Cockcroft Leadership Development Program	University-based year-long program with on-site intensives (in Columbia, SC) offered five times each year, supplemented with a leadership project.	Focus is on learning how to be an innovative health care leader and nurse leader from practice, education, and policy work with participants in the workshops. Costs include transportation and minimal registration fee.	www.sc.edu/ (see Center for Nursing Leadership)
National League for Nursing	Three programs housed in the Center for Transformational Leadership: • Leadership Development Program for Simulation Educators • Executive Leadership in Nursing Education and Practice Program (for those with 5 years of experience in a leadership position) • LEAD (for those who have experienced a rapid transition into a leadership role)	Includes face-to-face meetings, conference calls, webinars, and forum discussions throughout the 1-year programs. Cost ranges from $3,000 to $3,500.	www.nln.org/ (see professional development programs)

(continued)

TABLE 7.1 Examples of Selected Leadership Training Opportunities (*continued*)

LEADERSHIP DEVELOPMENT OPPORTUNITY	DESCRIPTION OF COURSE	TIME FRAME AND COST	CONTACT INFORMATION
Association of Nurse Executives	Various leadership development courses, including: • "Early Careerist," such as the Emerging Nurse Leader Institute • "Mid-Careerist," such as the Nurse Director Fellowship • "Executive," such as the Health Care Finance (workshop) and Harvard Business School course	Offerings range from 3-day short courses for $900 (e.g., Emerging Leader Institute) to year-long fellowships for $7,000 (e.g., Nurse Manager Fellowship) to $24,000 for the Harvard-based 1-year program for nurse executives.	www.aone.org/education

relate their challenges and respond to each other's questions, which often clarify an individual's thinking enormously. Feedback, engagement, and support from peers outside one's work environment offers a special, valuable viewpoint.

Leadership Project

Many think the purpose of the leadership project is to finish the work as a reflection of leadership skill. In fact, it is not the outcome that is most important, but rather the process and learning that occurs as the project journey unfolds. Leadership is about learning from one's missteps as well as successes. Any project is complicated and involves other people. It is inevitable that there will be lessons to be learned. If emerging leaders are open to examining themselves and their actions, growth is also inevitable. Such projects most often show participants how to set a vision, how to encourage others when they encounter obstacles, and how to coach others toward achieving success. Of course, not every project proceeds down a rosy path, and neither does the leadership journey.

DEVELOPING SELECTED AREAS OF LEADERSHIP SKILL

Not all leadership skills are required in every position; nor is every competency a good fit with each individual aspiring to be a leader. For instance, leaders at the top of the organization who are held accountable for the vision and implementation of longer range goals must have the ability to think strategically and, as we have discussed in other chapters, engage others in their organization. Hughes and Beatty (2005) described strategic thinking as requiring the ability to synthesize as well as analyze, nonlinear as well as linear thinking, visual as well as verbal skills, implicit and explicit expression, and that which engages the heart as well as the mind. Synthesis and analysis are different abilities, and some individuals are much better at one than the other; only a few are capable of both. All kinds of leaders are needed in an organization—the important thing is that you figure out what you are best at doing as well as what you enjoy!

Self-assessment of one's own strengths and areas less developed can be useful to both the emerging, developing leader and the seasoned leader as each continues his or her journey. Most professional leadership workshops and experiences do, in fact, include this as a part of their development curriculum. Courses use different assessment tools, but each tool will have some things in common. You will be asked questions about how you respond to different aspects of professional life in a variety of areas, such as how you:

- React to and manage change
- Communicate with your peers, your boss, and your subordinates
- Receive negative feedback
- Provide others with feedback
- Deal with conflict

There are hundreds of tools available for self-assessment. These tools take some time to complete, and there are no right or wrong answers. Some require a written manual to score, others provide you with immediate feedback. Yet others are more complicated and require a coach to explain the results. The advantage of programs that provide a coach is that he or she can help you focus on the positive feedback, without focusing on weaknesses. In addition, a coach can discuss with you how to approach working on some of the areas you are interested in strengthening, or those areas of most interest to your supervisor. Table 7.2 contains selected examples of leadership assessment tools. Several of these are associated with leadership theories discussed in earlier chapters.

TABLE 7.2. Selected Examples of Leadership Assessment Tools

LEADERSHIP ASSESSMENT TOOL	CONCEPTUAL COMPONENTS (SUBSCALES)	ITEMS	REFERENCES
Leadership practices inventory (**Kouzes & Posner, 2007**)	Model the way Inspire a vision Challenge the process Enable others to act Encourage the heart	30 items 5 subscales 10-point response format	www .leadershpchallenge .com

(continued)

TABLE 7.2. Selected Examples of Leadership Assessment Tools (*continued*)

LEADERSHIP ASSESSMENT TOOL	CONCEPTUAL COMPONENTS (SUBSCALES)	ITEMS	REFERENCES
Multifactor leadership questionnaire (MLQ-Form 5x) (**Bass & Avolio, 2004**)	Idealized influence Inspirational motivation Intellectual stimulation Individual consideration Contingent reward Active and passive management Laissez-faire	45 items 3 factors (Transformational, transactional, avoidant–passive)	www.mindgarden .com
Clinical leadership competency framework; self-assessment tool (**National Health Service, 2012**)	Demonstrating personal qualities Working with others Managing services Improving services Setting direction		www .leadershipacademy .nhs.uk
StrengthsFinder 2.0 (**Rath, 2007**)	34 themes and ideas for action, including relator, ideation, futuristic, etc. Based on one's core, which is calculated online An individual report is produced, providing a description of your top five strengths and specific suggestions for how to maximize your strengths and minimize any weaknesses	Assessment tool accessed by a code found at the end of Rath's book (2007) Assessment takes about 30 minutes	http://sf2. strengthsfinder .com/research

Reprinted with permission from Broome and Gilbert (2014b).

REFLECTION QUESTIONS

1. What kind of self-assessment of your own leadership skills have you engaged in?
2. How helpful was the feedback you received?
3. How did you use the insights you gained after completing the surveys to expand or strengthen the skills you needed?
4. What surprised you the most about what you learned?

CHALLENGES FOR LEADERS

Thus far we have been focusing on leadership strengths and how to develop yourself. Leadership is a journey; one filled with both opportunity and disappointments. Just as every leader must assess personal strengths, he or she must also reflect on abilities to deal with the inevitable challenges and failures that arise on the journey.

An important part of influence in health care is sharing your wisdom and experience with others who can learn from your successes and failures. So, do not forget what you have learned about clinical scholarship. It is your obligation as a leader to contribute to the discipline. That means presenting, writing, and publishing. In order for academic publications in health care to have meaning or application, they must be grounded in clinical practice and actual leadership experience. That is precisely why clinical scholarship is such an important part of your stewardship as a leader.

Take time to reflect on your practice and your leadership. Watch for influential things you are doing that might make a difference for someone else in a similar situation. Make friends with someone in an academic setting and work together to share your work with the discipline. This is part of your responsibility as a leader. Provide opportunities for your staff to become involved in research or demonstration projects in meaningful ways, and be sure that their contribution is noted appropriately. You are part of something greater than your organization; help your staff to see that, too. The world needs your influence, and you will be amazed at your ability to make a difference.

Professional activities that will enable you to share your experiences and mentor other emerging leaders are an important aspect of leadership. Your contributions to membership and participation on agency boards, editorial boards, governing boards of professional associations, and boards of nonprofit groups will all benefit such organizations. You, in turn, will learn a great deal and be able to bring that knowledge to your own organization.

One of the most difficult tasks of any leader who is involved at broader levels is how to bring back the knowledge one gains at those other "tables" working with other leaders. The challenge is to communicate the cues and insights and impressions one garners and frame them in ways others can hear. Of course, not all that you learn from such activities may have direct application to your own work, but your experiences can shape the way you think as a leader and how you influence goals and activities within your own organization. Broome finds it especially useful to develop written communication for others to read, reflect within groups, and then discuss as food for thought within her own organization, especially among peers inclined to support innovation.

DEALING WITH FEAR AND FAILURE

Fear and *failure* are terms not usually found in the table of contents of a leadership text. To teach leadership is usually to motivate, to paint the best and most hopeful picture, to instill fearlessness, and to draw on the assumption that you will not fail. But as expert clinicians today, leaders and managers who exhibit characteristics of transformational leadership hold more central positions in organizational networks of influence, and their direct reports are more influential in informal organizational networks (Bono & Anderson, 2005). In other words, transformational leaders tend to expand their influence and the influence of those whom they lead. As you make your own transformation from expert clinician to transformational leader, you enter a world of expectations. The world needs your expertise and preparation to improve health care, and facing fears in this context can be helpful.

Among the risks of breaking open the doors to find your own place as a transformational leader is discouragement when the cold water of reality splashes back in your face. Marshall (2011) called it the "Moses-off-the-mountain syndrome." You advance in education, you attend the workshop, you "go to the mountain" in your own pursuit of learning and reflection. You become singularly informed, educated, and impassioned. Then you unveil your latest inspired creation of ideas, and no one gets on board. It does not work. Review, regroup, and try again.

Leading can be lonely, but you have the capacity to continue toward your vision. Feed those who understand where you are going. Some days, you simply need to solve a problem. Or, you just need smart, quick action, and results. Other times, you need to spread innovations and new ways of thinking and acting.

Know this for certain: No leader who has accomplished anything has not had periods of fear or some major failure. Wheatley (2009, p. 81) assured that a "wild ride between hope and fear is unavoidable. Fear is the necessary consequence of feeling hopeful again." Hope and fear are born in the heart together. Wheatley continued, "Hope never enters a room without fear at its side. If I hope to accomplish something, I'm also afraid I'll fail. You can't have one without the other." Likewise, to be fearful is to hope that you will not fail. Wheatley (2009, p. 81) further admonished to replace fear and hope with the willingness to be insecure, to be vulnerable, to exchange "certainty for curiosity, fear for generosity." Be willing to treat plans and innovations as "experiments," to become less engaged in hope and fear and more willing to be engaged in discovery. Wheatley (p. 82) reminded that if we would remember that "we *are* hope, it becomes much easier to stop being blinded or seduced by hopeful prospects."

Every leader has met moments of failure. Do not ever think otherwise. Marshall remembers:

> When I could feel the ground sink beneath my feet. In my own experience of a perceived failure, I confessed to a friend and colleague that I could recall the very moment my core confidence cracked. It was a breathless, life-changing jolt for me to believe I had failed. My friend responded simply, "We *all* have cracks in our core confidence." She was right. I had lived a professional

REFLECTION QUESTIONS

Think of a recent experience in which you failed to accomplish what you set out to achieve.

1. When did it first occur to you that you would not be able to accomplish the goal?
2. How did it feel?
3. What factors do you think influenced the failure?
4. If that goal is still important to you, or to your organization, what kinds of different strategies would you use to achieve success?

life of one success upon another. I now know that every leader who has risked a better way has some healing wounds inside." (Marshall, 2011, p. 173)

The key is to learn from those failures and to find some oasis of strength and hope as you review the experience with another that you trust. And it is important to remember that although you may have played a role in the failure, it is highly likely that others around you also played a part. Just as success in never a solitary accomplishment, neither is a failure.

As you mature as a leader, you will find other leaders willing to share their own episodes of fear or failure. No truly successful leader has not known some defeat. It is often our best teacher. Do not allow fear or failure to rob you of curiosity and the willingness to risk. Instead find the lessons from which you can learn and grow.

SUSTAINING SELF AS LEADER

Caring for Self

Leadership is a lifelong pursuit. You have to care for yourself as you care for others. The first rule of servant leadership is self-mastery, and the first rule to have authentic or credible influence on the lives of others is to attend to one's own sense of being. The idea of work–life balance is a myth, so the priority must be on balancing energy. Manage personal resources to find what restores you and put some part of that restoration into each day (Barsh, Cranston, & Craske, 2008). Positions of leadership are often described as lonely. In a position of leadership, you have few lateral peers with whom you can exchange ideas and concerns on a daily basis. You are required to make difficult decisions that are sometimes unpalatable to others. You must keep confidences that should you disclose might explain and defend your actions and positions that may be misunderstood by some. Others may speak pejoratively about you, but you are restrained from saying anything about others. You generously announce the accomplishments of others but may not even mention your own latest award. These factors and others can create a sometimes lonely existence. It is therefore important to seek out confidantes and colleagues in similar positions with whom you can share and reflect.

Kibort (2005, p. 54) warned, "Get used to no thank-yous." It is an old adage that as a leader, if you are doing what you should, someone will be unhappy. In fact, the sooner you recognize this, the better you will adjust emotionally. No matter what you do, how hard you work, or how many people you communicate with, a few people will not be happy with what the organization or unit is doing and where you are going. You cannot possibly keep everyone happy, nor is that your job. An individual's satisfaction and happiness at work depend on many things—what is happening in the workplace and what is happening at home, how long he or she has been in the same job, temperament, and responses to change, among others.

Marshall recounted one example that occurred after she had worked for a year to develop a plan providing significant resources for some of her workers to acquire advanced education. She imagined that it would be among the greatest gifts in their lives. When it became a reality, she was amazed at the paucity of thanks—and treasured the few expressions that came. Broome had a similar experience when she strongly encouraged, and provided resources for, faculty to return for a doctorate. But in both cases, we were able to watch our workers blossom as leaders as they journeyed through their new educational programs and enjoyed the fruits of their opportunities. As a leader, you will work behind the scenes to advance the interests and careers of people who may well hold you in least regard, who may be unaware of their benefactor, but you will find fulfillment in your generative role as a leader. Here is a life lesson we have both learned: Much of the satisfaction from your accomplishments as a leader must come from a maturity that you may not even know you possess. It comes from within your vision and authentic caring for what you do and the people you serve. As you care for others, you must also find a way to care for yourself that preserves your own energy and facilitates positive influence on others.

Managing Stress. The physical and emotional effects of stress are well-known. If only knowledge about stress and self-awareness of how we feel when stressed were required to ameliorate its effects, we would all be in a continual state of serenity. Thus, you do not need to "know" more about stress. You know your own stressors and their effects. You know what they are in your own life: knot-in-the-stomach anxiety, overeating, overworking, or whatever it is for you.

But what do you do to reduce the effects of stress in your life? What works for you? Cryer, McCraty, and Childre (2003) proposed five steps for leaders to reduce the negative effects of stress:

1. Recognize and disengage, meaning to recognize the stomach knot and impose on yourself a "time out." Isolate and put aside the source of stress for a moment as if you are moving on to the next e-mail message. In an instant, switch mental gears.

2. Breathe through your heart. After recognizing and suspending the source of stress, shift your attention and focus like a laser to a familiar symbol, such as a specific part of your body. For example, consciously focus on your own heart, physically and emotionally, and breathe deeply.

3. Invoke a positive feeling. Turn your mind to an image in your life that only brings joy: the laughter of your child, "the smell of pine," new snow—whatever it is for you.

4. Ask yourself, "Is there a better alternative?" Take an objective view of the problem and consider another possible way to address it.

5. Note the change in perspective. Take the time to notice what it feels like now. Is your head clearer? Are you more generous? Are you willing to try it again?

In one recent study, Pipe et al. (2012) used techniques similar to those just described as part of an educational intervention with oncology staff and leaders and found they effectively promoted personal coping and enhanced well-being. The techniques can work for you.

Stress and Energy. By your own achievements, you have shown yourself to have energy and positive ambition. You have the energy to get things done, and you may actually derive energy from stress. One warning for the transformational leader is that "paradoxically, the energy that gets people going can also cause them to give up" (Gonzalez, 2016). One of the most attractive and effective characteristics of transformational leaders is their energy and enthusiasm, but if not tempered in reality and sensitivity, these can wear out the followers in an organization.

That dark side of highly energetic transformational leadership can ambush even the best leader or organization. If the leader does not tend to the care of self and others, or to the details of reality, boundless enthusiasm can wear down even the most devoted followers or staff. It is especially helpful for leaders to surround themselves with reality checkers, confidants, and transactional managers who can send a strong message when the leader may be marching so far ahead of the followers that he or she loses them. Part of caring for yourself as a leader is to be sure you have some colleagues and support staff who care about you, who can protect both the organization and you against yourself when you or the organization, or both, need it. Also, remember that transformational leaders see the big picture. Thus, every organization also needs someone to follow the details, add up the figures, and counts the beans.

Truly invested leadership takes all the energy of your being, all the time. You are always in charge and carry the burden of being the responsible one all the time. This can soon become physically and emotionally exhausting and depersonalizing. Moreover, you run the risk of forgetting who you are and where you and your organization are going. This exhaustion is rightly called *burnout*, because your sense of self is burned away and used up in an effort to be everything to everyone. Only by finding and sustaining a spiritual center can you reclaim yourself.

Identify which people, situations, or activities are toxic to your personal, emotional, social, and professional health and avoid them wherever possible. When you cannot avoid these folks, reframe an image and acquire a persona that allows you to be sensitive, but does not allow you to resent others in the organization. Keep in mind that you are being paid to do a job as the leader of a group, but that job does not include keeping everyone happy. Counter the stress and toxicity by exploring activities to relax, refresh, and restore you and your spiritual center. Then find ways to integrate those activities into your life on a regular basis. Is it a hobby? Is it beautiful music? Do you need to go fishing, skiing, or shopping? Take a nap or do yoga? Find time that is yours and hold it inviolate. If you travel professionally, invest in an extra personal day to go to a concert, a museum, an art gallery, or a ballgame. Find ways to see the personal joy in your work. Invite beauty, energy, and love, and they will be returned to you.

Use of Peer Networks and Career Coaches

Sometimes a leader simply wants to "do it myself," to get things done, but this usually does not work. Leaders must reach out to others when they would often like to just sit in a meeting and reflect. Or, they must bring people together to address something in which none of the parties is interested, but that is important to the organization. A leader usually has to find time to develop and sustain relationships both within and outside of the organization. Leaders who are embedded in their community and have lived there for years can turn to other leaders they know in other fields to seek advice when challenges and stress mount. At the very least they can bounce ideas off these peers and engage with them in activities designed to distract and relax.

Engaging a professional coach is an increasingly common method used now to help leaders new to a role develop their leadership, discuss options for action before they make a decision, and learn more about themselves. Authentic leaders (Broome, 2015; Laschinger, Wong, & Grau, 2013) are grounded in self-awareness, which is developed through self-reflection and feedback from others. In turn, they use this self-awareness to help mentor others in their careers. Coaches are helpful in this respect as they are almost always external to the organization, have no vested interests except that of the individual they are coaching, and bring a wealth of experience to the relationship. Unlike with a mentor, the relationship does not have a personal dimension. Professional coaches can be expensive and vary a great deal in their background and training, so it is important that the individual do sufficient research on the coach before committing or signing a contract. The length of time that you commit to coaching can span anywhere from 3 to 12 months, and the number of interactions, types of assessments, and other details should be outlined in a contract that describes the leader's goal for his or her own development, as well as input from supervisors to ensure alignment with the needs of the organization.

FINDING THE SPIRITUAL CENTER

It is possible that the most important thing you will do as a leader is to come to know yourself as a spiritual being. Your only consistent travel companion in this journey of life, work, and leadership is the self. As noted earlier, leadership at any level can be lonely at times, so one must find fulfillment in the company of the self. Furthermore, the person who is well acquainted with his or her whole self is able to build on personal strengths, acknowledge and improve on areas of personal weakness, and move beyond the self to lead, lift, and guide others to better service.

Finding the spiritual center is about finding meaning. Barsh et al. (2008, p. 35) reminded that meaning "provides energy and inspires passion. Without meaning, work is a slog between weekends. With meaning, any job can become a calling." A central finding of a landmark study of spirituality in the workplace by Mitroff and Denton (1999) was that people do not want to fragment or compartmentalize their lives to exclude meaning or spirituality from their work. Their second major finding was that few organizations provide successful models to integrate spirituality.

"Spirituality is a universal human phenomenon" (Allen & Marshall, 2010). Spiritual care of patients is a growing area of concern in health care. Indeed, the Joint Commission on Accreditation of Healthcare Organizations (2010) now requires health systems to address spiritual care. Attention to spirituality is associated with improved physical, psychological, and social health outcomes (Burkhart, Solari-Twadell, & Hass, 2008, p. 33). Spirituality "is the inclination to commune with a higher power beyond self, to find meaning within oneself, or to connect with something transcendent or metaphysical that is central to being spiritual. It is internal to the person . . . giving hope, promoting interconnectedness, and provid[ing] a sense of well-being" (Allen & Marshall, 2010, p. 233; Lubkin & Larsen, 2006). It implies a sense of transcendence, and it requires the time and space for personal reflection. It invites us to explore the deepest dimension of our uniqueness and potential for altruism as human beings (Wolf, 2004). It invites us to explore why we entered health care. It promotes a focus on values and a sense of community. It has been observed to help those within the organization to discover the human elements of the mission of the organization, break down silos that separate people, promote a balance of work and personal activities, uncover a perspective of health care from transactional to relational, and promote personal and leadership development (Wolf, 2004, p. 25). Spirituality may or may not be associated with religion and is not synonymous with religiosity (Burkhardt & Solari-Twadell, 2001). It is about sensitivity to the soul.

Moore (1992, 1994, p. 5) called the soul "that vast expanse, that universe of all of who we are." He explained, "Soul is not a thing, but a quality or a dimension of experiencing life and ourselves. It has to do with depth, value, relatedness, heart, and personal substance," rather than an object of religious belief. Get to know yourself, like yourself, and become interested in that person who is you. Moore (1992) reminded that "care of the soul begins with observance of how the soul manifests itself and how it operates," and that "we can't care for the soul unless we are familiar with its ways." Finding your spiritual center helps you to be honest, to embrace who you are, and to accept others. It empowers you to observe and reflect, to learn from, and to honor what you learn about yourself. It creates a confidence in authenticity and absolute honesty.

You can gain insight into the soul and who you are in a variety of ways. Take this short test to discover who you are. Ask yourself, "What do others believe about you that you don't think is true?" Is there some prickly inconsistency that you would like to smooth? Is your leadership persona a role you assume like a comfortable professional wardrobe, or one of which you tire and from which you seek relief? Ask yourself the next question, "What is your fatal flaw?" Is there something that others do not know about you that you dislike and want to change? Are you working on it? Is there someone who can help? Next question, "What is your benign flaw?" What is acceptable to others, but something you would like to change? Be cautioned not to look for errors and mistakes as points of self-condemnation, but instead value them, feel them, and bring them into your presence. Talk to yourself about them as if those faults, habits, or mistakes were errant charges that you can correct with gentleness. Mistakes and solutions, wounds and healing, regrets, and renewal of purpose are all part of the journey of finding the spiritual center as a leader.

On your way to fulfilling leadership, work to acquire your own repertoire of helpful habits to feed the spirit. The first helpful habit is to find an enduring faith—in God, a higher power, a positive energy, or a greater self; some form of faith that allows you to release custody of lingering problems at the end of the day to a greater metaphysical influence, allowing for rest and renewal so you can face them in the morning. The second habit of the spiritually centered leader is to love. Love here means to have meaningful, supportive relationships; to associate with nurturing people; and to avoid destructive, toxic people. Evidence is abundant on the value of social support in nearly every aspect of human life, including leading. Bolman and Deal (2001) reminded that every organization can be a bit like a family, either caring or dysfunctional (and perhaps some of both). To move toward a caring organization "begins with knowing—it requires listening, understanding, and accepting. It progresses through a deepening sense of appreciation, respect, and ultimately, love. Love is a willingness to reach out" (Bolman & Deal, 2001, p. 108).

Another aspect of leadership love is altruism. When one nurtures the sense of giving or charity without thought of reciprocation, somehow, the spirit of leadership is enlivened, and the leader assumes a position of strength, confidence, and humanity.

To sustain the spiritual self in leadership also requires a concerted attention to the physical self. Enormous energy is demanded of leaders in health care, which requires moderation in diet, activity, personal maintenance, and sleep. Positive health habits not only sustain the leader but also set a standard and model for colleagues and even patients. Similarly, leaders can do well by embracing beauty and aesthetics, humor, and congruency. Other specific spiritual practices include meditating, music, journeying to or designating sacred places, and prayer (Bolman & Deal, 2001; Porter-O'Grady & Malloch, 2007).

Because it seems so personal, inviting spirituality—however, it may be defined—into the leadership and work environment requires courage. Those who do it, however, note that it is worthwhile and conducive to creating an environment of respect, ethics, values, and integrity (Wolf, 2004). Leaders who promote spiritual exploration among workers and patients must be authentic. A spiritual focus cannot be feigned. You must inspire and model your best self. When you find your spiritual center, you will be amazed at your abilities to positively influence others. They will be drawn to you. You will enable your positional authority or power to become influence.

Becoming an effective, influential leader is an enriching journey. It begins with the first day you consider securing an official leadership position. It requires thoughtful preparation and self-assessment. It demands that leadership be viewed through the lens of making a difference and having influence. It includes constant self-assessment for growth and development of skills. It offers continuing challenges, and will prompt fears, failures, and associated courage. As you develop as a leader, care for yourself as you care for others. Look to networks and mentors for help. Mostly, find and nurture your best self. We have called that "best self" your spiritual center. Enjoy the journey—it is your time.

REFERENCES

Allen, D., & Marshall, E. S. (2010). Spirituality as a coping resource for African American parents of chronically ill children. *American Journal of Maternal-Child Nursing, 35*(4), 232–237.

Avoilo, B. J. & Bass, B. M. (2004). Multifactor Leadership Questionnaire: Manual and Sampler Set. Mind Garden, Inc. Redwood City, Ca.

Barsh, J., Cranston, S., & Craske, R. A. (2008). Centered leadership: How talented women thrive. *McKinsey Quarterly*, (4), 35–36.

Bolman, L. G., & Deal, T. E. (2001). *Leading with soul: An uncommon journey of spirit*. San Francisco, CA: Jossey-Bass.

Bono, J., & Anderson, M. (2005). The advice and influence networks of transformational leaders. *Journal of Applied Psychology, 90*(6), 1306–1314.

Broome, M. E. (2015). Leadership in science. *Nursing Science Quarterly, 28*(2), 164–166.

Broome, M. E., & Gilbert, J. (2014a). Developing and sustaining self. In J. Daly, S. Speedy, & D. Jackson (Eds.), *Leadership and nursing: Contemporary perspectives* (2nd ed., pp. 199–212). Sydney, Australia: Elsevier.

Broome, M., & Gilbert, J. (2014b). Developing and sustaining self. In J. Daly, S. Speedy, & D. Jackson (Eds.), *Leadership in nursing* (p. 203). Sidney, Australia: Elsevier.

Burkhardt, L., & Solari-Twadell, A. (2001). Spirituality and religiousness: Differentiating the diagnosis through review of the nursing literature. *International Journal of Nursing Terminologies & Classifications, 12*(2), 45–54.

Burkhart, L., Solari-Twadell, P. A., & Haas, S. (2008). Addressing spiritual leadership: An organizational model. *Journal of Nursing Administration, 38*(1), 33–39.

Cryer, B., McCraty, R., & Childre, D. (2003, July). Pull the plug on stress. *Harvard Business Review, 1–7.*

Gilbert, J. H., & Broome, M. E. (2015). Leadership in a complex world. In M. C. Sitterding & M. E. Broome (Eds.), *Information overload: Framework, tips, and tools to manage in complex healthcare environments.* Silver Spring, MD: American Nurses Association.

Gladwell, M. (2008). *Outliers: The story of success.* New York, NY: Little, Brown.

Gonzalez, T. A. (2016). *Transformational leadership.* Retrieved from http://changing minds.org/disciplines/leadership/styles/transformational_leadership.htm

Grenny, J., Patterson, K., Maxfield, D., McMillan, R., & Switzler, A. (2013). *Influencer: The new science of leading change.* New York, NY: McGraw-Hill.

Hughes, R., & Beatty, K. (2005). *Becoming a strategic leader.* Greensboro, NC: Center for Creative Leadership.

Joint Commission on Accreditation of Healthcare Organizations. (2010). *Joint Commission to allied health professionals.* Oakbrook, IL: Author.

Kibort, P. M. (2005, November/December). I drank the Kool-Aid—and learned 24 key management lessons. *Physician Executive, 31*(6), 52–55.

Kouzes, J. M., & Posner, B. Z. (2007). *The leadership challenge* (4th ed.). San Francisco, CA: Jossey-Bass.

Laschinger, H., Wong, C., & Grau, A. (2013). Authentic leadership, empowerment and burnout: A comparison in new graduates and experienced nurses. *Journal of Nursing Management, 21*(3), 541–543.

Lubkin, J. M., & Larsen, P. D. (2006). *Chronic illness: Impact interventions* (6th ed.). Sudbury, MA: Jones & Bartlett.

Marshall, E. S. (2011). *Transformational leadership in nursing: From expert clinician to influential leader.* New York, NY: Springer Publishing Company.

Martin, N. A., & Bloom, J. L. (2003). *Career aspirations and expeditions: Advancing your career in higher education administration.* Champaign, IL: Stipes.

McBride, A. (2011). *The growth and development of nurse leaders.* New York, NY: Springer Publishing Company.

Mitroff, I. I., & Denton, E. A. (1999). *A spiritual audit of corporate America: A hard look at spirituality, religion, and values in the workplace.* San Francisco, CA: Jossey-Bass.

Moore, T. (1992). *Care of the soul: A guide for cultivating depth and sacredness in everyday life.* New York, NY: HarperCollins.

Moore, T. (1994). *Soul mate: Honoring the mysteries of love and relationships.* New York, NY: HarperCollins.

National Health Service (2012). National Health Service Leadership Academy. Retrieved from www.leadershipacademy.nhs.uk.

Patterson, K., Grenny, J., McMillan, R., & Switzler, A. (2002). *Crucial conversations.* New York, NY: McGraw-Hill.

Pipe, T., Buchta, V., Launder, S., Hudak, B., Hulvey, L., Karns, K., & Pendergast, D. (2012). Building personal and professional resources of resilience and agility in the workplace. *Stress and Health, 28*(1), 11–22.

Porter-O'Grady, T., & Malloch, K. (2007). *Quantum leadership: A resource for health care innovation* (2nd ed.). Sudbury, MA: Jones & Bartlett.

Rath, T. (2007). Strengths Finder 2.0. New York, NY: The Gallup Press.

Stanley, T., Sitterding, M., Broome, M. E., & McCaskey, M. (2011). Engaging and developing research leaders in practice: Creating a foundation for a culture of clinical inquiry. *Journal of Pediatric Nursing, 26*(5), 480–488.

Switzler, A. (2016). Influencer: Change the way you change minds. *VitalSmarts*. Retrieved from https://www.vitalsmarts.com/press/2007/08/influencer-change-the-way-you-change-minds/

Sullivan, E. J. (2004). *Becoming influential: A guide for nurses.* Upper Saddle River, NJ: Prentice-Hall.

VitalSmarts: A twentyeighty company. (2016). Retrieved from https://www.vitalsmarts.com/

Wheatley, M. (2009, March). The place beyond fear and hope. *Shambhala Sun,* 79–83.

Wolf, E. J. (2004, March/April). Spiritual leadership: A new model. *Healthcare Executive,* 19(2), 23–25.

PART III

LEADING THE DESIGN OF NEW MODELS OF CARE

CHAPTER 8

Practice Model Design, Implementation, and Evaluation

Mary Cathryn Sitterding and Elaine Sorensen Marshall

We cannot solve our problems with the same thinking that created them.
—*Albert Einstein*

OBJECTIVES

- To describe factors influencing the need for care delivery redesign
- To discuss strategies and tactics influencing care model redesign and system change assessment
- To differentiate between evidence-based practice, practice-based evidence, and leader competencies necessary to implement evidence-based practice and practice-based evidence
- To describe patient and health care outcomes associated with practice model design
- To conduct self-evaluation of systems thinking competencies as they relate to practice model redesign and evaluation

MODELS OF CARE: EMBRACING THE SPIRIT OF INNOVATION

What exactly is driving the need for innovation in models of care delivery? Five key drivers have influenced and will continue to influence the need for innovation: (a) the patient's cross-continuum experience, (b) quality and safety, (c) workforce, (d) technology, and (e) cost.

Patients' Cross-Continuum Experience

The gap that exists between the manner in which health care decisions ought to be made and the way these decisions are actually made is remarkable. Nearly all patients expect to be in control of their medical and health decisions. Only 7% of adult, nonelderly patients want their physicians to be in control (Lynch, Perosino, & Stover, 2014). The idea of empowered patients and e-patients has emerged. Patient empowerment refers to patients who are "able to take charge of their health and their interactions with health care professionals," while e-patients are described as "those who are most technology savvy and engaged in digital health" (Moriates, Arora, & Shah, 2015, p. 239).

Some physicians and other health care providers perceive that information from the Internet leads to confusion and distress, and could result in potential harms through self-diagnosis or self-treatment (Ahmad, Hudak, Bercovitz, Hollenburg, & Levinson, 2006). Patients tend to be reluctant to approach their provider with information they have found on the Internet. But, it is clear that most Americans do search online for health information. This is the reality of our time.

The patient's active input into the experience of health care delivery has increased in significance exponentially. Measurement of what matters to patients is here to stay. Within the hospital setting, how well nurses and physicians communicate with patients, how well hospital staff member help patients to manage pain, and whether or not information is provided at discharge are publicly reported. These and other factors related to the patient experience, influence payer compensation. Efforts to provide patients and families with greater responsibility for health care spending through consumer-directed health plans have become progressively popular as a potential way to promote cost savings. Shared decision making may be a tool to empower patients to take a more active role in their care, and may help to improve the value and quality of care (Moriates et al., 2015). The Affordable Care Act (ACA) encourages the used of shared decision making in health care. The ACA authorized the creation of the Patient-Centered Outcomes Research Institute (PCORI), enabling funding of research-related to shared decision making involving patients as part of patient-centered research priorities (Caramenico, 2012).

Quality and Safety

More than 15 years ago, *To Err Is Human,* a seminal document published by the Institute of Medicine (IOM), startled health care providers, payers, and consumers with devastating facts associating preventable hospital deaths with health care delivery (IOM, 1999). Updates provided in a systematic review published by James (2013) suggested that the early estimates of the effects of patient error were low. For example, James (2013) proposed that the true number of premature deaths associated with preventable harm to patients was more than 400,000 per year. Further, serious harm seems to be 10- to 20-fold more common than lethal harm.

Significant accomplishments since the publication of the IOM's 1999 report include reductions in hospital-acquired conditions, adverse drug events, untoward surgical event rates, and device failures. Despite progress, patient safety and quality remain among the most important public health issues. Increased attention on patient safety has been exhibited by a national focus, research funding, and the creation of an entire new field of study with extensive published results. Additionally, the business case for safety, increased transparency, team training and teamwork, development of coalitions of hospitals and health care systems dedicated to patient safety, and health information technology have all been accomplished following publication of the IOM report.

A key change driving accomplishments in patient safety is senior leadership engagement (including the development of specialty positions such as medication and safety officers), public awareness, measurement and improved detection, and academic research. Results have demonstrated the effectiveness of interventions, including funding and practice bundles to reduce infection, creative staffing and education, adoption of national patient safety-related guidelines, evidence-based practices, development of the business cases, media involvement, legislation and regulations to create incentives, focus on system not individual, patient–family engagement, transparency, medication safety, and smart applications technology (National Patient Safety Foundation, 2015).

Despite increased focus on quality and patient safety since the IOM report in 1999, a multitude of harms has been revealed beyond mortality. For example, one in ten hospitalized patient experiences an adverse event, such as a health care-acquired infection, pressure ulcer, preventable adverse drug event, or a fall (U.S. Department of Health and Human Services Agency for Healthcare Research & Quality [USHHS AHRQ], 2014). One in two surgeries includes a medication error and/or an adverse drug event (Nanji, Patel, Shaikh, Seger, & Bates, 2015), and more than 700,000 outpatients are treated in the emergency department every year for adverse events caused by a medication (Budnitz et al., 2006). More than 12 million patients each year suffer a diagnostic error in outpatient care, half of which are estimated to potentially cause harm (Singh, Meyer, & Thomas, 2014). Approximately one-third of Medicare beneficiaries in skilled nursing facilities experience an adverse event, half of which are preventable (U.S. Office of Inspector General, 2014).

Barriers to change include inadequate definitions or concepts of patient safety and avoidable versus unavoidable harm, measurement challenges and a paucity of research evidence for prevention, potential need for increased governmental oversight, culture of nonreporting, need for individual accountability and transparency, lack of funding, fragmented care delivery system, isolation of professional specialties, lack of leadership at all levels, need for education for young professionals, poor physician staffing and repayment structures, and need for incentives. There is less focus on ambulatory populations despite larger numbers of patients, errors in outpatient settings, and delays in diagnosis in the ambulatory setting (National Patient Safety Foundation, 2015). The entire traditional culture of care is ripe for redesign to prevent error and promote quality.

Workforce

Workforce health, safety, and shortages significantly influence the need for innovation in care delivery redesign. Workforce safety is associated with patient safety. Inadequate workforce safety results in the likelihood that the team will make errors or fail to follow safe practices (LLI, 2013). Hospitals have been described as among the most hazardous job sites in the United States. The U.S. Occupational Safety and Health Administration (OSHA, 2013) reported the rate of hospital work-related incidents at seven injuries or illnesses per every 100 full-time employees, a rate described as twice that of private industries.

The health care workforce shortage is another important factor related to patient quality and safety. It is a global problem. The World Health Organization estimated a global shortage of well over four million physicians and nurses (Scheffler, Liu, Kinfu, & Dal Poz, 2008; WHO, 2006). Overall, a major increase and reliance upon community health workers and paraprofessionals in the developing world (Crisp & Chen, 2014), and creative use of auxiliary staff in the United States, have occurred.

Costs associated with nursing care are remarkable. Nursing labor costs make up 30.1% of all hospital expenditures annually (Welton, 2011). In the next 10 to 15 years, approximately one-third of the nursing professionals will reach retirement age. Although the actual supply of nurses has continued to grow, it has not kept pace with the significant increase in demand for nurses (American Association of Colleges of Nursing [AACN], 2016). Primary factors influencing demand include (a) increasing demands for baccalaureate-prepared nurses across settings, (b) slow growth in supply, and (c) aging of the workforce.

The impact of increasing demand and decreasing supply of registered nurses (RNs) and rapid aging of the nursing workforce means that by the year 2020 there will be 20% fewer nurses than needed in the U.S. health care system. This translates into an unprecedented shortage of more than 400,000 RNs (Buerhaus, Staiger & Auerbach, 2000; U.S. Department of Labor and Bureau of Labor Statistics, 2015). Recruitment, retention, and innovation in understanding and expediting nursing expertise will be a central challenge given the aging nursing workforce and related losses to retirement, increasing ratio of newly licensed novice RNs, and shortage of nurse educators (Bleich et al., 2009).

Technology

What are the benefits and barriers of technology to care delivery, and how might this information shape new models of care? The deployment of new technology is a driving force behind rising health care costs. Predictive models of health and societal care requirements for the next quarter-century suggest a staggering shift in complexity of care requirements influenced by advanced population age and multimorbidity. This will raise the cost of care. Cost-effectiveness analysis provides a means of measuring the value of new technology and considering value in relation to societal willingness to pay for new and expensive technology.

eHealth has many definitions, but usually refers to the processes of health care service delivery by the use of interactive technology (Oh, Rizo, Enkin, & Jadad, 2005). Ideally, eHealth would improve the flow of information and improve communication among health care providers, patients, and others.

The telehealth platform and a highly monitored home environment can serve as an adjunct to traditional health services, enabling people to receive care in their homes instead of in a hospital, and offering a healing environment at a lower cost, within the comforts of their home. Studies are showing a reduction in readmissions from this model, which gives patients and families the tools they need to participate in their own recovery and wellness, while giving care teams the oversight they need to care for their patients and connect in meaningful ways (DiSanzo, 2014).

Yet, health information technology (IT) usability and effectiveness is imperfect at best. Metzger, Welebob, Bates, Lipsitz, and Classen (2010) described in a simulation study, a computerized physician order entry system in which 62 hospitals failed to identify 52% of potentially fatal errors. Furthermore, Schiff and colleagues (2016) found that 79.5% of all erroneous orders were entered with 28% easily placed, and another 28.3% placed with only minor workarounds and no warnings. Health IT has also been shown to contribute to clinician burnout (Babbott et al., 2014). Health IT usability testing is not uniformly conducted (Ratwani, Fairbanks, Hettinger, & Benda, 2015), thus explaining clinician resistance, use of workarounds, and low satisfaction.

Cost

What if banking, home building, automobile manufacturing, shopping, or airline travel were like health care? What have we learned about the cost of health care in the United States? How will that knowledge inform new models of care? A report from the IOM (2013, p. 5) included the following creative reminder to promote rethinking of how health care is funded:

- If banking were like health care, automated teller machines (ATM) transactions would not take seconds but perhaps days or longer as a result of unavailable or misplaced records.
- If home building were like health care, carpenters, electricians, and plumbers each would work with different blueprints, with very little coordination.
- If automobile manufacturing were like health care, warrantees for cars that require manufacturers to pay for defects would not exist. As a result, few factories would seek to monitor and improve production line performance and product quality.
- If shopping were like health care, product prices would not be posted, and the price charged would vary widely within the same store, depending on the source of payment.
- If airline travel were like health care, each pilot would be free to design his or her own preflight safety check, or not to perform it at all.

Hospital costs total more than $850 billion per year, almost 33% of all U.S. health care spending, with charges averaging $4,300 a day for hospitals in the United States (Costs of Care, 2016). The United States spends at least twice as much per capita per year, approximately $8,500, as any other developed nation. The IOM (2013) report titled *Best Care at Lower Cost* addressed the phenomenal waste of our nearly $3 trillion annual health care expenditures. Some factors that contribute to such costs include medications heavily promoted despite limited evidence regarding efficacy, unnecessary procedures and surgeries, variation in the cost of instrumentation during surgery, and complications associated with surgery (Topol, 2015).

New care design is imperative given the issues of patient experience, quality and safety, workforce, technology, and cost. Incremental innovation is insufficient to achieve radical change. Disruptive innovation will be required. We must accelerate our efforts to meet the needs of those we serve and with whom we serve. An understanding of implications for professional practice models and the practice environment is important in order to advance such needed innovation.

Professional Practice Models

Professional practice models are described as "the driving force of nursing care; a schematic description of a theory, phenomenon, or system that depicts how nurses practice, collaborate, communicate, and develop professionally to provide the highest quality of care for those served by the organization (e.g., patients, families, communities). Professional practice models illustrate the alignment and integration of nursing practice with the mission, vision, and values that nursing has adopted" (American Nurses Credentialing Center [ANCC], 2014, p. 74).

Foundational elements of professional practice are nursing autonomy and control over practice as well as collaborative relationships. Hoffart and Woods (1996) defined a professional practice model as a system (structure, process, and values) that supports RN control over the delivery of nursing care and the environment in which care is delivered. They asserted that a professional practice model has five subsystems, which are as follows:

1. Values (nurse autonomy, nurse accountability, professional development, high-quality care)
2. Professional relationships (teamwork, collaboration, consultation)
3. A patient care delivery model (primary care and case management)
4. A management approach (decentralized decision making, expanding the scope of nurse manager responsibilities; structure changes to support professional practice)
5. Compensation, rewards (recognized professional achievement and contribution toward organizational goals)

The terms *professional practice model* and *care delivery model* are used interchangeably. However, care delivery models or systems, in contrast to professional practice models, have been described as "integrated within the professional practice model and promote continuous, consistent, efficient, and accountable delivery of nursing care. The care delivery system is adapted to meet evidence-based practice standards, national patient safety goals, affordable and value-based outcomes, and regulatory requirements" (ANCC, 2013, p. 41). In one concept analysis, Camicia et al. (2013) described attributes of a practice model. Common themes among practice models include change, empowerment, improving nursing practice, improving outcomes, strengthening practice, and colleagueship (Camicia et al., 2013).

Innovative Practice Models

Joynt, Kimball, and associates (Joynt & Kimball, 2008, pp. 3–5; Kimball, Joynt, Cherner, & O'Neil, 2007) performed a large-scale study of innovative care delivery models throughout the United States. Most of the criteria for inclusion provide a guide for evaluation of effective new models for nursing. They include innovation in provider roles and teams, interdisciplinary activities, sustainability and replicability, and demonstrate impact on patient or business outcomes. Among the 60 new care delivery models examined, the majority of which were not-for-profit acute care hospitals located in urban or suburban areas, Joynt and Kimball (2008) identified eight common elements:

1. Elevated roles for nurses, with nurses as care integrators
2. Migration to interdisciplinary care with a team approach
3. Bridges across a continuum of care
4. Movement toward recognition of the home as setting for care
5. Targeting high users of health care, such as the elderly
6. Sharpened focus on the patient
7. High use of technology in care delivery
8. Focus on results, such as outcomes, quality of care, and cost

The study represents a beginning of the important dialogue to invent, examine, and share care delivery models that work.

Some models feature the role of the RN to create safe passage for the patient in the health care system. For example, *Synergy* (Everett & Broome, 2001) is the patient-centered common data model at IU Health. It is represented at the core of professional practice, depicting the organization of nursing care and the mechanisms of high quality, efficiency, and effectiveness.

Synergy is a differentiated nursing practice care delivery model. The model matches the RN competencies and academic preparation with the patient's care requirements. It is based on the premise that synergy occurs and outcomes are optimized when a patient's needs and characteristics are matched with a nurse's (or many nurses') competencies.

Patient characteristics considered in the appropriation of care include resiliency, vulnerability, stability, complexity, resource availability, participation in care, participation in decision making, and predictability. Complementary nurse competencies include clinical judgement, advocacy, caring practices, collaboration, systems thinking, response to diversity, clinical inquiry, and facilitator of learning.

Safe passage at the point of care is created when RN characteristics are perfectly and strategically matched to meet the patient's care requirements. Many leaders believe this is accomplished through application of the *Synergy* (Everett & Broome, 2001) care delivery model incorporating Benner's novice to expert model for development (see Benner, 1984). Nursing work is conducted within a cognitively and relationally demanding environment where the average nurse is interrupted every 3 minutes and completes more than 50% of his or her tasks in less than 30 seconds (Cornell, Riordan, Townsend-Gervis, & Mobley, 2011; Sitterding, Broome, Everett, & Ebright, 2012; Sitterding, Ebright, Broome, Patterson, & Wuchner, 2014). The *Synergy* model promotes safe passage by enabling situation awareness through an explicit understanding of unit-based patient characteristics that signal the nurse when to notice and react to patient characteristics.

Transforming Care at the Bedside

Improvement and results orientation in care delivery model innovation are illustrated in numerous models, including the Institute for Healthcare Improvement (IHI) *Transforming Care at the Bedside* (TCAB) care delivery project. The IHI launched a large collaborative project funded by the Robert Wood Johnson Foundation (RWJF) to "transform care at the bedside" in hospitals. Several positive outcomes have been reported, and the project has provided a foundation for continued work toward "safe and reliable care, vitality and teamwork, patient-centered care, and value-added care processes" (IHI, 2010). TCAB promotes front-line participation in transformative change, the integration of the voices of patients and their family, and ongoing learning and improvement. Among participating TCAB organizations, specific outcomes have been positive and include:

- Average number of falls with moderate or greater injury per 1,000 patient days decreased by 52% from 2005 to 2007
- Average number of codes (cardiac arrest) per month decreased by 33% from 2005 to 2007
- Voluntary nurse turnover decreased to less than 5% from 2003 to 2007
- Patient satisfaction scores increased from 2005 to 2007
- Average 30-day readmission rate decreased by 29% from 2006 to 2007
- Proportion of time nurses spent in direct care increased from 47% in 2005 to 50% in 2007 (Hassmiller & Rutherford, 2016)

Coordination of Care. Coordination of care is a core element described in models of care delivery. In a study commissioned by the IOM, more than nine million Medicaid and dual Medicare/Medicaid patient claims records of five states were analyzed to determine patterns and costs associated with uncoordinated care. Approximately 10% of patients demonstrated extreme patterns of uncoordinated care and accounted for 30% of program costs. Uncoordinated care patients accounted for 46% of drug costs, 32% of medical costs, and 36% of total costs for this population. On average, patient costs for those experiencing uncoordinated care were 75% higher than matched patients whose care was coordinated. Owens (2010) suggested that enhanced care coordination could reduce costs by 35%. The projected annual savings associated with enhanced care coordination is estimated at $135.5 billion for national and public plans and $240.1 billion for combined public and private payment plans (American Nurses Association [ANA], 2012).

Care coordination has been defined by the IHI, the National Quality Forum (NQF), and the AHRQ. Writing for the IHI (2010), Craig, Eby, and Whittington (2011) defined: "the best coordination model is one in which a patient experiences primary care as delivered by an integrated, multidisciplinary team that includes at least one care coordinator staff person." The NQF defined care coordination as "a function that helps ensure people, functions, and sites are met over time" (NQF, 2006). The AHRQ defined care coordination as "the deliberate organization of patient care activities between two or more participants (including the patient) involved in a patient's care to facilitate the appropriate delivery of health care services" (McDonald et al. 2010). Care coordination models of delivery include the following: (a) acute care coordination models, (b) care coordination as described involving transition, (c) community-based care coordination, (d) care coordination for children with special health needs, (e) care coordination of mental health care, and (f) primary care medical home models of care coordination (ANA, 2012).

Transition in Care Cross-continuum transition in care (TCM) models of care delivery recognized and described by the American Academy of Nursing (AAN) Edge Runner program focus on transitional care led by master's-prepared advanced practice nurses (APNs) in conjunction with the patient's entire health care team, targeting high-risk patients at risk for poor postdischarge outcomes in order to improve them. The model is described as an evidence-based innovative model of hospital-to-home care in which APNs work to ensure a smooth transition from hospital care to home care. The program assures that APNs (a) establish a relationship with patients and their families soon after hospital admission; (b) design the discharge plan in collaboration with the patient, the patient's physician, other involved providers, and their family caregivers; and (c) implement the plan in the patient's home following discharge, substituting for traditional skilled nursing follow-up. Outcomes associated with the TCM model of care include the following:

• Since 1991, when compared with standard care, the TCM has demonstrated longer intervals before initial rehospitalizations, fewer rehospitalizations overall, shorter hospital stays, and better patient satisfaction.

- In a 4-year trial (1997–2001) involving a group of elderly patients hospitalized with heart failure, the APN care model cut hospitalization costs by more than $500,000, compared with a group receiving standard care—for an average savings of approximately $5,000 per Medicare patient.
- One project demonstrated efficacy in translating the evidence-based innovation into practice, in partnership with a major insurer (Aetna) targeting Medicare Advantage consumers (2005–2007). The program was offered as an ongoing benefit for high-risk members in transition from acute care to home in a select market (AAN, 2012; RWJF, 2009).
- An ongoing clinical trial (2005 to present) in hospitalized, cognitively impaired older adults and their family caregivers has revealed similar savings in health resource utilization, with health, quality of life, and cost analyses ongoing.

Notably, the TCM is recognized as an exemplary model for care delivery coordination (Naylor, Aiken, Kurtzman, & Olds, 2010). The TCM model has demonstrated improved quality and cost outcomes for high-risk, cognitively intact and impaired older adults when compared with standard care in the following outcomes: reductions in preventable hospital readmissions for both primary and coexisting health conditions; improvements in health outcomes; enhanced patient experience with care; and a reduction in total health care costs (AAN, 2014).

Coordination of care means the primary care provider takes responsibility for management of patients' health needs across the care continuum. In an international survey of patients with complex care needs, patients in the United States who had a primary care provider reported some of the best care coordination experiences. However, in the United States, those patients with complex care needs, who could benefit most from care coordination, were least likely to report having a regular primary care provider (Schoen et al., 2011).

Models for the Future. Arguably, the time has come for new more effective models. New models must include recognition of a set of interdisciplinary values and relationships among representatives of all disciplines. They need to include

REFLECTION QUESTIONS

1. How would you describe the models you have experienced as a nursing professional, as a family member, or as a patient; that is, professional practice models, shared decision-making models, care delivery models, improvement-focused models?
2. What value-based empirical outcomes have you noticed in the models you have experienced? Value to whom?
3. How would you assess the professional practice model and care delivery model within your service setting?
4. How would you incorporate the voices of key stakeholders in your assessment and care model redesign?

patients and consumers as integral members of planning teams. New models will consider care coordination across all settings, including community-based and home environments. Models will recognize use of evidence and technology and focus beyond productivity and effectiveness toward excellence.

Transformational leadership will be required to positively influence professional practice models. Excellence in practice model redesign, implementation, and evaluation will depend on you and the next generation of transformational leaders.

CARE MODEL DESIGN AND SYSTEM CHANGE

There is, perhaps, not a single person in the United States who will argue that our health care system does not need change or redesign at some level. The U.S. health care system is ranked among the highest in cost and lowest in outcomes on almost any scale among those of developed countries. Our health care system has been the brunt of criticism from popular media to the federal government itself (Hacker, 2007; Oberlander, 2007). Myriad factions, each with its own self-interest, and the mere weight of the complexity of all aspects of the system, seem to overwhelm hopes of immediate or fundamental change.

Assessing the Environment

How might you assess the environment for professional practice, including care delivery? Nearly as important as environment for patient care is the concept of the work environment for the clinician. For the past 30 years, leaders in nursing have been investigating work environments that support nursing practice, recruitment, and retention, and are beginning to identify how such factors are important to patient outcomes (Aiken, Sochalski, & Lake, 1997; Ives Erickson et al., 2004; Kramer & Hafner, 1989; Lake, 2002; McClure, Poulin, Sovie, & Wandelt, 2002). From some of this work has emerged the concept of Magnet® hospitals, which have been officially recognized to provide positive environments for professional nursing practice. Work environments that support professional nursing practice include the following:

- Magnet hospital recognition
- Preceptorships and residencies
- Differentiated nursing practice
- Interdisciplinary collaboration

The American Association of Colleges of Nursing (AACN) (2002) has outlined the specific hallmarks of the environment that supports professional nursing practice:

- **Manifest a philosophy of clinical care emphasizing quality, safety, interdisciplinary collaboration, continuity of care, and professional accountability.**

For example, nursing staff have meaningful input into policy development and operational management of issues related to clinical quality, safety, and clinical outcomes evaluation; and nurse staffing patterns have an adequate number of qualified nurses to meet patients' needs, including consideration of the complexity of patient care.

- **Recognize contributions of nurses' knowledge and expertise to clinical care quality and patient outcomes.** For example, the organization differentiates the practice roles of nurses based on educational preparation, certification, and advanced preparation; and the organization has a compensation and reward system that recognizes role distinctions among staff nurses and other expert nurses (e.g., based on clinical expertise, reflective of nursing practice, education, or advanced credentialing).

- **Promote executive-level nursing leadership.** For example, the nurse executive participates as a member of the governing board and has the authority and accountability for all nursing or patient care delivery, financial resources, and personnel.

- **Empower nurses' participation in clinical decision making and organization of clinical care systems.** For example, there is a decentralized, unit-based program or team organizational structure for decision making, and a demonstrated leadership role for nurses in performance improvement of clinical care and the organization of clinical care systems.

- **Maintain clinical advancement programs based on education, certification, and advanced preparation.** For example, financial rewards are available for clinical advancement and education; and peer review, patient, collegial, and managerial input is available for performance evaluation on annual or routine basis.

- **Demonstrate professional development support for nurses.** For example, professional continuing education opportunities are available and supported; specialty certification and advanced credentials are encouraged, promoted, and recognized; and APNs, nurse researchers, and nurse educators are employed and utilized in leadership roles to support clinical nursing practice.

- **Create collaborative relationships among members of the health care provider team.** For example,
  - Professional nurses, physicians, and other health care professionals practice collaboratively and participate in standing organizational committees, bioethics committees, the governing structure, and the institutional review processes;
  - Professional nurses have appropriate oversight and supervisory authority of unlicensed members of the nursing care team; and
  - An interdisciplinary team peer review process is used, especially in the review of patient care errors.

- **Utilize technological advances in clinical care and information systems.** For example, documentation is supported through appropriate application of technology to the patient care process; and appropriate equipment, supplies, and technology are available to optimize the efficient delivery of quality nursing care.

Assessing the Organization

One classic and popular perspective for assessing an organization is through Peter Senge's (1990) lens of "the learning organization." Senge asserted that because people are designed for learning, so must be the organizations in which they work. He suggested that the first level of organizational learning is adaptive learning, which is about coping. However, a higher level of learning is generative learning, which is about expanding capacities and capabilities. Generative learning requires a broader perspective, in which leaders are not the authoritative "charismatic decision makers" but rather "designers, teachers, and stewards" (p. 9). Senge outlined a principle of creative tension whereby members of the organization are able to see the idealistic vision of where and what they want to be, while at the same time recognizing the "current reality" and telling the truth about where they are. Senge explained that leading in an environment of creative tension is different than traditional problem solving. Rather than trying to escape, avoid, or reduce some aspect of the current reality by solving a problem, the leader in a learning organization uses the creative tension to create positive changes in the current realities according to the direction of the organizational vision. In other words, it is a difference in perspective that moves the leader and the organization from repairing what is wrong to inventing what works.

Still another perspective is offered by Bulger (2003), who called for a vision of "healer-clinicians" in "the therapeutic institution." He developed an assessment tool called the Organization Therapeutic Index for health care institutions that measures the following constructs:

- Scientific and technical competence
- Understanding suffering and pain, death, and dying
- Appreciating the placebo effect
- Expanding health care roles and responsibilities
- Communicating dignity and respect
- Demonstrating organizational loyalty to patients
- Making the patient part of the health care team
- Emphasizing teamwork and collaboration
- Taking the environment into account
- Affirming cultural sensitivity and workforce diversity
- Working with the community

Unfortunately, the assumptions of the measure are based almost exclusively on the discipline of medicine in large hospital systems.

Lukas et al. (2007, p. 309) evaluated 12 U.S. health care systems to identify essential elements necessary for enduring transformation of patient care. They found the following five critical factors: (a) impetus to transform, (b) leadership commitment to quality, (c) improvement initiatives that actively engage staff in meaningful problem solving, (d) alignment to achieve consistency of organization goals with resource allocation and actions at all levels of the organization, and (e) integration to bridge traditional intraorganizational boundaries among individual components.

Innovation may happen within or external to the system. Four key elements can drive change within the system by affecting its components:

1. Mission, vision, and strategies that set its direction and priorities
2. Culture that reflects its informal values and norms
3. Operational functions and processes that embody the work done in patient care
4. Infrastructure such as IT and human resources that support the delivery of patient care (Lukas et al., 2007)

Transformational change within the system is iterative and happens over time across the organization. Christensen (1997) referred to evolutionary changes as "sustaining innovations." Sustaining innovations are usually introduced by current industry leaders who continue to develop and focus on improved processes consistent with their established values. They develop improved products and services within the context of their history and tradition. More challenging is radical and revolutionary change called "disruptive innovations." Examples of these include the telephone disrupting the telegraph, semiconductors disrupting vacuum tubes, cellular phones disrupting fixed telephone lines, and perhaps retail medical clinics disrupting the traditional physician's office. Health care systems are poised to be ambushed by disruptive innovation. As leaders in health care, we need to brace ourselves for disruptive innovations that will threaten the way we have been doing business.

Some hope is on the horizon for organizations that are prepared. First, they must create new organizational structures or capabilities within their own boundaries to develop new processes. Second, they could spin out independent organizations to develop new processes and values to solve new problems. Or, finally, they might acquire or collaborate with a different organization whose processes and values match the need of the new task (Christensen & Overdorf, 2000). These suggestions further underscore the urgency for interdisciplinary and cross-discipline collaboration in health care. We need to collaborate, not only nurses with physicians, but also nurses with engineers, nurses with humanists, and physicians with who-knows-who-else.

A writer for the *New York Times* (Rae-Dupree, 2009) reminded that two key factors in current health care systems, the general hospital and the physician's practice, are largely based on business models over 100 years old. These systems are built on a foundation of fee-for-service based on treating illness. Some integrated systems are preparing to deal with disruptive innovations that will fundamentally change health care practice.

Redesign Assessment and Managing Change

Practice model redesign begins with an assessment of the professional practice model, care delivery model, and health care environment. Collaborative assessment including all key stakeholders is imperative as involvement in the assessment of need will dramatically influence adoption of the next generation practice model. Redesign should include all key stakeholders—those influenced by and operating within the redesigned model, including disciplines outside of nursing, consumers (patients and families), and payers. Box 8.1 challenges you to begin this redesign process. Consider the ANCC Magnet® Recognition Model (2014) as a framework to evaluate sources of transformational leadership, structural empowerment, exemplary professional practice, and new knowledge evidence. Consider the concepts from the TCAB or TCM models described earlier in this section. Consider the framework offered by the AACN (2002). Consider

BOX 8.1. LEARNING ACTIVITY: PRACTICE MODEL REDESIGN

Scenario: It's 2025. One-third of the nursing workforce has reached retirement age. New graduates have doubled over the past few years; however, the days are long gone when a new graduate selected one role within one setting and remained in that role and that setting for more than 3 years. Transformational nurse leaders are in high demand and are expected to positively influence acquisition or sustainability of Magnet designation, with particular prioritization monitoring the workforce and mitigating knowledge loss given the typical 3-year turnover rates experienced in U.S. hospitals. The volume and complexity of health care needs and expectations among baby boomers have crippled many organizations practicing traditional eminence-based medicine. A Magnet system of hospitals in the Midwest is recruiting transformational leaders. You are one of their top three candidates. Your final interview is with the system chief nurse executive (CNE), chief executive officer (CEO), chief financial officer (CFO), and patient–family advisory representative (PFAR). They present you with the following challenge:

> We are interested in disrupting our existing care delivery model. We would like to redesign and pilot within our geriatric service area and, in particular, those older than the age of 65 diagnosed with chronic illness. No, we do not have a geriatric unit. Your assignment is to span the boundary between units and sites of care delivery, ensuring care delivery for persons older than the age of 65 who have evidence of at least one admission in the past year with congestive heart failure, chronic obstructive pulmonary disease, or diabetes. Your assignment also includes the interdisciplinary workforce providing care for this population. We are proud to have achieved a number of awards but believe that we owe it to the community we serve to do better in coordinating their care delivery. You can be as creative as necessary regarding human and material resources given you maximize the role of the RN and all assignments are within licensed scope of practice. A few simple rules are as follows:
>
> * You must remain budget neutral.
> * Your plan must be patient-centric and reflect the ideas of those closest to the point of care delivery.
> * Target empirical outcomes must reflect the triple aim of quality and safety, cost-effectiveness, and the patient–family experience.

Take the challenge. Embrace the opportunity to redesign and transform. It's your turn to design.

TABLE 8.1 Practice Model Evaluation Parameters

PRACTICE MODEL EVALUATION PARAMETER (Each Evaluated from 1 To 10 According to Evidence Provided)
American Nurses Credentialing Center (ANCC) or hospital recognition
Preceptorships and residencies
Differentiated nursing practice
Interdisciplinary collaboration
Clinical care emphasizing quality, safety, interdisciplinary collaboration, continuity of care, and professional accountability philosophy
Contributions of nurses' knowledge and expertise recognized
Executive-level nursing leadership promoted
Shared leadership at the point of care and organizational level
Clinical advancement programs based on education, certification, and advanced preparations
Professional development support for nurses
Collaborative relationships among members of the health care provider team
Utilization of and technological advances in clinical care and information systems

collaborative development of an assessment tool referencing key concepts previously discussed in this chapter and illustrated in Table 8.1.

EVIDENCE-INFORMED PRACTICE

No organizational or systemwide change can be effective or enduring without the wise and appropriate use of evidence. By now, evidence-based practice should be a way of life. Its value has been well demonstrated in all aspects of health care and proven to be so critical to patient care outcomes that the leader who is not inspirational in its universal application is irresponsible. It is fundamental to clinical practice, and it is an essential role for leaders to assure its universal implementation. The basic tenets of effective use of evidence must be part of the daily discourse of the transformational leader. The leader can facilitate the examination and use of evidence from all disciplines. No single profession, practice, or area of study owns all helpful information for health care.

Advancing Evidence-Based Practice

Unfortunately, despite universal recognition of the importance of evidence-based practice, it continues to require the vigilance of a bold leader to implement and ensure its practice throughout the entire organization. Marchionni and Ritchie (2008) outlined specific organizational factors needed to support the implementation of evidence-based practice, including a culture of learning and transformational leadership. Practice leaders and managers can support specific evidence-based projects and decision making, facilitate measurement of quality and safety, use outcome measures to evaluate quality, and support exemplars at the point-of-service level of care (Newhouse & Johnson, 2009). Smooth and pervasive use of evidence in practice requires some degree of change or transformation of the entire system, culture, leadership characteristics, evaluation methods, and professional environment (Cummings, Estabrooks, Midodzi, Wallin, & Hayduk, 2007; Newhouse, 2007, 2009).

Leaders in clinical practice can inspire and promote the use of evidence in practice by linking with academic settings that foster collaboration with students and faculty. APNs can model the use of evidence in daily patient care. Each setting has its unique characteristics that must be considered in the application of evidence. Implications of context and culture are especially important, since evidence-based practice is not a solitary act of practice but an initiative that requires an entire community of committed clinicians. For example, conditions in rural and community hospitals may require unique and inventive infrastructures to support evidence-based practice (Burns, Dudjak, & Greenhouse, 2009; Sossong et al., 2009; Vratny & Shriver, 2007).

Recruit everyone at all levels into the role of implementing evidence-based practice in a context of shared accountability and shared governance (Melnyk, 2007; Melnyk & Fineout-Overholt, 2014; Newhouse, 2009; Waddell, 2009). Pervasive use of evidence in practice certainly requires the support of leadership, but it must also be claimed, integrated, and practiced with a sense of autonomy and creativity at the point of care (Schulman, 2008; Strout, Lancaster, & Schultz, 2009) and throughout the system.

Although significant descriptive work has been done to highlight the strategic role of leaders and managers, and the literature offers abundant case examples (Cullen, Greiner, Greiner, Bombei, & Comried, 2005; MacRobert, 2008; Marchionni & Ritchie, 2008), there is little empirical hypothesis testing or theory testing regarding the best practice for leadership oversight or strategies to implement and sustain evidence-based practice (Gifford, Davies, Edwards, Griffin, & Lybanon, 2007). Factors influencing adoption of evidence at the point of care delivery include, characteristics of the evidence (newly developed or revised guideline or protocol), availability of practice, prompts that trigger the adoption of evidence, the perceived advantage of adopting the evidence from the perspective of the end user, and mindful communication with all key stakeholders. including opinion leaders, change champions, core groups of influence, and academic detailing (Pittman & Sitterding, 2012).

The advent of the doctor of nursing practice (DNP) degree launches the opportunity for the clinician prepared at the highest level to guide other health care providers in practice inquiry. DNPs are prepared to lead systematic inquiry regarding the realities and complexities of practice, the challenges of translating discovery research into practice, and effective integration of evidence into individual, community, and population-based health care. The DNP focuses on providing leadership for evidence-based practice. This requires competence in translating research, evaluating evidence, applying research in decision making, and implementing viable clinical innovations to change practice. Considerable emphasis is placed on a patient population perspective, including how to obtain assessment data on populations or cohorts and how to use data to make decisions about and evaluate programs (AACN, 2015).

Practice-Based Evidence

A growing methodological turn on the concept of evidence-based practice is practice-based evidence. Horn and Gassaway (2007, p. S50) described practice-based evidence as a "rigorous, comprehensive" research methodology "that fills gaps in information needed by clinical and health policy decision makers." Horn and colleagues (Tunis, Stryer, & Clancy, 2003; Westfall, Mold, & Fagnan, 2007) have led the charge to point out weaknesses in traditional methods of evidence-based practice to answer all clinical, leadership, and policy questions. Rather than performing randomized controlled trials, practice-based evidence proposes the use of practical clinical trials. Characteristics include comparing clinically based, existing alternative interventions actually in practice rather than introducing new interventions; large and diverse study populations rather than selected criterion-based samples; recruitment of samples from heterogeneous practice settings rather than from matched, controlled settings; and data collection from a broad and vast range of outcomes rather than selected, isolated variables. In other words, methods of practice-based evidence study what is actually practiced in a large number of situations, by collecting huge data sets of detailed information on as many variables as possible to compare the effectiveness of interventions and identify what actually works in practice. Furthermore, variables of study are drawn from the perspective of an inclusive multidisciplinary team of researchers, practitioners, and others who have direct experience with the issues to be studied, and the method depends on local knowledge. Rather than *efficacy* measured by evidence-based approaches, practice-based methods measure *effectiveness*. What might be considered as confounding and irrelevant variables in a randomized controlled study would be considered relevant, included, and controlled statistically in the practice-based method. The method resembles a kind of epidemiological method largely within institutional acute care environments. From this method have been developed several measures of severity indices used in clinical practice (Horn et al., 2002). The practice-based evidence approach has demonstrated effectiveness in identifying best practices on a range of clinical situations, including pediatric bronchiolitis (Willson, Landrigan, Horn, & Smout, 2003), stroke rehabilitation (Conroy, DeJong, & Horn, 2009), and pressure ulcer treatment (Bergstrom et al., 2005).

Practice-based evidence is informed by what is referred to as *big data*, a huge collection of data that is unmanageable by traditional evidence-based means. One of the first published incidents of using big data to influence decision making by physicians was in 2011 at Lucile Packard Pediatric Hospital, Stanford, where Dr. Frankovich searched through her medical records of pediatric lupus patients to determine whether or not to prescribe anticoagulant medication. Because there were no published guidelines and scant literature on the subject, she resorted to analyzing the patterns revealed in her collection of medical charts. Practice-based or big data research in nursing enables the discipline to use large data sets to examine important health care quality questions, looking for hidden patterns in the data informing hypothesis generation versus hypothesis testing. Brennan and Bakken (2015) assert that nursing needs big data and big data needs nursing.

Practice-based evidence reveals patterns shared by thousands and can inform hypotheses that in turn can be answered through the analytical evaluation of multiple data streams (big data). The term *big data* refers not only to the volume of data, but also to other characteristics, such as variety, velocity, veracity, and value.

Data science is defined as systematic study of the organization and use of digital data in order to accelerate discovery, improve critical decision-making processes, and enable a data-driven economy (Ahalt et al. 2014). Practice-based steps or the process and structure for data science inquiry are as follows: (a) obtain, (b) scrub, (c) explore, (d) model, and (e) interpret (see Table 8.2). Together, these steps form the acronym OSEMN, pronounced as *awesome* (Mason & Wiggins, 2010).

The roles of nurses at various levels in data science are proposed as follows: (a) baccalaureate-prepared nurses expected to implement data policies, contribute to knowledge development from the bedside, and contribute to devising pathways of informed practice; (b) master's-prepared and doctorally prepared APNs expected to oversee and implement data policies, initiate knowledge development from the bedside, and devise pathways of informed practice; (c) data-intensive PhD-prepared nurses expected to conduct inquiry into basic nursing phenomena supported by data science methods; and (d) doctorally prepared nurse data scientists expected to generate new methods informed by the discipline's phenomena of concern and knowledge-building traditions (Brennan & Bakken, 2015).

The characteristic of variety refers to the type of data such as images or data that comes in a continuous flow (e.g., electronic medical records). Veracity of the data is determined by whether the data are able to be validated, traced or unanticipated conditions. Velocity of the data refers to the speed at which data are generated and received, while value is the potential of the data for contributing to important scientific discoveries (Brennan & Bakken, 2015).

Practice-based evidence shows promise in public health and certainly is helpful to policy leaders, yet, the practice-based evidence method needs to be further developed in those areas. All nurses are responsible for providing evidence-based practice. Not every nurse will be or should be a data nurse scientist, but all nursing practice should be informed by evidence and

TABLE 8.2 Practice-Based Evidence: OSEMN Model Steps

DATA SCIENCE STEP	STEP DESCRIPTION
Obtain: pointing and clicking does not scale	Without any data, there is little data science you can do. So, the first step is to obtain data. Unless you are fortunate enough to already possess data, you may need to do one or more of the following: • Download data from another location (e.g., a web page or server) • Query data from a database or application program interface (API; e.g., MySQL or Twitter) • Extract data from another file (e.g., an HTML file or spreadsheet) • Generate data yourself (e.g., reading sensors or taking surveys)
Scrub: the world is a messy place	It is not uncommon that the obtained data has missing values, inconsistencies, errors, weird characters, or uninteresting columns. In that case, you have to *scrub*, or clean, the data before you can do anything interesting with it. Common scrubbing operations include: • Filtering lines • Extracting certain columns • Replacing values • Extracting words • Handling missing values • Converting data from one format to another
Explore: you can see a lot by looking	Once you have scrubbed your data, you are ready to explore it. This is where it gets interesting, because here you will get really into your data. We show you how the command line can be used to • Look at your data • Derive statistics from your data • Create interesting visualizations
Models: always bad, sometimes ugly	If you want to explain the data or predict what will happen, you probably want to create a statistical model of your data. Techniques to create a model include clustering, classification, regression, and dimensionality reduction.
Interpret: the purpose of computing is insight, not numbers.	The final and perhaps most important step in the OSEMN model is interpreting data. This step involves: • Drawing conclusions from your data • Evaluating what your results mean • Communicating your result

OSEMN, obtain, scrub, explore, model, and interpret.

Source: Mason and Wiggins (2010).

data science. The role of the nurse leader will be to facilitate all nurses learning their role in the use of data and evidence in driving excellence in care delivery.

Evidence-based practice and practice-based evidence recommendations in and of themselves are insufficient to translate evidence to the point of care delivery. Process improvement models are necessary to translate the evidence or new knowledge. Steps in process improvement include the following: (a) interdisciplinary team formation (representing expertise on the topic, those expected to implement the evidence, and the voice of those influenced by the evidence—patients and families); (b) development of a key driver diagram (identification of factors influencing adoption of the evidence); (c) development and implementation of interventions matching the key driver diagram; and (d) measurement representing the rate and effectiveness of adoption.

Using Evidence for Leadership

Just as research indicates the need to integrate evidence-based practice throughout health care practice, conventional wisdom suggests that evidence can drive leadership. But that is not always the case. Likely in no other area of clinical practice are individual characteristics, preferences, and situations more complex and unique than in the context of leadership. Nevertheless, evidence informs leadership.

Indeed, a growing number of health care leaders prefer the term evidence-*informed*, rather than evidence-*based*, practice in leadership and policy (Best et al., 2009; Bowen & Zwi, 2005; Chalkidou, Walley, Culyer, Littlejohns, & Hoy, 2008; Fretheim, Oxman, Lavis, & Lewin, 2009; Lavis, Oxman, Moynihan, & Paulsen, 2008; Lavis, Paulsen, Oxman, & Moynihan, 2008a, 2008b; Rycroft-Malone, 2008). Certainly, appropriate evidence and use of data are critical to most aspects of leadership practice (Brandt et al., 2009), but caution is warranted in wholesale development or use of formal or standardized protocols for leadership.

First, empirical evidence based on controlled trials is simply not available or sufficient to mandate a particular formula for a specific leader's decision making in a particular situation or setting. Second, leadership is objective and artful, intellectual and emotional, evidence-based and creative risk taking. There are helpful guidelines, studies, experts, cases, competencies, and anecdotes, but effective leadership will not follow neatly from a database of clinical trials and outcomes (Arndt & Bigelow, 2009). Leadership is empirical and metaphysical, positivistic and interpretive. It happens always in the natural setting rather than a controlled environment. Data are important to successful leadership, but leading is often about meaning more than measurement. People function in a place of context, meaning, and stories. Thus, the wise leader balances use of data from evidence, appropriate technologies, and educated talents of instinct.

Technology: Informatics, Electronics, and Other Tools

Modern use of evidence always includes some aspect of technology. Sometimes, the very word *technology* feels like either some wolf in the wilderness waiting to ambush our comfort in the status quo or the next great gadget to make life easier. Indeed, in too many cases, technologies continue to be "underused, misused, or overused" (Fitzpatrick et al., 2010, p. 16). The truth is that technology has always been part of the work of leadership in health care. Although we all seem to have an image of what technology means, there is not a clear definition. It generally refers to the application of science and scientific invention to practice. It includes the tools and machines used to monitor, care for, and treat patients; clinical information systems; communication systems; databases for patient classification; education systems; clinical evidence; and even personnel management.

Informatics and Health Care. Informatics is the science and application of gathering, using, manipulating, storing, retrieving, and classifying information. Broadly, it may include artificial intelligence, computer science, information science, cognitive science, social sciences, and health care sciences. It focuses on how data are structured and organized to support knowledge building and decision making. The goal of informatics is to store and integrate data in order to provide accurate, accessible, and useful information. Just as it is hard to imagine professional leadership and practice without using informatics, it is nearly impossible to imagine future possibilities for applications of informatics to support leadership and health care.

Informatics and technology for consumers already provide information access, distance support groups, communication resources, and direct care by telehealth. New areas of expertise continue to emerge among health care providers. One can only imagine what the future may hold for consumer health care using informatics. On the horizon are personal access to medical records and databases, customized diagnosis, and personal prescriptions and treatments. Informatics is critical to define, represent, and apply nursing and health care knowledge across care settings, as well as to provide large data sets to promote the discovery of new knowledge. Kossman and Brennan (2008, p. 417) described the significance of health information technology (IT) for nursing leaders:

> Effective [health information technology] systems support nurse leaders by collecting and analyzing data pertinent to nursing practice, quality, and outcomes. This fosters benchmarking and best practices identification. Financial and administrative databases offer useful information but are not sufficient for nursing decisions. [For example], the Nursing Minimal Data Set and Nursing Management Minimal Data Set identify essential data necessary to characterize nursing practice.

Such data sets collect, identify, and provide information related to demographics, service, and health care data; environment and financial elements;

and other provider-sensitive data to improve patient outcomes. Access and management of information have broken down barriers across countries, across distance, across disciplines, and across roles. But as a leader, never forget that it is human beings who create knowledge, and *knowledge* is very different from *information*, and *wisdom* is a step beyond knowledge.

Although technology and informatics are pervasive throughout health care, the industry continues to fall well behind others in the effective, cross-disciplinary, or global use of available technologies. Porter-O'Grady and Malloch (2008, p. 181) further chided:

> It is a travesty of both time value and duplication that each health care institution establishes its own policies, practices, protocols, and procedures without access either to each other or to regional and national databases where a repository of this information is available to all. There is simply no hope of establishing regional or national standards of excellence in practice and clinical care if no one accesses the virtual community where these processes can be located.

Historically, neither health care providers nor business or leadership experts have been prepared with competencies in informatics. That will change for the next generation of advanced clinicians, especially among nurses with a DNP degree (Trangenstein, Weiner, Gordon, & McArthur, 2009). Westra and White-Delaney (2008) have begun the work to identify the unique knowledge and skills required for the health care leader. The list should certainly include some degree of computer skills, informatics knowledge, and some informatics skills. At this point, leaders must recognize the significance of informatics to health care, identify specific needs and opportunities for their applications, and develop new expertise and collaborate with experts specifically qualified to support desired outcomes.

Electronic Health Records. One important aspect of the use of informatics in health care that has lagged far behind is the still-emerging electronic health record (EHR). It is ironic and unfortunate that health care is among the last industries to effectively use electronic technology for client records.

Computerized medical records were available over 40 years ago (Ausman, 1967; Schenthal, Sweeney, & Nettleton, 1961; Thompson, Classen, & Haug, 2006). Analysis of early studies revealed that use of the EHR saved 24% of documentation time of nurses in hospitals, but did not reduce documentation time especially for physicians (Poissant, Pereira, Tamblyn, & Kawasumi, 2005), apparently hampering its adoption. Other studies have demonstrated as much as 90% reduction in medication errors associated with transcription, and 30% to 50% reduction in errors associated with prescribing. Other evidence indicates that such record systems increase use of preventive care, reduce use of laboratory tests, track drug utilization, improve detection of infections, reduce patient length of stay in hospitals, and even reduce mortality risks (Thompson et al., 2006). Of course, the EHR will not eliminate errors altogether. Already, we have identified errors of data entry and data retrieval (Ash, Berg, & Coiera, 2004), but if we are able to generalize the use of an electronic record, a whole new range of opportunities would likely open to transform care in ways yet unknown. Possibilities to improve access to patient information across settings, to develop electronic decision support measures to improve safety and care, and to create entirely new care models await the full implementation of the EHR.

Telehealth and Telemedicine. *Telehealth* and *telemedicine* are terms that are also commonly used, often without specific definition. Telehealth has been defined as "the use of electronic information and telecommunications technologies to support long-distance clinical health care, patient and professional health-related education, public health, and health administration" (U.S. Health Resources and Services Administration, 2001). Telemedicine is now generally considered synonymous with telehealth. Telehealth continues to have amazing promise to extend the benefits of excellent health care to populations without access and to extend educational opportunities to clinicians beyond restraints of distance and resources. In rural, underserved areas, telehealth can offer immediate feedback, decrease isolation, and extend health and lifesaving benefits not otherwise possible. As the promise of telehealth becomes a reality, it requires the most creative and effective leaders to maneuver through a variety of challenges, such as licensure and practice across state or national boundaries, access and insurance coverage to patients, fair reimbursement to providers, scrutiny of liability and other legal issues, patient privacy, fair distribution of resources and services, assurance of interprofessional collaboration, standard patient documentation systems, and a world of other issues yet unknown. Telehealth must be practiced outside traditional paradigms, so all of our thinking related to what we have always done will be challenged. Rae-Dupree (2009) observed that the idea that technology decreases the provider–patient relationship is a myth. It actually enhances it. Overcoming perceptions of this mismatch between technology and relationships will require thoughtful and effective leadership.

Technology and Simulation. Use of simulation for clinical preparation as well as practitioner development is another mode that continues to grow. Simulation laboratories are now pervasive all over the country in medical and nursing schools as well as health care organizations. These expensive extensions of practice preparation and development are an attractive focus for community donors as they provide a tangible product of the investment and an impressive "high-tech" image of the future. They are used to train practitioners in skills. At first, such laboratories focused on teaching skills and procedures on individual high-fidelity mannequins. Now, the trend is to create specific simulated clinical sites, such as the simulated intensive care unit, labor and delivery unit, or even homes and community centers. The centers provide safe environments for skill practice and feedback. Although these simulation centers are often shared among disciplines, we have yet to see much truly integrated, collaborative use. There is a growing movement toward using such centers to train care teams in collaboration and communication. The future waits for the use of such simulation centers to promote leadership development.

Technologies on the Horizon. Regardless of its form, it is clear that technology will continue to change the face of health care practice and leadership. It will provide entrepreneurial opportunities beyond current imagination. One example is the growth of genetic identification of disease propensity now, followed by technological advancement in the development of genetically informed individualized medications and treatments. Patient assessment, interventions, and communications will become more technological than mechanical, and mass customization will become as prevalent in health care as it is currently in online shopping. As technology continues to advance and change communication modes, choice and access will shift control of health care decisions toward the patient and community, and finally, we will begin to see consumers as central members of our professional care teams.

Our models of care of the future will move away from traditional clinical practice, practitioner-based designs to information-based, consumer-access models "that inform, empower, and actualize the consumer to take individual action with regard to his or her health status" (Porter-O'Grady, 2001, p. 66). Other technology and tools of the future that will change health care as we know it are out there, about to happen, and yet unknown. Innovative technologies on the immediate horizon include the legacy of the Human Genome Project, which has forever changed the timing, processes, and ethics of the entire process of care, from history and diagnosis to prevention, therapies, and interventions. We have only to imagine (or perhaps cannot even imagine) the technologies that will change health care, change how we manage health care, and change us as leaders.

Implications of Technology for Leadership. Technology and information access and management have changed the lives of leaders. Leaders play a critical role in the selection and adoption of technology in care services. For example, the clinical leader must collaborate and interact closely with providers at the point of care first to learn what technology is needed and then to assure that the appropriate technology is employed. This requires orchestration of input and feedback from staff nurses and other direct care providers. Furthermore, the leader must cultivate close relationships with IT experts and personnel as well as technology vendors to assure the appropriate integration and support for the technology. Finally, the leader must be the frontline translator of the needs, uses, and outcomes of technology to the highest levels of health care administration to assure understanding and resources for the use of technology. Indeed, the leader must interpret such data across disciplines as well as up and down from patient to care provider to business administrator. Always, the purpose of technology in health care is, first, to improve the quality of care and, second, to assure effective business performance of the organization.

Instant access and communication have blurred the lines between personal and professional lives and expectations. Leaders are called upon to guide organizations through the overwhelming information and incredible velocity of change. Furthermore, the leader's promotion and management of the use of technology can be an important recruitment factor as nurses and other health care workers are drawn to work environments that effectively employ technology (Fitzpatrick et al., 2010). On the other hand, Wheatley (2006, p. 29) warned:

> Unlike past organizational change efforts, knowledge management is truly a survival issue. Done right, it can give us what we so desperately need—organizations that act with intelligence. Done wrong, we will, like lemmings, keep rushing into the future without using our intelligence to develop longer-term individual and organizational capacity. To continue blindly down our current path, where speed and profits are the primary values, where there is no time to think or reflect, is suicidal.

We have learned how to retrieve, store, and manage information. We are learning how to convert information to knowledge. It is in the human capacity to apply and wisely use the technologies and information, to reflect on what matters, to project how things can be better. But, when will we learn how to transform information to knowledge and knowledge to wisdom?

Productivity and Effectiveness

We use technology to seek, store, and measure results. But measurement of productivity in health care is a special challenge. Although we are in the business of healing, health care is an industry, a business that measures outcomes and expects accountability and productivity. Increases in cost, wide variations in quality, more diverse and better informed patients and consumers, and public and business concerns regarding value for investment have provoked a greater interest in productivity and effectiveness in health care in general across the United States. Value is what the customer receives for the price paid. To promote efficiency and productivity, Womack and Jones (2005, p. 60) proposed the concept of "lean consumption," which is when a business provides the full value that customers expect with the "greatest efficiency and least pain." It requires integrated and streamlined processes and attention to meeting the needs of the customer or patient.

Traditionally, productivity refers to the amount or quality of output per unit of input, a return on investment, or worker efficiency. It is easy to measure the productivity of a machine or even the productivity of labor to produce a product. Health care outputs are more vexing. To a large health care system in today's market-oriented culture, productivity may mean its margin of the market. To a hospital worker, productivity may be the timely accomplishment of the day's duties. Ultimately, the productivity of a national health care system must be measured by the health of all its citizens.

From a management and human resources perspective, productivity usually refers to productive hours of human labor, most often referred to as full-time equivalents (FTEs), or staff workload used in some formula of output. In acute care systems, outputs are usually measured in some measure related to patient census, acuity levels, patient throughputs, or procedures performed. Other measures include staff turnover related to manager effectiveness.

There are several formal quality and productivity programs. Among the most popular are Six Sigma and Lean. These programs are focused toward manufacturing production but are growing in use in large health care systems and hospitals (Shankar, 2009). Their goal is to improve quality and decrease cost, with a focus on work processes. Six Sigma is "a disciplined data-driven approach and methodology for eliminating defects" (Lean Enterprise Institute, 2016; Pepper & Spedding, 2010). The program uses jargon such as "champion" for leaders and awards "belts" (e.g., "green belt" and "master black belt" status). The management approach is driven by outcomes data, usually financial, and based on projects to improve processes by controlling variation and improving predictability. Lean is "a systematic approach to identifying and eliminating eight "wastes" through continuous improvement by following the product at the 100 percent pull of the customer" (Lean Enterprise Institute, 2016; Pepper & Spedding, 2010). Systems measure productivity by reducing waste of time and human resources for a "lean" journey of the patient across care settings facilitated by efficient coordination of care (Kim, Spahlinger, Kin, Coffey, & Billi, 2009). Principles are that all work is process, that process flow can be optimized, and that employee flexibility increases productivity and reduces waste. The eight wastes of lean are waiting, defects, extra processing, inventory, excessive motion, transportation, overproduction, and underutilized employees. An increasing number of such outcomes-based measures are considered in a context of productivity.

The long-term value of such programs in human healing organizations remains to be determined. Effectiveness is reflected by accomplishment of mission, goals, and outcomes and satisfaction by all concerned, including and especially the people we serve. The danger of a focus on efficiency, in its usual sense, in health care is its potential effects on quality and patient satisfaction, not to mention pushing out the goals of healing and well-being, which have some human subjective, reflective, and social characteristics that challenge productivity measurement. Productivity and effectiveness must ultimately refer to a focus on value.

The Mayo Clinic Policy Center (2007) identified six action principles to assure productivity in health care for the future: (a) develop a definition of value based upon the needs and preferences of patients, measureable outcomes, safety, and service, compared with the cost of care over time; (b) pay providers based on value and develop a methodology for allocating finite resources; (c) create competition around results through pricing and quality transparency; (d) hold all sectors in health care accountable for reducing waste inefficiencies; (e) create a trusted mechanism to synthesize scientific and clinical information in an impartial and rigorous way for both consumers and providers; and (f) encourage formation of integrated systems to deliver effective and appropriate care.

The future will require increased knowledge, facility, and creativity by all leaders in health care regarding how to integrate important business and market principles into the enterprise of healing. We will need to move beyond safety and efficiency toward value and excellence. The leader who promotes productivity and fosters effectiveness continually sends a message of clear intention of what is expected and when it must be produced. He or she instills a sense of ownership of goals, processes, and outcomes. Even detractors must know the goals, the work, and the desired outcomes of the organization. In business, effectiveness is often associated with the concept of execution. Execution is the action of getting things done. It requires careful match of people with processes and tasks that come together for highest performance and best results. All does not always go as planned, but the leader guides the team through continuous improvement and recovery. The leader is also the key person to clearly articulate desired outcomes in a manner that can be identified and measured. Why do some good organizations fall short of acceptable productivity and effectiveness? Leaders, beware of some habits that can quash the spirit to produce. Over-planning and over-measuring can kill the spirit, especially in health care. We are in it because we want to help people. We need time to reflect, to cherish our contact with those we serve, and to create. Over-planning, over-processing, and "over-proceduring" can be devastating. Good leaders hold people accountable, then guide them toward success, recognize that success, and celebrate it.

Effective practice design and management for the future will consider innovative models, embracing an entrepreneurial context. Such designs must include continual assessment at the local unit and entire systems level, decisions based on evidence, effective use of technology in all areas of patient care, and creative ways of measuring effectiveness that improve the efficiency of the system while promoting environments of healing.

EVALUATION OF NEW MODELS OF CARE DELIVERY

Improving Patient and Health Care Outcomes

Patient and health care outcomes generally refer to the results of our practices on structure, process, or products. The modern origin of the concept of outcomes management is attributed to Paul Ellwood (1988), who referred to outcomes management as "a technology of the patient experience." His basic principles included an emphasis on established standards, measurement of patient functional status and well-being and disease-specific clinical outcomes, collecting outcome data from the broadest reach, and analysis and dissemination to health care decision makers.

Over the past three decades, Ellwood's work has been quoted and emulated broadly. In the beginning, outcomes referred to the "five Ds of death, disability, disease, discomfort, and dissatisfaction" (American College of Emergency Physicians [ACEP], 2009; HSRG, 1992; White, 1967). They have evolved to include clinical outcomes, functional status, satisfaction, and cost (ACEP, 2009; Lonborg, 1995; Nelson, Mohr, Batalden, & Plume, 1996).

Unfortunately, even with all the rhetoric and guidelines, the focus on outcomes in health care continues to be relatively unintegrated into our daily operational activities. It is to be hoped that current efforts on safety and quality are changing this outlook. Never underestimate the influence of the quality of leadership on patient outcomes. West et al. (2002) found significant correlations between leaders' management of employees and patient mortality in hospitals. Positive leadership practices included clarifying work objectives, identifying training needs, and providing feedback on performance, with focus on achieving organizational goals and improving individual performance and satisfaction. Wong and Cummings (2007) reviewed studies attempting to relate nursing leadership and patient outcomes, finding positive relationships among transformational leadership styles, patient satisfaction, and reduced adverse events. But research on leadership in health care has been largely descriptive and related to the styles or traits of the leaders.

Meade (2005, p. 5) reported the results of a study of seven health care facilities identified as "high-performing" organizations. High performance was defined as showing statistically significant progress sustained over 3 years on the following criteria: "increases in patient satisfaction ratings, increases in employee satisfaction ratings, reductions in employee turnover, increases in market share, financial return, or other growth indicators, and improvements on self-selected quality indicators." Meade (2005, p. 3) also identified the most influential factors in the success of high-performing health care organizations. The first, most important factor was commitment of the executive and senior leadership and leadership direction, alignment, and commitment to the vision and mission of the organization (Ulrich, Zenger & Smallwood, 2013). Achievement of positive health care outcomes requires vision, passion, and example at the highest levels. Second, was leadership evaluation and accountability. Meade argued for a "no excuses" environment where leaders would be evaluated and rewarded according to outcomes performance. Third was support for leadership development throughout the organization. You cannot expect leaders and managers at all levels to function without development as leaders themselves. This is part of the stewardship of generativity of leaders. Managers benefit from development specifically focused to prepare them as leaders. The fourth factor to achieve positive outcomes was open communication and formal opportunities for such communication throughout the organization. Finally, high-performing organizations nurtured a culture where everyone knew that patient-centered care and positive patient outcomes were the "right thing to do," that they "should" be doing what made sense for patients. Such organizations also reported a more friendly and helpful atmosphere, more collaboration and teamwork, and more regard for each other within the organization as well as for patients themselves.

Barriers to involving an entire organization into monitoring patient-centered outcomes are generally culture related. They include cultural cynicism about the value of outcomes measurement, resistance to change, beliefs that the status quo is sufficient, lack of accountability, or poor leadership skills among managers (Meade, 2005). With few exceptions, outcomes systems have been confined to acute care settings, although the concept of health care outcomes actually probably began in public health with community reporting systems. Clardy, Booth, Smith, Nordquist, and Smith (1998) provided a model to measure public health mental health services across an entire state.

Outcomes have become the language of education and health care. Whenever an idea or concept grows in organizations, it develops theories; coins its own language, jargon, and meanings; attracts structures; and soon becomes a world of its own. Soon, citizens of that world begin to use only the language of the new world, speak only to each other, and build systems and processes around themselves. Do not let this happen in the endeavor to pursue positive outcomes in health care. Allow some positive deviance to break open the thinking once in a while. Allow independent examples of success to flourish, and learn from them to improve the entire organization. Sometimes, solutions are in plain sight but just need a new way of looking at them. We need new practices outside the tradition. Look at old problems in new ways. To do that is a hallmark of the complexity theory and transformational leadership. Sternin (2007) argued that such positive deviance has changed some of the world's most pressing problems. The unfortunate rhetorical assumption related to outcomes is that there *is* actually an *outcome*, or destination, to care. The reality is that health care is an ongoing, iterative process to promote health, relieve suffering, and encourage healing. The inspiring leader keeps that vision ahead of the work with a healthy perspective that outcomes are markers on a continuing road toward excellence and improved health.

Quality Improvement and Customized Care: Currency of Customers and Clients

Safety and quality may be the most common areas of discussion and action in health care today. They are critical to individual patient care and for the very survival of health care systems.

Continuous quality improvement is the official jargon for creating an institutional culture that examines processes and systems of care to ensure quality of care. Unfortunately, all too often, the focus on measuring quality stops at safety, or the absence of harm, rather than on elevation of standards beyond safety to excellence. Increased public scrutiny has pushed efforts toward improved quality throughout various types of health care systems (Advisory Board, 2004; Arnold et al., 2006). Arnold et al. (2006, p. 215) noted that chief nursing executives now spend the majority of their time on issues of quality, compliance, and patient safety requirements: "As regulatory requirements become increasingly intense and consumer expectations heighten, quality and compliance-related pressures mount." Nursing leaders have begun to fill that leadership gap to make quality one of the most important current issues in all health care situations.

Brooks (2008) outlined a number of official databases or standards directed specifically at quality for nursing practice. We suspect you are familiar in your own agency with at least one of these. They include the National Database for Nursing Quality Indicators, the Veterans Administration Outcomes Database, the National Voluntary Consensus Standards for Nursing Sensitive Care from the Joint Commission on Accreditation of Healthcare Organizations, and the standards of Transforming Care at the Bedside from the IHI and Robert Wood Johnson

Foundation. Much of the focus among these efforts is on hospital care, but similar issues of quality pervade health care throughout our communities.

The National Quality Forum (NQF, 2004) outlined 15 "nursing-sensitive" measures now generally used in acute care institutions as indicators of quality. The measures are divided into three areas: patient-centered outcome measures, nursing-centered intervention measures, and system-centered measures. *Patient-centered outcome measures* include failure to rescue (or death among surgical inpatients with treatable serious complications), pressure ulcer prevalence, patient falls prevalence, falls with injury, restraint prevalence, urinary catheter-associated urinary tract infections, central line catheter-associated infections, and ventilator-associated pneumonias. *Nursing-centered intervention measures* include counseling patients with acute myocardial infarction, heart failure, or pneumonia regarding smoking cessation. *System-centered measures* include skill mix among RNs, practical nurses, and unlicensed personnel; nursing care hours per patient day; measures of nurse involvement in system governance and professional relationships; and voluntary turnover of nurse employees. Obviously, the list reflects important measures for patient survival, but if a stranger from another planet with superior health care visited our system, would that stranger find these measures as minimum for safety or as measures of excellence in healing? We are moving in the right direction with the focus toward improvement of care, and such efforts are making a difference in nursing performance and patient outcomes. But again, the challenge of leaders of the next level is to move performance to higher levels of excellence and healing.

Benchmarking. There are several mechanisms by which leaders may engage the organization in pursuit and evaluation of quality. One common way for leaders to confirm, measure, or monitor quality is benchmarking. Benchmarking is a method of comparing aspects of performance with similar organizations. It is usually done to provide information for strategic planning or to improve the processes, productivity, and quality of services. It allows you to make a professional comparison of the quality of your own setting with that of others anywhere in the world (Hollingsworth, 2008). Indeed, engagement in benchmarking activities in itself is a step toward improvement of quality. There is a difference between benchmarking and adopting industry standards or regulatory guidelines. Benchmarking is a voluntary, thoughtful, and selective activity of identifying peer organizations or organizations that you aspire to emulate on a specific process or outcome. You are then able to set specific goals related to the benchmark findings. The following are some of the steps outlined by Hollingsworth (2012, pp. 49–50) for successful benchmarking:

1. Identify benchmarking partners.
2. Determine what constitutes the benchmark calculation or data source.
3. Gather information from peer sources.
4. Compare actual data to benchmark data.

5. Identify variances and calculate gaps in performance.
6. Identify ideas for improvement, set goals, and develop and implement an action plan.

Benchmarking is most commonly done in hospitals and educational settings, but the principles apply to other settings such as primary care or public health.

Magnet Designation. Magnet designation is another mark of quality. It has been recognized for more than 25 years as a "hallmark of excellence" for quality and professional nursing in hospitals (Wolf, Triolo, & Ponte, 2008). Magnet status is sponsored by the American Nurses Credentialing Center of the American Nurses Association.

Basic criteria, or "forces of magnetism," include quality of nursing leadership, organizational structure, management style, personnel policies and programs, professional models of care, quality improvement, consultation and resources, autonomy, community supportive partnerships, nurses as teachers, image of nursing, collegial nurse–physician relationships, and professional development. Magnet hospitals have consistently scored high on support to nursing practice, nursing workload, and nurse satisfaction (Lacey et al., 2007). Application of Magnet principles has spread abroad (Aiken, Buchan, Ball, & Rafferty, 2008; Chen & Johantgen, 2010) but has yet to move to practice settings outside hospitals. The fundamental shift between the 2008 and 2013 model was an emphasis on empirical outcomes. For organizations applying for Magnet designation, evidence of empirical outcomes as sources of evidence for transformational leadership, structural empowerment, exemplary professional practice, and new knowledge are required. Outcomes are defined as "quantitative and qualitative evidence related to the impact of structure and process on the patient, the nursing workforce, the organization, and the consumer. These outcomes are dynamic and measureable and may be reported at the individual unit, department, population, or organizational level" (ANCC, 2014, p. 4).

Baldrige National Quality Award. Another example of a specific external measure of quality for hospitals is the Malcolm Baldrige National Quality Award, a federal award (sponsored by the American Society for Quality [ASQ]) to health care organizations. It evaluates how organizations meet particular standards on leadership; strategic planning; customer and market focus; measurement, analysis, and knowledge management; human resource focus; process management; and results (ASQ, 2016). The standards include strategic business principles, core values, and role modeling of leaders in principles that ultimately promote quality, such as "planning, communication, coaching, development of future leaders, review of organizational performance, and staff recognition" (Baldrige National Quality Program & National Institute of Standards and Technology, 2008; Goonan & Stoltz, 2004; Kurtzman & Jennings, 2008a, p. 241).

National Quality Forum. The NQF is a private, nonprofit organization that develops strategies for quality measurement and reporting in health care. Its mission is to set national priorities and goals for performance improvement, endorse national consensus standards for measuring and publicly reporting on performance, and promote the attainment of national goals through education and outreach programs (NQF, 2009). It has exerted considerable recent influence on performance, influencing initiatives of pay-for-performance, which is a paradigm that began with the Centers for Medicare and Medicaid Services whereby third parties reimburse health care providers based on quality and efficiency rather than on services and procedures, only. This approach requires health care agencies to monitor and report data on specific measures with standards that must be met in order to receive payment reimbursement (Gelinas, 2008). Third parties are beginning to withhold payment for conditions related to poor care quality and paying for performance on safety and quality. The movement has begun to change the culture of quality in patient care.

Other Quality Initiatives. Brooks (2008, p. 146) further proposed four key trends that will shape the future of quality and safety in nursing practice: "(1) transparency; (2) 100K Lives Campaign and standards of care; (3) pay-for-performance/pay-for-reporting; and (4) patient centeredness and coordination of care" (Reinertsen, 2006). Transparency refers to the trend of health care agencies toward publishing outcome data. Such publication is thought to increase competition on measures of quality. The 100K Lives Campaign refers to an initiative begun in 2005 and involving more than 2,600 health care organizations to reduce national hospital deaths by 100,000. It is part of the move toward transparency to improve quality of care. Patient centeredness and coordination of care include accountability for quality processes within entire patient care systems and coordination of patient care across settings.

A variety of individual demonstration movements across the country have begun to make a difference. One example is the Hospital Quality Incentive Demonstration, whereby hospitals are rewarded financially for top performance on specific outcomes. The Physician Group Practice Demonstration provides for physician groups to be rewarded for innovative proactive patient care and disease management in specific areas to reduce health care costs. Also, the Hospital Consumer Assessment of Health Plans Survey is designed to measure and standardize data on patient satisfaction. Private health care systems and advocate organizations have joined the movement, with a range of initiatives to change the culture toward incentives for quality and efficiency.

The recent Transforming Care at the Bedside project (IHI, 2010) was a major national effort to address issues of quality, safety, and reliability; vitality of nursing engagement and teamwork; patient-centered care; and value-added care processes in hospitals. It specifically targeted medical–surgical units in a large number of hospitals across the country (IHI, 2010; "Program Enables 50 New Initiatives," 2004; Rutherford, Lee & Greiner, 2004; "Transforming Care at the Bedside," 2005). Specific, broad targets were impressive (Rutherford et al., 2004, p. 4):

- There are no unanticipated deaths.
- No needless pain and suffering occurs.
- Clinicians, staff, and students will say, "I contribute to an effective care team within a supportive environment that nurtures my professional career/ growth and continually strives for excellence."
- Patients will say, "They give me exactly the help I want (and need) exactly when I want (and need) it."
- Unnecessary documentation is eliminated, reducing total documentation by 50%.
- Clinicians spend 70% of their time in direct patient care.

Measures to monitor achievement of targets include, "adverse events, unanticipated deaths, patient falls, unplanned returns to the intensive care unit, pressure ulcer prevalence, hospital-acquired pneumonia prevalence, care team satisfaction, voluntary turnover, patient and family satisfaction, percentage of time spent in direct patient care, percentage of time spent in documentation, percentage of time spend in value-added work, and costs per diagnosis-related group for the top three diagnoses of patients" (Rutherford et al., 2004, p. 4). Results have been highly positive and vary from situations of critical care (Donahue, Rader, & Triolo, 2008) to general medical–surgical patient care (Lorenz, Greenhouse, Miller, Wisniewski, & Frank, 2008; Upenieks, Needleman, et al., 2008; Viney, Batcheller, Houston, & Belcik, 2006), focusing on specific patient choices (Scott-Smith & Greenhouse, 2007) as well as multihospital systems (Martin et al., 2007).

Such trends toward quality offer important opportunities for leadership, particularly in nursing. Similar initiatives need to be tested in settings beyond hospitals. Transformational nurse leaders must have a foundation in understanding the interdisciplinary aspects of care in continuous quality improvement processes, and in patient-centered care. The next challenge is to create systems in which quality of care is integrated as second nature into all aspects of health care, including primary care and community health care. As the leader, remember that the tools for quality management are "the means, not the end." Kibort (2005, p. 54) reminded, "Remember they are just tools. Learn to use a few of them well. And stick to the fundamentals."

Nearly always, an initiative for quality improvement means leadership in change and change management; whether it is a change of procedure or process, change of product, or change of culture. Weber and Joshi (2000) noted that understanding change is most critical to successful quality improvement initiatives. It is important for the leader to understand the following eight critical strategies to manage change for quality improvement:

1. Develop a vision for change.
2. Focus on the change process.

3. Analyze which individuals in the organization must respond to the proposed change and what barriers exist.
4. Build partnerships between physicians and administration.
5. Create a culture of continuous commitment to . . . [quality].
6. Ensure that . . . [quality] begins with leadership.
7. Ensure that change is well communicated.
8. Build in accountability for change [and quality]. (Weber & Joshi, 2000, p. 388)

As previously discussed, we must be continually aware, in an environment of increased public and regulatory scrutiny and associated reporting requirements, to distinguish between competence in compliance and excellence. Every other industry is moving toward customized service. Patients are becoming accustomed to know what they want and to expect care specific to their needs. Nursing leadership, in particular, can create new paradigms and care models that frame productivity as value-added care. This vision of care "goes beyond direct care activities and includes team collaboration, physician rounding, increased communication, and patient centeredness . . . [in order to] improve efficiency, quality, and service," for example (Upenieks, Akhaven, & Kotlerman, 2008, p. 294). Excellence in quality represents not only a minimum standard of care but superb care.

Kurtzman and Jennings (2008a, p. 241) suggested the need to develop "quality literacy," calling for leaders to acquire and advance understanding of principles of quality, "both conceptually and practically." This includes, the development of a business case that includes a set of standard performance measures to highlight nursing's influence on quality. The business case must provide "clear, unambiguous, quantifiable evidence of the primacy of nursing's contribution." Evidence is the rule of the day. As a leader, you must speak the language and provide the data to support the work that you know leads to excellence.

An innovative study of leaders in 370 hospitals in all 50 states revealed that specific attributes of transformational leadership are related to both quality improvement and knowledge management, resulting in better patient outcomes (Gowen, Henagan, & McFadden, 2009). Another study in England found that specific leadership activities of training personnel, team working, and appraisal of hospital staff were directly related to patient mortality (West et al., 2002). To lead the charge in authentic quality of care, leaders must create and communicate a specific plan, gather appropriate data, use the data in specific evidence-based decision making, provide training and education to all members of the work team, and reward excellent performance (Kurtzman & Jennings, 2008b).

Knowledge and processes of quality improvement in health care have expanded to become recognized as a science with its own emerging body of knowledge. Cronenwett (2010) outlined its characteristics. It "considers local context, or what outcomes are achieved in what settings with what roles and processes, and it requires knowledge of [the specific] discipline, local culture, quality improvement methods and measures, and how to manage change." Furthermore, specific methods for reporting and publishing work on quality improvement have been proposed (Howell, Schwartz, O'Leary, & McDonnell, 2015).

In all the efforts to accelerate quality initiatives, we must not forget the viewpoint of patients themselves. Jennings and associates (Jennings & McClure, 2004; Kurtzman & Jennings, 2008a, p. 241) warned that since most current indicators of quality in all of our lists and recommendations are developed and driven by data needs for compliance to "payers and purchasers, accreditors, and other policymakers," Aspects of care that are most meaningful to clinicians, patients, and family members may not be reflected in these measures. Consequently, while enormous measurement "activity" may be taking place, nurse executives must ask themselves, "What are we gaining from this activity and does it reflect the aspects of care that are most vital? How can we use the findings from the measurement efforts to make improvements in the quality of patient care?"

Quality and customized service are the currency of consumers across society today. People have become accustomed to demanding quality and to having service for particular individual needs. Providers of a service such as health care cannot afford to overlook the personal meaning of that service to those who need it and receive it.

Although most of the published work on quality reflects practice in acute care, in any position or any setting, as a leader, you will devote considerable attention to quality. The public now demands it. There is an amazing array of resources for leaders in standards, structures, and processes to test, evaluate, and improve quality. The vigilance and hard work required to sustain formal activities in quality improvement are enormous. In the midst of all the work, remember that you are the transformational leader. Look beyond the work "activity" to the vision and meaning of improving lives and promoting healing. Quality "work" can be exhausting if it is not ultimately meaningful to patients and providers and born from passion and inspiration. That reflects the true challenge to leaders.

Assessing and Managing Risk. Risk is the other side of safety and quality.

There are two aspects to risk management. One is to reduce risk to patients in particular situations, such as taking measures to reduce infection transmission or to prevent pressure ulcers. The other part of risk management is to prevent incidents for which the institution may be held liable or to provide an environment for patients and workers that reduces loss to the organization (Pozgar, 2011). With the increased attention to patient safety, risk to patients and to organizations has risen to the forefront of health care. Legal issues can become entangled with risk management. Risk managers have become invaluable in helping to assess issues, develop interventions, and evaluate outcomes to prevent and reduce risks to patient safety and to the organization as well as to interpret legal implications. Risk management encompasses an entire body of knowledge and experts. The effective leader recognizes and works effectively with others who have such expertise.

Depending on the size of the organization, either the risk manager or you as leader are responsible for developing and enforcing systems to identify, report, and communicate incidents that expose individual or organizational risk.

Risk managers develop policies and procedures that address issues related to risk, such as confidentiality, informed consent, product performance, and sentinel events. They work closely with clinicians, managers, and quality management experts. Major areas of stewardship in risk management include loss prevention and reduction, claims management, financial risk, and compliance with regulatory and accrediting organizations (Dearman, 2009).

It has become the responsibility of the leader to ensure the effectiveness of systems and to change the culture toward a systems perspective and transparency. Most important to reduce adversarial and litigious responses to risk is transparency, to be genuine with patients and families, and to meet their expectations. Patients and families expect reliable, competent care each and every time.

Assuring High Reliability. The populations we serve expect highly reliable performance. High reliability encompasses several components illustrated within teams and organizations that anticipate and contain hazards (see Figure 8.1). Hazard anticipation is influenced by a preoccupation with failure, reluctance to simplify, and a sensitivity to operations. Hazard containment is influenced by an environment enabling deference to expertise and resilience (Weick & Sutcliff, 2011).

Hazard anticipation and hazard containment describe high reliability behaviors. Preoccupation with failure (things going wrong), sensitivity to operations (staffing patterns), and reluctance to simplify are components enabling hazard anticipation. In contrast, resilience and deference to expertise enable hazard containment. Each of these components is critically necessary for

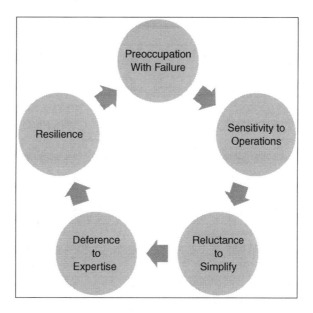

FIGURE 8.1 Components of highly reliable performance.

risk anticipation and management. (For a detailed discussion defining and describing each of the components of high reliability, see Weick & Sutcliff, 2011).

Highly reliable performance relies on higher levels of mindfulness at the point of care delivery. Although highly reliable performance is difficult, it is not necessarily expensive and can be instilled through changes to existing structures (e.g., human resources practices that reward and support interpersonal competence and learning; consistent leader rounding and follow up on what has been heard; selecting people who operate well under difficult conditions), as well as by changing conversations (e.g., infusing higher levels of honesty, respect, and trust into interactions) and through the questions we ask (e.g., "What do we need to look out for? What is a different assumption we could make about this problem? Where does the relevant expertise reside, and how can I draw upon it when I need it? How do we know we need to stop and adjust?"). Operating in a highly reliable manner through processes of mindful organizing (Vogus & Sutcliffe, 2007) can also benefit employees through increasing commitment, lowering emotional exhaustion, and reducing turnover (Vogus, Cooil, Sitterding, & Everett, 2014).

High reliability is a developmental process that needs to be kept alive. You are never done becoming highly reliable and sustaining high reliability. It needs to be continuously achieved. High reliability is best thought of as an ongoing process of organizing rather than a stable structure of an organization.

Key components of effective risk management include effective policies and procedures, documentation of patient care and other clinical activities, and timely and transparent reporting of critical incidents. Effective risk management requires leadership at the highest level of ethical behavior. The transformational leader engages the expertise of risk managers and lawyers as appropriate to manage and contain risk for patients, employees, and the organization. Such a leader also has the values and principles that provide the foundation for effective assessment, management, and reduction of risk.

SYSTEMS THINKING COMPETENCIES: LEADERSHIP IN ACTION

Organizations with high reliability that can ensure quality care, low-risk environments, and a patient-centered focus demand transformational leaders. These competencies are well described by the American Organization of Nurse Executives (2016) and include communication and relationship building, knowledge of the health care environment, leadership, professionalism, and business skills. Moreover, Hughes et al. (2014) described leadership competencies important in systems thinking. Such competencies include business acumen, strategic acting and thinking, organizational decision making, managing conflict, impact and influence across the system, building collaborative relationships, promoting organizational transition, adaptability and agility, initiating organizational innovation, and demonstrating vision. Table 8.3 contains questions to guide your own self-assessment of these competencies.

TABLE 8.3 Systems Thinking Survey

SYSTEMS THINKING COMPETENCY	SURVEY QUESTION
Business acumen	To what extent do I understand the perspectives of different areas in the business and have a firm grasp of external conditions affecting the organization?
Strategic planning	To what extent do I develop long-term objectives and strategies? Am I effective at translating vision into realistic business strategies?
Organizational decision making	To what extent do I make timely decisions? Do I really understand complex issues? Do I develop solutions that effectively address problems?
Managing conflicting perspectives	To what extent do I recognize that every decision has conflicting interests and constituencies? Am I able to balance short-term payoffs with long-term improvement?
Act systematically	To what extent do I understand the political nature of the organization and work appropriately within it? How effective am I at establishing collaborative relationships and alliances throughout the organization?
Influence across the organization	To what extent am I good at inspiring and promoting a vision? Am I able to persuade and motivate others? Do I skillfully influence superiors? Am I able to delegate effectively?
Build collaborative relationships	To what extent do I know how to build and maintain working relationships with coworkers and external parties? Do I negotiate and handle work problems without alienating people? Do I understand others and get their cooperation in nonauthority relationships?
Promote organizational transition	To what extent do I support strategies that facilitate organizational change initiatives and position the business for the future?
Adapt to new conditions	To what extent can I adapt to changing business conditions and remain open to new ideas and new methods?
Initiate organizational innovation	To what extent am I visionary, able to seize new opportunities, and consistently generate new ideas? Do I introduce and create needed change even in the face of opposition?
Demonstrate vision	To what extent do I understand, communicate, and stay focused on the organization's vision?

Source: Hughes, Beatty, and Dinwoodie (2014, p. 268).

BEYOND PATIENT SAFETY TO PRACTICE EXCELLENCE

Safety is the most basic and essential expectation of effective health care. It is simply to "minimize risk of harm to patients and providers through both system effectiveness and individual performance" (Cronenwett, 2010; Cronenwett et al., 2007, p. 122). Reason demands that it be the right of anyone receiving care. Cipriano (2008, p. 6) confirmed that attention to patient safety requires systems thinking. She asserted that, first, we must remove individual fear from the system, changing the question from "Who did this and what did the person do wrong?" to "What is the flaw in the system or process that provided the opportunity for error?" Thus, "eliminating fear and blame encourages people to report mistakes and allows creativity to flourish" to reduce errors and improve safety. She explained this in the context of the complex adaptive system of health care.

Conditions are changing. Nurses are quickly taking the lead to launch initiatives that improve patient safety. For example, the Quality and Safety Education for Nurses consortium, sponsored by the Robert Wood Johnson Foundation (Cronenwett, 2010; Cronenwett et al., 2007), has begun a major national effort to prepare health professionals, especially nurses, to lead in shaping professional identity among students and practitioners by committing to continuous improvement of quality care and patient safety. The project has begun to articulate specific knowledge, skills, and attitudes needed to promote patient care quality and safety. Specific goals, or competencies, of the project include patient-centered care; teamwork and collaboration; evidence-based practice; commitment to quality improvement, including use of data to monitor outcomes of care processes; safety; and informatics, or use of "technology to communicate, manage knowledge, mitigate error, and support decision-making" (Cronenwett, 2010).

Borrowing from other high-risk industries such as airlines, health care facilities are moving away from scrutinizing and condemning individual actions to emphasizing how to build safety into the entire complex system. This shift requires a change of assumptions, interprofessional collaboration, new views of policy, and universal transparency. Indeed, an expanded body of knowledge and a new realm of research on systems and patient safety are quickly emerging.

Another key aspect of safety that has recently come to the forefront for nursing leadership is that of employee and nurse safety. Rogers (1997) outlined five areas of risks or hazards for nurses and other health care workers: biological and infectious disease risks, chemical hazards, environmental hazards, physical risks, and psychological risks. The American Nurses Association has launched several initiatives to raise professional, social, and policy consciousness about health, safety, and quality for nurses and health care leaders, including its Healthy Work Environment program, which maintains that the workplace should be safe, empowering, and satisfying (ANA, 2016). A healthy work environment is not merely the absence of real and perceived threats to health, but a place of physical, mental, and social well-being. Other safety initiatives at ANA include bullying and violence prevention; chemicals, drugs, and biohazard safety; safe patient handling and mobility; safe staffing; and sharps safety. Leaders in health care today, especially those who most closely oversee patient care, are diligently searching for ways to assure the safety of patients. We are researching, creating plans, impaneling experts, and funding programs focused specifically on safety—but let us remember that safety is only the beginning. When will safety become second nature, the rightful outcome of every patient, family, and provider experience? When will safety be the everyday stipulation and reality of our work, and when will the focus of our practice move beyond safety to excellence? Your charge as a leader is to help to create the answers to these questions.

We must ask ourselves why major national panels must take official positions on patient safety, while we flutter to spend time and resources to design new models for safety. Think of it: *safety*—among the most basic needs. In other words, we are still trying to simply do no harm. Huge resources are now devoted to designing systems to prevent us from giving the wrong medication or the wrong dose to the wrong patient. We are developing programs with targets to avoid needless deaths in our system—a *health care* system, a system in which people enter unaware and with every right to expect that there is no possibility they will be harmed or killed by the system. When can we move from safety to excellence and healing? The answer must come from the next generation of leaders.

REFERENCES

Advisory Board. (2004). Enhancing nursing business performance (pp. 2–24). Washington DC: The Advisory Board Company.

Ahalt, S., Bizon, C., Evans, J., Erlich, Y., Ginsberg, G., Krishnamurthy, A., & Wilhelmsen, K. (2014). *Data to discovery: Genomes to health. A white paper from the National Consortium for Data Science.* Chapel Hill, NC: Renaissance Computing Institute. Retrieved from http://data2discovery.org/dev/wp-content/uploads/2014/02/NCDS-Summit-2013.pdf

Ahmad, F., Hudak, P. L., Bercovitz, K., Hollenburg, E., & Levinson, W. (2006). Are physicians ready for patients with Internet-based health information? *Journal of Medical Internet Research, 8*(3), e22.

Aiken, L. H., Buchan, J., Ball, J., & Rafferty, A. M. (2008). Transformative impact of Magnet designation: England case study. *Journal of Clinical Nursing, 17*(24), 3330–3337.

Aiken, L. H., & Sochalski, J., & Lake, E. T. (1997). Lower Medicare mortality among a set of hospitals known for good nursing care. *Medical Care, 32*(8), 771–787.

American Academy of Nursing. (2012, March 5). *The imperative for patient, family, and population centered interprofessional approaches to care coordination and transitional care.* Washington, DC: Author. Retrieved from http://www.aannet.org/assets/docs/PolicyResources/aan_care%20coordination_3.7.12_email.pdf

American Academy of Nursing. (2014). Making transitional care more effective and efficient. *Raise the Voice: Edge Runner.* Washington, DC: Author. Retrieved from http://www.aannet.org/edge-runners--making-transitional-care-more-effective---efficient

American Association of Colleges of Nursing. (2002). Hallmarks of the professional nursing practice environment. *Journal of Professional Nursing, 18*(5), 295–304.

Association of Colleges of Nursing. (2015, August). *The doctor of nursing practice: Current issues and clarifying recommendations.* Report from the Task Force on the Implementation of the DNP. Washington DC: AACN.

American Association of Colleges of Nursing. (2016). *Hallmarks of the professional nursing practice environment.* Washington, DC: Author. Retrieved from http://www.aacn.nche.edu/publications/white-papers/hallmarks-practice-environmen.

American Association of Critical-Care Nurses, & American Association of Critical-Care Nurses. (2011). *The AACN synergy model for patient care.* Retrieved from www.aacn.org

American College of Emergency Physicians. (2009). *Quality of care and outcomes management movement.* Retrieved from http://www.acep.org/practres.aspx?id=30166

American Nurses Association. (2012, June). *White paper: The value of nursing care coordination.* Retrieved from http://www.nursingworld.org/carecoordinationwhitepaper

American Nurses Association. (2016). *Healthy work environment.* Retrieved from http://www.nursingworld.org/MainMenuCategories/WorkplaceSafety/Healthy-Work-Environment

American Nurses Credentialing Center. (2014). *Magnet recognition program manual.* Silver Spring, MD: Author.

American Organization of Nurse Executives. (2016). AONE: The voice of nursing leadership. Retrieved from http://www.aone.org/

American Society for Quality (2016). Malcolm Baldrige National Quality Award. Retrieved from http://asq.org/learn-about-quality/malcolm-baldrige-award/overview/overview.html

Arndt, M., & Bigelow, B. (2009). Evidence-based management in health care organizations: A cautionary note. *Health Care Management Review, 34*(3), 206–213.

Arnold, L., Drenkard, K., Ela, S., Goedken, J., Hamilton, C., Harris, C., . . . White, M. (2006). Strategic positioning for nursing excellence in health systems: Insights from chief nursing executives. *Nursing Administration Quarterly, 30*(1), 11–20.

Ash, J. S., Berg, M., & Coiera, E. (2004). Patient care information system-related errors. *Journal of the American Medical Informatics Association, 11*(2), 104–112.

Ausman, R. K. (1967). Automated storage and retrieval of patient data. *American Journal of Surgery, 114*(1), 159–166.

Babbott, S., Manwell, L. B., Brown, R., Montague, E., Williams, E., Schwartz, M., . . . Linzer, M. (2014). Electronic health records and physician stress in primary care: Results from the MEMO Study. *Journal of the American Medical Informatics Association, 21*(e1), e100–e106.

Baldrige National Quality Program & National Institute of Standards and Technology. (2008). *Health care criteria for performance excellence.* Gaithersburg, MD: National Institute of Standards and Technology.

Benner, P. (1984). *From novice to expert: Excellence and power in clinical nursing practice.* Menlo Park, CA: Addison-Wesley.

Bergstrom, N., Horn, S. D., Smout, R. J., Bender, S. A., Ferguson, M. L., Taler, G., & Voss, A. C. (2005). The National Pressure Ulcer Long-Term Care Study: Outcomes of pressure ulcer treatments in long-term care. *Journal of the American Geriatrics Society, 53*(10), 1721–1729.

Best, A., Terpstra, J. L., Moor, G., Riley, B., Norman, C. D., & Glasgow, R. E. (2009). Building knowledge integration systems for evidence-informed decisions. *Journal of Health Organization and Management, 23*(6), 627–641.

Bleich, M. R., Cleary, B. L., Davis, K., Hatcher, B. J., Hewlett, P. O., & Hill, K. S. (2009). Mitigating knowledge loss: A strategic imperative for nurse leaders. *Journal of Nursing Administration, 39*(4), 160–164.

Bowen, S., & Zwi, A. B. (2005). Pathways to "evidence-informed" policy and practice: A framework for action. *PLOS Medicine, 2*(7), e166.

Brandt, J. A., Edwards, D. R., Sullivan, S. C., Zehler, J. K., Grinder, S., Scott, K. J., & Maddox, K. L. (2009). An evidence-based business planning process. *Journal of Nursing Administration, 39*(12), 511–513.

Brennan, P., & Bakken, S. (2015). Nursing needs big data and big data needs nursing. *Journal of Nursing Scholarship, 47*(5), 477–484.

Brooks, J. (2008). Continuous quality improvement. In H. R. Feldman, M. Jaffe-Ruiz, M. L. McClure, M. J. Greenberg, & T. D. Smith (Eds.), *Nursing leadership: A concise encyclopedia* (pp. 145–149). New York, NY: Springer Publishing Company.

Budnitz, D. S., Pollock, D. A., Weidenbach, K. N., Mendelsohn, A. B., Schroeder, T. J., & Annest, J. L. (2006). National surveillance of emergency department visits for outpatient adverse drug events. *Journal of the American Medical Association, 296*(15), 1858–1866.

Buerhaus, P. I., Staiger, D. O., & Auerbach, D. I. (2000). Implications of an aging registered nurse workforce. *Journal of the American Medical Association, 283*(22), 2948–2954.

Bulger, R. J. (2003). *The quest for therapeutic institutions.* Washington, DC: Association of Academic Health Centers.

Burns, H. K., Dudjak, L., & Greenhouse, P. K. (2009). Building an evidence-based practice infrastructure and culture: A model for rural and community hospitals. *Journal of Nursing Administration, 39*(7/8), 321–325.

Camicia, M., Chamberlain, B., Finnie, R. R., Nalle, M., Lindeke, L. L., Lorenz, L., . . . McMenamin, P. (2013). The value of nursing care coordination: A white paper of the American Nurses Association. *Nursing Outlook, 61*(6), 490–501.

Caramenico, A. (2012, June 19). Patient-centered care, shared decision-making gets $30M in funding. *FierceHealthcare.* Retrieved from http://www.fiercehealthcare.com/search/site/Patient%20centered%20care%2C%20shared%20decision%20making%20gets?solrsort=score%20desc&include-pr=0&site-filter=0

Chalkidou, K., Walley, T., Culyer, A., Littlejohns, P., & Hoy, A. (2008). Evidence-informed evidence-making. *Journal of Health Services Research & Policy, 13*(3), 167–173.

Chen, Y. M., & Johantgen, M. E. (2010). Magnet hospital attributes in European hospitals: A multilevel model of job satisfaction. *International Journal of Nursing Studies, 47*(8), 1001–1012.

Christensen, C. (1997). *The innovator's dilemma.* Boston, MA: Harvard Business School.

Christensen, C. M., & Overdorf, M. (2000). Meeting the challenge of disruptive change. *Harvard Business Review, 78*(2), 66–77.

Cipriano, P. (2008). Improving health care with systems thinking. *American Nurse Today, 3*(9), 6.

Clardy, J. A., Booth, B. M., Smith, L. G., Nordquist, C. R., & Smith, G. R. (1998). Implementing a statewide outcomes management system for consumers of public mental health services. *Psychiatric Services, 49*(2), 191–195.

Conroy, B. E., DeJong, G., & Horn, S. D. (2009). Hospital-based stroke rehabilitation in the United States. *Topics in Stroke Rehabilitation, 16*(1), 34–43.

Cornell, P., Riordan, M., Townsend-Gervis, M., & Mobley, R. (2011). Barriers to critical thinking: Workflow interruptions and task switching among nurses. *Journal of Nursing Administration, 41*(10), 407–414.

Costs of Care (2016). *Cost framework.* Retrieved from http://www.costsofcare.org/costframework/

Craig, C., Eby, D., & Whittington, J. (2011). Care coordination model: Better care at lower cost for people with multiple health and social needs. IHI Innovation Series white paper. Cambridge, MA: Institute for Healthcare Improvement. Retrieved from http://www.ihi.org/resources/pages/ihiwhitepapers/ihicarecoordinationmodel whitepaper.aspx

Crisp, N., & Chen, L. (2014). Global supply of health professionals. *New England Journal of Medicine, 370*, 950–957.

Cronenwett, L. (2010, January). *Quality and safety implications for doctoral programs in nursing.* Paper presented at the meetings of the American Association of Colleges of Nursing, Captiva Island, FL.

Cronenwett, L., Sherwood, G., Barnsteiner, J., Disch, J., Johnson, J., Mitchell, P., . . . Warren, J. (2007). Quality and safety education for nurses. *Nursing Outlook, 55*(3), 122–131.

Cullen, L., Greiner, J., Greiner, J., Bombei, C., & Comried, L. (2005). Excellence in evidence-based practice: Organizational and unit exemplars. *Critical Care Nursing Clinics of North America, 17*(2), 127–142.

Cummings, G. G., Estabrooks, C. A., Midodzi, W. K., Wallin, L., & Hayduk, L. (2007). Influence of organizational characteristics and context on research utilization. *Nursing Research, 56*(4), S24–S39.

Dearman, V. (2009). Risk management and legal issues. In L. Roussel & R. C. Swansburg (Eds.), *Management and leadership for nurse administrators* (5th ed., pp. 470–493). Sudbury, MA: Jones & Bartlett.

DiSanzo, D. (2014, January 14). Op/Ed: Hospital of the future will be a health delivery network, *U.S. News & World Report Health.* Retrieved from http://health.usnews.com/health-news/hospital-of-tomorrow/articles/2014/01/14/oped-hospital-of-the-future-will-be-a-health-delivery-network

Donahue, L., Rader, S., & Triolo, P. K. (2008). Nurturing innovation in the critical care environment: Transforming care at the bedside. *Critical Care Nursing Clinical of North America, 20*(4), 465–469.

Ellwood, P. M. (1988). Outcomes management: A technology of patient experience. *New England Journal of Medicine, 318*(23), 1549–1556.

Everett, L. Q., & Broome, M. E. (2001). Academic-practice partnerships tool kit. Washington DC: AACN.

Fitzpatrick, M. A., Grant, S., McCue, P. O., O'Rouke, M. W., Reck, D. L., Shaffer, F. A., & Simpson, R. (2010). Nurse leaders discuss the nurse's role in driving technology decisions. *American Nurse Today, 5*(1), 16–19.

Fretheim, A., Oxman, A. D., Lavis, J. N., & Lewin, S. (2009). SUPPORT tools for evidence-informed policymaking in health 18: Planning monitoring and evaluation of policies. *Health Research Policy and Systems, 7*(Suppl. 1), S18.

Gelinas, L. S. (2008). National Quality Forum. In H. R. Feldman, M. Jaffe-Ruiz, M. L. McClure, M. J. Greenberg, & T. D. Smith (Eds). *Nursing leaership: A concise encyclopedia* (pp. 392–397). New York, NY: Springer Publishing Company.

Gifford, W., Davies, B., Edwards, N., Griffin, P., & Lybanon, V. (2007). Managerial leadership for nurses' use of research evidence: An integrative review of the literature. *Worldviews on Evidence-Based Nursing, 4*(3), 126–145.

Goonan, K. J., & Stoltz, P. K. (2004). Leadership and management principles for outcomes-oriented organizations. *Medical Care, 42*(4), III31–38.

Gowen, C. R., Henagan, S. C., & McFadden, K. L. (2009). Knowledge management as a mediator for the efficacy of transformational leadership and quality management initiatives in U.S. health care. *Health Care Management Review, 34*(3), 129–140.

Hacker, J. S. (2007). Healing our Sicko health care system. *New England Journal of Medicine, 357*(8), 733–735.

Hassmiller, S. B., & Rutherford, P. (2016). *Raise the Voice: Edge Runner: Transforming care at the bedside.* American Academy of Nursing. Retrieved from http://www.aannet. org/edge-runners--transforming-care-at-the-bedside

Health Services Research Group (1992). Outcomes and the management of health care. *Canadian Medical Association Journal, 147,* 1775–1780.

Hoffart, N., & Woods, C. Q. (1996). Elements of a nursing professional practice model. *Journal of Professional Nursing, 12*(6), 354–364.

Hollingsworth, N. (2012). Benchmarking. In H. R. Feldman, M. J. Greenberg, M. Jaffe-Ruiz, A. B. McBride, T. D. Smith, & R. Alexander, *Nursing leadership: A concise encyclopedia.* (2nd ed.). (pp. 49–50). New York, NY: Springer Publishing Company.

Horn, S. D., & Gassaway, J. (2007). Practice-based evidence study design for comparative effectiveness research. *Medical Care, 45*(10), S50–S57.

Horn, S. D., Torres, A. Willson, D., Dean, J. M., Gassaway, J., & Smout, R. (2002) Development of a pediatric age- and disease-specific severity measure. *Journal of Pediatrics, 141*(4), 496–503.

Howell, V., Schwartz, A., O'Leary, J., & McDonnell, C. (2015). The effect of the SQUIRE (Standards of Quality Improvement Reporting Excellence) guidelines on reporting standards in the quality improvement literature: A before and after study. *BMJ Quality & Safety, 24*(6), 349–351.

Hughes, R. L., Beatty, K. C., Dinwoodie, D. L. (2014). *Becoming a strategic leader: Your role in your organization's enduring success* (2nd ed.). San Francisco, CA: Jossey-Bass.

Hussey, P. S., Anderson, G. F., Osborn, R., Feek, C., McLaughlin, V., Millar, J., & Epstein, A. (2004). How does the quality of care compare in five countries? *Health Affairs, 23*(3), 89–99.

Institute for Healthcare Improvement. (2010). *Transforming care at the bedside.* Retrieved from http://www.ihi.org/search/pages/results.aspx?k=Transforming+healthcare +at+the+bedside

Institute of Medicine. (1999). *To err is human.* Washington DC: National Academies Press.

Institute of Medicine. (2013). *Best care at lower cost: The path to continuously learning health care in America.* Washington, DC: National Academies Press. Retrieved from http:// www.nap.edu/read/13444/chapter/3

Ives Erickson, J., Duffy, M., Gibbons, P., Fitzmaurice, J., Ditomassi, M., & Jones, D. (2004) Development and psychometric evaluation of the professional practice environment scale. *Journal of Nursing Scholarship, 36*(3), 279–284.

James, J. T. (2013). A new, evidence-based estimate of patient harms associated with hospital care. *Journal of Patient Safety, 8*(3), 122–128.

Jennings, B. M., & McClure, M. L. (2004). Strategies to advance health care quality. *Nursing Outlook, 52*(1), 17–22.

Joynt, J., & Kimball, B. (2008). *Innovative care delivery models: Identifying new models that effectively leverage nurses.* Princeton, NJ: Robert Wood Johnson Foundation.

Kibort, P. M. (2005, November/December). I drank the Kool-Aid—and learned key management lessons. *Physician Executive, 31*(6), 52–55.

Kim, C. S., Spahlinger, D. A., Kin, J. M., Coffey, R. J., & Billi, J. E. (2009). Implementation of lean thinking: One health system's journey. *Joint Commission Journal on Quality and Patient Safety, 35*(8), 406–413.

Kimball, B., Joynt, J., Cherner, D., & O'Neil, E. (2007). The quest for new innovative care delivery models. *Journal of Nursing Administration, 37*(9), 392–398.

Kossman, S. P., & Brennan, P. F. (2008). Nursing informatics. In H. R. Feldman, M. Jaffe-Ruiz, M. L. McClure, M. J. Greenberg, & T. D. Smith (Eds.), *Nursing leadership: A concise encyclopedia* (pp. 416–419). New York, NY: Springer Publishing Company.

Kramer M., & Hafner, L. P. (1989). Shared values: Impact on staff nurse job satisfaction and perceived productivity. *Nursing Research, 38*, 58–64.

Kurtzman, E. T., & Jennings, B. M. (2008a). Capturing the imagination of nurse executives in tracking the quality of nursing care. *Nursing Administration Quarterly, 32*(3), 235–246.

Kurtzman, E. T., & Jennings, B. M. (2008b). Trends in transparency: Nursing performance measurement and reporting. *Journal of Nursing Administration, 38*(7/8), 349–354.

Lacey, S. R., Cox, K. S., Lorfing, K. C., Teasley, S. L., Carroll, C. A., & Sexton, K. (2007). Nursing support, workload, and intent to stay in Magnet, Magnet-aspiring, and non-Magnet hospitals. *Journal of Nursing Administration, 37*(4), 199–205.

Lake, E. T. (2002). Development of the practice environment scale of the nursing work index. *Research in Nursing & Health, 25*(3), 176–188.

Lavis, J. N., Oxman, A. D., Moynihan, R., & Paulsen, E. J. (2008). Evidence-informed health policy 3: Interviews with the directors of organizations that support distribution in British Columbia. *Implementation Science, 17*(3), 55.

Lavis, J. N., Paulsen, E. J., Oxman, A. D., & Moynihan, R. (2008a). Evidence-informed health policy 1: Synthesis of findings from a multi-method study of organizations that support the use of research evidence. *Implementation Science, 17*(3), 53.

Lavis, J. N., Paulsen, E. J., Oxman, A. D., & Moynihan, R. (2008b). Evidence-informed health policy 1: Survey of organizations that support the use of research evidence. *Implementation Science, 17*(3), 54.

Lean Enterprise Institute. (2016). *What is lean?* Retrieved from http://www.lean.org/WhatsLean/.

Lonborg, R. (1995). Measuring patient satisfaction over the entire episode of care. Congress on Health Outcomes and Accountability, Washington DC.

Lorenz, H. L., Greenhouse, P. K., Miller, R., Wisniewski, M. K., & Frank, S. L. (2008). Transforming care at the bedside: an ambulatory model for improving the patient experience. *Journal of Nursing Administration, 38*(4), 194–199.

Lukas, C. V., Holmes, S. K., Cohen, A. B., Restuccia, J., Cramer, I. E., Shwartz, M., & Charns, M. P. (2007). Transformational change in health care systems: An organizational model. *Healthcare Management Review, 32*(4), 309–320.

Lynch, W., Perosino, K., & Stover, M. (2014). *Altarum Institute survey of consumer health care opinions*. Washington, DC: Altarum Institute. Retrieved from http://altarum.org/sites/default/files/uploaded-related files/Spring_2014_Survey_of_Consumer_Health_Care_Opinions.pdf.

MacRobert, M. (2008). A leadership focus on evidence-based practice: Tools for successful implementation. *Professional Case Management, 13*(2), 97–101.

Marchionni, C., & Ritchie, J. (2008). Organizational factors that support the implementation of a nursing best practice guideline. *Journal of Nursing Management, 16*(3), 266–274.

Martin, S. C., Greenhouse, P. K., Merryman, T., Shovel, K., Liberi, C. A., & Konzier, J. (2007). Transforming care at the bedside: Implementation and spread model for single-hospital and multihospital systems. *Journal of Nursing Administration, 37*(10), 444–451.

Mason, H., & Wiggins, C. (2010). A taxonomy of data science. *Dataists*. Retrieved from http://www.dataists.com/2010/09/a-taxonomy-of-data-science/

Mayo Clinic. (2007, January). *Improving productivity in healthcare: Effectiveness, efficiency, and value: Executive summary.* Retrieved from http://www.mayoclinic.org/health-policycenter/forum2-summary.html

McClure, M., Poulin, M., Sovie, M., & Wandelt, M. (2002). *Magnet hospitals: Attraction and retention of professional nurses.* Kansas City, MO: American Nurses Association.

McDonald, K. M., Schultz, E., Albin, L., Pineda, N., Lonhart, J., Sundaram, V., . . . Malcolm, E. (2010). *Care coordination measures atlas* (AHRQ Publication No. 11-0023-EF). Rockville, MD: U.S. Department of Health and Human Services Agency for Health Care Research and Quality.

Meade, C. M. (2005). Organizational change processes in high performing organizations: In-depth case studies with healthcare facilities. *Alliance for Health Care Research,* 5–28.

Melnyk, B. M. (2007). The evidence-based practice mentor: A promising strategy for implementing and sustaining EBP in healthcare systems. *Worldviews on Evidence-Based Nursing, 4*(3), 123–125.

Melnyk, B. M., & Fineout-Overhold, E. (2014). *Evidence-based practice in nursing and healthcare: A guide to best practice.* (3rd Ed.). Riverwoods, IL: Wolters Kluwer Health.

Metzger, J., Welebob, E., Bates, D. W., Lipsitz, S., & Classen, D. C. (2010). Mixed results in the safety performance of computerized physician order entry. *Health Affairs, 29*(4), 655–663.

Moriates, C., Arora, V., & Shah, N. (2015). *Understanding value-based healthcare.* New York, NY: McGraw-Hill.

Nanji, K. C., Patel, A., Shaikh, S., Seger, D. L., & Bates, D. W. (2016). Evaluation of peri-operative medication errors and adverse drug events. *Journal of the American Society of Anesthesiologists, 124*(1), 25–34.

National Patient Safety Foundation. (2015). *Free from harm: Accelerating patient safety improvement fifteen years after To Err Is Human.* Boston, MA: Author.

National Quality Forum (2004). National voluntary consensus standards for nursing sensitive care: An initial performance measure set. Washington DC: Author. Retrieved from http://www.qualityforum.org/Publications/2004/10/National_Voluntary_Consensus_Standards_for_Nursing-Sensitive_Care__An_Initial_Performance_Measure_Set.aspx

National Quality Forum (2006). NQF endorsed definition and framework for measuring care coordination. Available at http://www.qualityforum.org/Project_Pages/Care_Coordination_Measures.aspx

National Quality Forum (NQF). (2009). *Mission and vision.* Washington, DC: Author. Retrieved from http:// www.qualityforum.org/About_NQF/Mission_and_Vision.aspx

Naylor, M., Aiken, L., Kurtzman, E., & Olds, D. (2010). *Nursing's contributions to care coordination and transitional care: State of the science.* Princeton, NJ: Robert Wood Johnson Foundation.

Nelson, E. C., Mohr, J. J., Batalden, P. B., & Plume, S. K. (1996). Improving healthcare, Part 1: The clinical value compass. *Joint Commission Journal on Quality Improvement, 22*(4), 243–258.

Newhouse, R. P. (2007). Creating infrastructure supportive of evidence-based nursing practice: Leadership strategies. *Worldviews on Evidence-Based Nursing, 4*(1), 21–29.

Newhouse, R. P. (2009). Nursing's role in engineering a learning healthcare system. *Journal of Nursing Administration, 39*(6), 260–262.

Newhouse, R. P., & Johnson, K. (2009). A case study in evaluating infrastructure for EBP and selecting a model. *Journal of Nursing Administration, 39*(10), 409–411.

Oberlander, J. (2007). Learning from failure in healthcare reform. *New England Journal of Medicine, 357*(17), 1677–1680.

Oh, H., Rizo, C., Enkin, M., & Jadad, A. (2005). What is eHealth? A systematic review of published definitions. *Journal of Medicine & Internet Research, 7*(1), e1. Retrieved from http://apps.himss.org/ihf/docs/ihfjournal/what_is_ehealth.pdf

Owens, M. K. (2010). Costs of uncoordinated care. In P. L. Yong, R. S. Saunders, & L. A. Olsen (Eds.), *The health care imperative: Lowering costs and improving outcomes: Workshop series summary.* Washington, DC: National Academies Press.

Pepper, M. P. J., & Spedding, T. A. (2010). The evolution of lean Six Sigma. *International Journal of Quality & Reliability Management, 27*(2), 138–155.

Pittman, J., & Sitterding, M. (2012). WOC nurse and practice innovation. *Journal of Wound, Ostomy, and Continence Nursing, 39*(5), 488–491.

Poissant, L., Pereira, J., Tamblyn, R., & Kawasumi, Y. (2005). The impact of electronic health records on time efficiency of physicians and nurses: A systematic review. *Journal of the American Medical Informatics Association, 12*(5), 505–516.

Porter-O'Grady, T. (2001). Beyond the walls: Nursing in the entrepreneurial world. *Nursing Administration Quarterly, 25*(2), 61–68.

Porter-O'Grady, T., & Malloch, K. (2008). Beyond myth and magic: The future of evidence-based leadership. *Nursing Administration Quarterly, 32*(3), 176–187.

Pozgar, G. D. (2011). *Legal aspects of healthcare administration* (11th ed.). Sudbury, MA: Jones & Bartlett.

Program enables 50 new initiatives in four months: "Transforming care at the bedside" program. (2004). *Health Care Benchmarks & Quality Improvement, 11*(9), 100–101.

Rae-Dupree, J. (2009, February 1). Disruptive innovation applied to healthcare. *New York Times,* BU3.

Ratwani, R. M., Fairbanks, R. J., Hettinger, A. Z., & Benda, N. C. (2015). Electronic health record usability: Analysis of the user-centered design processes of eleven electronic health record vendors. *Journal of the American Medical Informatics Association, 22*(6), 1179–1182.

Reinertsen, J. L. (2006). Quality and safety: Quality is now strategic. In Society for Healthcare Strategy and Market Development of the American Hospital Association and American College of Healthcare Executives. *Futurescan: Healthcare trends and implications 2006–2011* (pp. 20–24). Chicago, IL: Health Administration Press.

Robert Wood Johnson Foundation. (2009, March). Nursing's prescription for a reformed health system: Use exemplary nursing initiatives to expand access, improve quality, reduce costs, and promote prevention. *Charting Nursing's Future, 2009*(9), 1. Retrieved from http://www.aannet.org/assets/docs/RaisetheVoice/rwjf_charting%20nursing%20future_mar09.pdf

Robert Wood Johnson Foundation. (2014, May 1). *Survey: Physicians are aware that many medical tests and procedures are unnecessary, see themselves as solution,* Princeton, NJ: Author. Retrieved from http://www.rwjf.org/en/library/articles-and-news/2014/04/survey--physicians-are-aware-that-many-medical-tests-and-procedu.html

Rogers, B. (1997). As I see it: Is health care a risky business? *American Nurse, 29,* 5–6.

Rutherford, P., Lee, B., & Greiner, A. (2004). *Transforming care at the bedside. IHI innovation series white paper.* Boston, MA: Institute for Healthcare Improvement.

Rycroft-Malone, J. O. (2008). Evidence-informed practice: From individual to context. *Journal of Nursing Management, 16*(4), 404–408.

Scheffler, R.M, Liu, J. X., Kinfu, Y., & Dal Poz, M. R. (2008). Forecasting the global shortage of physicians: An economic and needs-based approach. *Bulletin of the World Health Organization, 86* (7), 516-523B.

Schenthal, J. E., Sweeney, J. W., & Nettleton, W. (1961). Clinical application of electronic data processing apparatus: II. New methodology in clinical record storage. *Journal of the American Medical Association, 178*(3), 267–270.

Schiff, G. D., Amato, M. G., Eguale, T., Boehne, J. J., Wright, A., Koppel, R., ... Seger, A. C. (2016). Computerized physician order entry-related medication errors: Analysis of reported errors and vulnerability testing of current systems. *British Medical Journal of Quality & Safety, 25*(5), 315–319. Retrieved from http://qualitysafety.bmj.com/content/early/2015/01/16/bmjqs-2014-003555

Schoen, C. Osborne, R., Squires, D., Doty, M., Pierson, R. & Applebaum, S. (2011). New 2011 survey of patients with complex care needs in eleven countries finds that care is often poorly coordinated. *Health Affairs, 30*(12), 2437–2448.

Schulman, C. S. (2008). Strategies for starting a successful evidence-based practice program. *AACN Advanced Critical Care, 19*(3), 301–311.

Scott-Smith, J. L., & Greenhouse, P. K. (2007). Transforming care at the bedside: Patient controlled liberalized diet. *Journal of Interprofessional Care, 21*(2), 179–188.

Senge, P. M. (1990). *The art and practice of the learning organization* (pp. 3–11). New York, NY: Doubleday.

Shankar, R. (2009). *Process improvement using Six Sigma: A DMAIC guide.* Milwaukee, WI: ASQ Quality Press.

Singh, H., Meyer, A., & Thomas, E. (2014). The frequency of diagnostic errors in outpatient care: estimations from three large observational studies involving US adult populations. *BMJ Quality & Safety, 10,* 1136.

Sitterding, M. C., Broome, M. E., Everett, L. Q., & Ebright, P. (2012). Understanding situation awareness in nursing work: A hybrid concept analysis. *Advances in Nursing Science, 35*(1), 77–92.

Sitterding, M. C., Ebright, P., Broome, M., Patterson, E. S., & Wuchner, S. (2014). Situation awareness and interruption handling during medication administration. *Western Journal of Nursing Research, 36*(7), 891–916.

Sossong, A. E., Cullen, S., Theriault, P., Stetson, A., Higgins, B., Roche, S., & Patillo, D. (2009). Renewing the spirit of nursing: Embracing evidence-based practice in a rural state. *Nursing Clinics of North America, 44*(1), 33–42.

Sternin, J. (2007). *Positive deviance: Moving from intractable problems to successful outcomes.* Allentown, NJ: Plexus Institute.

Strout, T. D., Lancaster, K., & Schultz, A. A. (2009). Development and implementation of an inductive model for evidence-based practice: A grassroots approach for building evidence-based practice capacity in staff nurses. *Nursing Clinics of North America, 44*(1), 93–102.

Thompson, D. I., Classen, D. C., & Haug, P. J. (2006). EHRs in the fourth stage: The future of electronic health records based on the experience at Intermountain Healthcare. *Journal of Healthcare Information Management, 21*(3), 49–60.

Topol, E. (2015). *The patient will see you now: The future of medicine is in your hands.* New York, NY: Basic Books.

Trangenstein, P. A., Weiner, E. E., Gordon, J. S., & McArthur, D. (2009). Nursing informatics for future nurse scholars: Lessons learned with the doctorate of nursing practice (DNP). *Studies in Health Technology & Informatics, 146,* 551–555.

Transforming care at the bedside: Using a team approach to give nurses—and their patients—new voices in providing high-quality care. (2005). *Quality Letter in Health Care Leadership, 17*(11), 1–8.

Tunis, S. R., Stryer, D. B., & Clancy, C. M. (2003). Practice clinical trials: Increasing the value of clinical research for decision making in clinical and health policy. *Journal of the American Medical Association (JAMA), 290*(12), 1624–1632

Ulrich, D., Zenger, J., & Smallwood, N. (2013). *Results-based leadership.* Boston, MA: Harvard Business Press.

Upenieks, V. V., Akhavan, J., & Kotlerman, J. (2008). Value-added care: A paradigm shift in patient care delivery. *Nursing Economics, 26*(5), 294.

Upenieks, V. V., Needleman, J. Soban, L., Pearson, M. L., Parkerton, P., & Yee, T. (2008). The relationship between the volume and type of transforming care at the bedside innovations and changes in nurse vitality. *Journal of Nursing Administration, 38*(9) 386–394.

U.S. Department of Health and Human Services Agency for Healthcare Research and Quality. (2014, April 16). *Outpatient diagnostic errors affect 1 in 20 U.S. adults, AHRQ study finds.* Rockville, MD: Author. Retrieved from http://www.ahrq.gov/news/newsroom/press-releases/2014/diagnostic_errors.html

U.S. Department of Labor Bureau of Labor Statistics. (2015). *Occupational outlook handbook: Registered nurses job outlook.* Retrieved from http://www.bls.gov/ooh/healthcare/registered-nurses.htm#tab-6

U.S. Health Resources and Services Administration. (2001). *Report to Congress on telemedicine.* Washington, DC: Author.

U.S. Office of Inspector General. (2014, February). *Adverse events in skilled nursing facilities: National incidence among Medicare beneficiaries.* Washington, DC: Author.

Viney, M., Batcheller, J., Houston, S., & Belcik, K. (2006). Transforming care at the bedside: Designing new care systems in an age of complexity. *Journal of Nursing Care Quality, 21*(2), 143–150.

Vogus, T. J., Cooil, B., Sitterding, M., & Everett, L. Q. (2014). Safety organizing, emotional exhaustion, and turnover in hospital nursing units. *Medical Care, 52*(10), 870–876.

Vogus, T. J., & Sutcliffe, K. M. (2007). The impact of safety organizing, trusted leadership, and care pathways on reported medication errors in hospital nursing units. *Medical Care, 45*(10), 997–1002.

Vratny, A., & Shriver, D. (2007). A conceptual model for growing evidence-based practice. *Nursing Administration Quarterly, 31*(2), 162–170.

Waddell, A. W. (2009). Cultivating quality: Shared governance supports evidence-based practice. *American Journal of Nursing, 109*(11), 53–57.

Weber, V., & Joshi, M. S. (2000). Effecting and leading change in health care organizations. *Joint Commission Journal on Quality and Patient Safety, 26*(7), 388–399.

Weick, K. E., & Sutcliffe, K. M. (2011). *Managing the unexpected: Resilient performance in an age of uncertainty* (Vol. 8). Hoboken, NJ: John Wiley & Sons.

Welton, J. M. (2011). Hospital nursing workforce costs, wages, occupational mix, and resource utilization. *Journal of Nursing Administration, 41*(7/8), 309–314.

West, M. A., Borrill, C., Dawson, J., Scully, J., Carter, M., Anelay, S., . . . Waring, J. (2002). The link between the management of employees and patient mortality in acute hospitals. *International Journal of Human Resource Management, 13*(8), 1299–1310.

Westfall, J. M., Mold, J., & Fagnan, L. (2007). Practice-based research—"Blue Highways" on the NIH roadmap, *Journal of the American Medical Association (JAMA), 297*(4), 403–406.

Westra, B. L., & White-Delaney, C. (2008, November). Informatics competencies for nursing and health care leaders. *AMIA Annual Symposium Proceedings, 2008*, 804–808.

Wheatley, M. J. (2006). *Leadership and the new science: Discovering order in a chaotic world* (3rd ed.). San Francisco, CA: Berrett-Kohler.

White, K., (1967). Improved medical statistics and health systems. *Public Health Reports, 82*, 847–854.

Willson, D. F., Landrigan, C. P., Horn, S. D., & Smout, R. J. (2003). Complications in infants hospitalized for bronchiolitis or respiratory syncytial virus pneumonia. *Journal of Pediatrics, 143*(5), 142–149.

Wolf, F., Triolo, O., & Ponte, P. R. (2008). Magnet recognition program: The next generation. *Journal of Nursing Administration, 38*(4), 200–204.

Womack, J. P., & Jones, D. T. (2005, March). Lean consumption. *Harvard Business Review, 83*(3), 58–68.

Wong, C. A., & Cummings, G. G. (2007). The relationship between nursing leadership and patient outcomes: A systematic review. *Journal of Nursing Management, 15*(5), 508–521.

World Health Organization. (2006). The world health report 2006: Working together for health. Geneva, Switzerland: Author.

CHAPTER 9

Creating and Shaping the Organizational Environment and Culture to Support Practice Excellence

Megan R. Winkler and Elaine Sorensen Marshall

There are two ways of being creative. One can sing and dance. Or one can create an environment in which singers and dancers flourish.
—*Warren G. Bennis*

OBJECTIVES

- *To describe the importance of organizational environments and cultures and how these relate to positive patient, health care provider, and organizational outcomes*
- *To provide an overview of the components of and ways to create a culture of practice excellence in a health care organization*
- *To identify particular approaches to building safe environments for all individuals within a health care system*
- *To describe mentoring approaches to support the next generation of health care leaders*

Environment and culture matter. They matter to patients, health care providers, and other health care staff. The importance of place and culture as dynamic aspects of individual health and behavior is not new (Alter, 2013; Cummins, Curtis, Diez-Roux, & Macintyre, 2007). Who we are is inextricably related to where we are (Torkington, 2012) and, thus, signifies the critical implications of the landscapes for the health and well-being of patients, families, staff, and providers. The challenge for the health care leader is to assure not only that the complex holistic links between people and their environment are recognized but that organizational environments and cultures are built to enhance health and healing for all.

Many challenges and obstacles abound to successfully build and manage such environments in health care systems (Dixon-Woods, McNicol, Martin, 2012; Parmelli et al., 2011). Several of these challenges, in part, relate to the rapid cultural and structural evolution of U.S. hospitals from the authoritarian—yet caring—local landmarks of progress, science, and technical procedures to the much more corporate and complex systems they are today. These changes require a shift in organizational leadership—from top-down approaches focused on control to leadership approaches that create conditions and environments that foster relationships and collaboration for productive, adaptive outcomes (Ford, 2009; Shi & Singh, 2015).

This chapter introduces some of the ways leaders can nurture the relationships and build the conditions to promote best care for patients and families and best working conditions for providers and staff. Specifically, we review how to build and maintain a culture of practice excellence, how to build safe environments for all people to thrive, and interpersonal and organizational techniques useful to develop the future leaders of health care. As these strategies are examined, it is important to have a basic understanding of the diverse settings where nursing leaders serve.

SETTINGS FOR CURRENT AND FUTURE HEALTH CARE

The reality is that the future point of service in health care continues to extend beyond the hospital setting. This challenges our traditional thinking that persists in viewing hospitals as the center of the health care system infrastructure. Given this, it is valuable to consider the growing diversity of practice settings. Reviewing the breadth of purpose of care settings from prevention to curative, and their unique challenges moving forward, helps us think about the potential adaptations needed in leadership. Different settings present specific purposes and complexities and multiple ways for leaders to support and shape culture and environment.

Primary Care Environments

Primary care can be viewed as the first level of contact for people entering the health care system. It is best conceptualized as an approach to providing health care rather than a list of specific services (Shi & Singh, 2015). Within the U.S. health care system, primary care environments are of growing focus and concern. Among issues of the shortage of primary care physicians (Bodenheimer, Grumbach, & Berenson, 2009; Kane et al., 2009; Petterson et al., 2012), the national steps made for all Americans to possess health insurance and access to care, and an increasingly entrepreneurial approach among large health systems to acquire small, independent primary care practices (Sealover, 2015), primary care has been firmly placed in the conversations of today's greatest health care challenges.

The role of nursing in U.S. primary care remains one of both opportunity and relative adversity. Across the United States, more than 55,000 primary care nurse practitioners ([NPs]; advance practice nurses or APNs) stand poised with the preparation to alleviate provider shortages and inadequate access to patients (U.S. Agency for Healthcare Research and Quality [USAHRQ], 2014). Yet, in as many as 28 states, serious limitations on scope of practice and regulation parity with medicine continue (National Council of State Boards of Nursing, 2016; Pearson, 2009; Phillips, 2015). At present, APNs comprise approximately 20% of the primary care workforce (USAHRQ, 2014), and consistently demonstrate similar or better outcomes than their physician colleagues across a range of health indicators (Buerhaus, DesRoches, Dittus, & Donelan, 2015; Hing, Hooker, & Ashman, 2011; Newhouse et al., 2011; Stanik-Hutt et al., 2013). Yet, "increasing the number of NPs alone will not address the deficiencies in primary care delivery because many policy and practice setting barriers affect NPs' ability to offer services at the full range of their educational preparation and competencies" (Poghosyan, Boyd, & Clarke, 2016, p. 146). Moreover, disagreement proliferates between physicians and APNs regarding their respective roles in primary care (Donelan, DesRoches, Dittus, & Buerhaus, 2013) and how patients and the public perceive and view these roles (American Academy of Family Physicians, 2012; Budzi, Lurie, Singh, & Hooker, 2010). These and other unique challenges, such as roles and responsibilities of registered nurses in primary care, ways to facilitate collaboration with physicians (McInnes, Peters, Bonney, & Halcomb, 2015), and the role of nurses in patient-centered medical homes (American Academy of Nurse Practitioners [AANP], 2016b; American Nurses Association [ANA], 2010; Carver & Jessie, 2011; Robezneiks, 2012) are critical for leaders to address as they strive to provide the best preventive, acute, and chronic care to patients and families.

Community and Rural Settings

Community nursing leadership claims an inspiring history from the moment Lillian Wald set out to establish Henry Street Settlement and officially launched public health nursing. Today's community-based nursing centers, from school-based clinics and academic outreach centers to faith-based organizations, represent this legacy. Such centers serve the poor, underserved, and marginalized in both urban and rural settings and are led by practitioners who understand how these circumstances are produced from the social determinants of health. As it is expected that the need for such centers will only increase, the need for leadership is critical to identify the best way to care for people and populations who live in these diverse settings.

It is important to remember that the population of much of our nation, and the world, resides in rural environments, and each setting presents its own unique challenges for leadership. Such challenges include a decreasing ability of rural hospitals to survive financially, unique patient populations and aging communities, limited services, patient acuity and volume issues, workforce shortages, nurse staffing problems, and communication challenges—to name a few (Hall & Owings, 2014; Hunsberger, Baumann, Blythe, & Crea, 2009; MacDowell, Glasser, Fitts, Nielsen, & Hunsaker, 2010; Montour, Baumann, Blythe, & Hunsberger,

2009). In these communities, rural residents generally have poorer health status and less access to professional care than do urban families (Smith, Humphreys, & Wilson, 2008; Wallace et al., 2010; Weaver, Geiger, Lu, & Case, 2013). Moreover, practitioners and leaders in rural settings are often isolated by distance among areas of service from colleagues, thus limiting mutual leadership support.

Yet, despite these challenges, there are great opportunities for rural health care leaders to optimize resources to improve health in their communities. Personal, cultural, and family attachments to rural communities are often strong, demonstrated by some as an exceptional attachment to community and a sense of home (Hayes, 2006). Tapping into this loyalty and attachment to place may be an important clue as leaders seek to address some of the previously listed staffing and infrastructure challenges. Leaders and practitioners will also require a generalist approach to care, along with creativity, flexibility, and a broad knowledge base, to meet the distinct and varied needs of these communities (Montour et al., 2009). Furthermore, leaders need their own support systems and should strive to overcome their geographical distance by collaborating with leaders from other settings. Reaching out and connecting to other leaders can help facilitate (a) the development of mutual support, as leaders in other rural settings may experience similar issues (Hall, Weaver, Handfeld-Jones, & Bouvette, 2008); (b) partnerships for additional services, as larger care systems may be able to provide specialized care to patients via telehealth (American Hospital Association, 2011); and (c) assistance in implementing some of the core leadership competencies in rural health settings, such as understanding designated reimbursement mechanisms and developing leadership skills for dealing with multidisciplinary management teams (Robertson & Cockley, 2004).

Home as Place for Care

The patient or family home is another environment of care where leadership seeks definition. Home has special meaning for each person, group, and population, and is not necessarily confined to a domicile but may be perceived as a family, neighborhood, community, cultural or ethnic group, or nation. The meaning of home is diverse, ranging from a discrete place of personal power, security and safety, togetherness, or self-reconciliation to a transitional process of nesting to achieve integration of person with place (Molony, 2010). While some have proposed a model that recognizes home as significant to home health care (Williams, 2004), what continues to be missing is a definition of home as a center for health care, healing, and caregiving (Marshall, 2008).

Home is where health care began—it was the place where babies were born, where the sick received care, and where the dying and bereaved were comforted. Physicians and nurses aided as guests in homes, and family members were the primary caregivers (Marshall, 2008). Eventually, science and technology formalized health care, and moved it from homes to institutions. Hospitals have been the center of care through most of the 20th century. However, care is again beginning to shift back to the home in response to increasing costs and efficiency of medical treatments; shortened hospital stays; increasing informal treatment of chronic illness and disabilities; decreased institutionalization for mental illness, physical disabilities, and the aging population; and the growing palliative care and hospice movements (Boughton & Halliday, 2009; Henriksen, Joseph, Zayas-Caban, 2009; Marshall, 2008). This shift demonstrates important improvements in patient outcomes, such as in pain and wound care (Data. Medicare.gov, 2015), but is simultaneously met with cuts in payment rates for home health care services from policy makers and a continued fragmented approach to home health payment from Medicare that emphasizes volume over value (Lee & Schiller, 2015). In addition, care is once again assigned to family members. As portions of care, time, and financial responsibility are reallocated in some capacity to these caregivers (Dybwik, Tollali, Nielsen, & Brinchmann, 2011; Marshall, 2008), a number of consequences may result for family caregivers' own well-being and financial security (American Association of Retired Persons Public Policy Institute, 2009; Dybwik et al., 2011).

Therefore, the implications of the home environment for care are greater than one might imagine for health care leaders across all settings. The patient or family home is part of the entire spectrum of patient care and healing. Attention to the complex implications of the home environment for care is imperative to promote clinical practice interventions, policy, and leadership that recognizes all aspects of the family and health environment; accepts all aspects of the patient and family experience; supports patient and family strength and resilience; reduces informal caregiver burden; reduces financial hardship on the family and household; preserves the privacy and sanctity of home; and promotes the general health of all members of the community. How leaders address the patient's home is an indicator of their vision and sensitivity to all environments and settings for care.

Health Care Practice Settings and Beyond

Despite the increasing shift in care to the home and community, the large majority of nurses (63.2%) continue to provide care in hospital settings (U.S. Health Resources and Services Administration, 2013), and federal projections predict that the demand for registered nurses in hospitals will climb 36% by 2020 (American Association of Colleges of Nursing, 2015). As a result, many of you may find yourselves leading in these inpatient and outpatient hospital-based settings. Leadership at the executive level in these settings requires multiple skills and knowledge of the health care environment to implement strategic operations and to guide and execute cultural changes. For those who find themselves in the highest ranked administrative positions—such as a vice president, chief nursing officer, or chief executive officer—leadership is critical, as these individuals are responsible not only for developing strategies to promote practice excellence in clinical care, education, and research but also for simultaneously ensuring that strategies and practices are consistent with the organization's mission, vision, and values (Hader, 2009).

Beyond the settings of health care are many others where expert clinicians may find themselves taking leadership roles—for example, at insurance firms, to create more affordable and accessible insurance for their customers (Campaign for Action, 2015); or in academic institutions, to help educate the next generation of nurses, APNs, and health care leaders. Further, with increased knowledge of legal and political issues, expert clinicians are ideally poised to shape national and even international health policy (Bahadori & Fitzpatrick, 2009). Indeed, it is the leaders who are informed by clinical practice who are the ones who will continue to make a significant difference in health care reform to meet the needs of American and global citizens. Innovative opportunities abound in areas and settings not yet imagined. Whole new industries, models, and environments wait to be invented to prevent illness, relieve suffering, and promote healing—and it may be your clinical expertise and leadership that helps to create or sustain these groundbreaking approaches to health care.

CREATING AND SUSTAINING A CULTURE OF EXCELLENCE IN CARE DELIVERY AND PROFESSIONAL SUPPORT

Among the many important areas a leader in health care must influence, the shaping and preservation of an organizational culture of excellence is one of the most fundamental. Culture includes nearly every aspect of our lives. It involves the values, knowledge, beliefs, and attitudes that are shared within a social group and learned through processes of social interaction. It assists us in making sense of the behavior of others and helps us to know what behaviors are appropriate or accepted in various life domains (Schein, 2012). In health care organizations:

> Culture rules. The point of service is driven by the culture of the patient population, and the system is driven by the culture of its community, which gives it purpose, and the culture of its members or workers, who give it focus. These constituencies converge to drive the system to thrive. (Porter-O'Grady & Malloch, 2015, p. 60)

Health care organizational cultures possess highly unique features. Individuals and populations of patients (indeed, the very experience of being a patient) contribute their own subculture to the entire gestalt of the organization. The significant interchange, characterized by an intimacy and urgency known only to health care leaders, caregivers, and patients, creates a supernal uniqueness to the culture. Such a culture merits the most rigorous scrutiny, best thinking, and most devoted commitment to it truly becoming a culture of excellence for patient caring and healing.

And, just as important as the culture of excellence created for patient care is the culture of excellence created for supporting those who give their lives to promote health and provide care for the suffering. The environment must be as healthy for those who work as it is for those who are served. For the past 30 years, leaders in nursing have been investigating work environments that support nursing practice, recruitment, and retention (Kramer & Hafner, 1989). They have begun to identify how such factors are critical not only to workforce outcomes, such as productivity, turnover/burnout, and satisfaction (Aiken et al., 2011b; Baernholdt & Mark, 2009; Gunnarsdottir, Clarke, Rafferty, Nutbeam, 2009; Lewis & Malecha, 2011; Warshawsky & Sullivan Havens, 2011), but to the patient outcomes, such as reduced falls and medication errors, quality care, hospital-acquired infections, and mortality (Aiken et al., 2011a, 2011b; Duffield et al., 2011; Wong, Cummings, & Ducharme, 2013).

Culture of Excellence

To understand whether a culture of excellence needs to be built, leaders in health care must first understand what a culture of excellence might look like. One model that is helpful in conceptualizing this is the American Nurses' Credentialing Center (ANCC) Magnet® Model. In this model, a culture of excellence has five connected components:

1. Transformational leadership
2. Structural empowerment
3. Exemplary professional practice
4. New knowledge, innovations, and improvements
5. Empirical outcomes

Each component possesses several crucial elements, some of which include (a) having strategically positioned nursing leadership advocating on behalf of staff and patients; (b) creating decision-making structures and processes that facilitate the influence of direct care to boardroom nurses on the organization's operations and patient care practices; (c) ensuring effective and efficient care is provided through interprofessional collaboration to produce high-quality patient outcomes; (d) integrating research and evidence-based practice to generate innovations and improvements in clinical care and organizational processes; and, (e) obtaining reliable and valid empirical measurements of quality outcomes related to leadership and patient care (ANCC, 2016).

It is important to distinguish that we refer here to the *ANCC Magnet Model*, rather than *Magnet Status*—a recognition limited to hospital-based organizations providing acute care services. Despite data demonstrating that Magnet Status hospitals show a 14% lower mortality risk, 12% lower fail-to-rescue rates, a more highly educated nursing workforce, and better work environments than non-Magnet hospitals (Kelly, McHugh, & Aiken, 2011; McHugh et al., 2013), other research demonstrates better outcomes in terms of patient care, staffing, and nurse satisfaction among non-Magnet facilities (Goode, Blegen, Park, Vaughn, & Spetz, 2011). Several explanations for these variations may exist, but one to consider is that leaders do not necessarily need Magnet recognition to implement the important components of practice excellence from the Magnet Model. Striving to build a culture of excellence rather than obtaining a particular status allows leadership to avoid viewing the Magnet Status as a destination, as "too often the standards are treated as a maximum possible achievement instead of a continuing journey toward nursing excellence" (Summers & Summers, 2015, para. 2).

Moreover, accepting the ANCC Magnet Model as a framework for building and sustaining of a culture of excellence carries a simultaneous risk of over-simplifying this goal and the process to get there. Therefore, it is crucial that leaders—even those of Magnet-recognized facilities—judiciously examine the limitations and gaps of the model (Summers, 2012; Summers & Summers, 2015). Transformational leaders consider how they can move their organizations to fill these important gaps and continue to improve patient health and provider well-being beyond that required of the recognition. Individual standards of excellence and unique initiatives toward the highest standards are the hallmarks of transformational leaders.

Creating and Sustaining a Culture of Excellence

Building or supporting any culture, let alone one of excellence, takes a reorientation on the part of health care leaders—to first recognize the presence and power of an organization's culture. Regardless of the qualifications of the leader, no proposed mission, vision, or strategy for change that is not consistent with the existing organizational culture has a chance of success. Why? Because *culture eats strategy and structure for breakfast every day* (Kibort, 2005; Wesley, 2014). Despite our common orientation to "solve problems" as leaders (and as health care providers) (Ross, 2011), culture has a way of defending against anything that changes its tradition or comfort and will fight at every turn to maintain itself (Wesley, 2014). Thus, as a transformational leader, you must identify an organization's culture; recognize that many of its characteristics, strengths, and challenges are likely long-standing; and, understand that creating sustainable changes in the organizational culture is one of the most important approaches to achieving any outcomes you desire.

Second, effective organizational leaders realize that we are often uncon-scious of the organizational cultures in which we work. Values, assumptions, beliefs, patterns of behavior, and relationships are often woven so deeply into the organization that we may take them for granted. "We get so deeply entrenched in the cultures that we are a part of that we don't even realize how much they are informing the way *we* do things" (Ross, 2011, p. 184) and how our behaviors and actions contribute to the perpetuation of the orga-nizational culture's norms and values. This level of unawareness can create even greater challenges for leaders as they attempt to make cultural changes. The transformational leader is informed, visionary, and able to see beyond and outside self and setting.

Ross (2011) proposed an organizational change model that is highly helpful in thinking about this continual process of constructing cultural change.

Resistant organizational cultures can confine leaders to tactical and operational decisions, preventing them from directing energy toward vision or strategic decisions. Therefore, having strategies available to use in creating and sustaining cultural change is crucial for any organizational leader. While Ross (2011) developed this phase-oriented process specifically to promote organizational diversity and inclusion, it is presented here as a way of creating a change in culture to one of practice excellence.

Ross (2011) explained that to create change we must first shift consciousness in how we approach the work of creating a culture of excellence. A positive, favorable vision, or collective identity, that is integrated into the fabric of the organization must first be developed—not by leaders in solitude, but rather by collecting a group of staff members who represent a microcosm of the organization. Once a vision is created of where the organization wants to go toward practice excellence, the next phase is to comprehend where the organization is at present. All too often, "we are oriented toward finding the things we can do rather than really working to understand the system that is in place and the ways that various aspects of that system affect one another" (Ross, 2011, p. 180).

Assessing the culture of an organization can be a lengthy process but is vital. Transformational leaders listen and engage organizational members in honest exchange and generative dialogue. This is facilitated by communication methods, such as inviting all to participate in negotiations, building upon previous ideas, clarifying ideas, and affirming alternative ideas proposed by others (Thomas, Sargent, & Hardy, 2011). Effective leaders also create other avenues for assessment and evaluation of the organization's history, mission and values, legends, stories, culture, environment, and other leverage points. They observe who and how people enter the organization, how people learn within the organization, and how people fail or thrive in the organization. Leaders learn from their followers, value them, and then build on their experiences.

In addition to other phases required for cultural change (e.g., strategic planning, building new systems and structures, and overcoming "this-is-the-way-we-do-it-here" syndromes), providing stakeholder education and development, developing trust, and moving a culture of excellence from one created to one sustained requires an ongoing structure in place to measure accountability to the vision and its goals. Organizational cultures are not fixed elements; thus, consistent feedback as to how the cultural change is progressing or regressing is key. Moreover, regeneration, which is regular renewal of the organizational culture by acknowledging accomplishments and building upon them, is important to keeping the culture energetic, vibrant, and ready to react to the needs of the workforce, patients, and community (Ross, 2011).

Organizational cultures are always creating themselves—whether you are aware or unaware of their existence or want them to or not. But leadership does matter (Kibort, 2005). Therefore, the important question for leaders is, "Will you consciously create the culture in your organization, or will it unconsciously create itself while you try to survive it?" (Ross, 2011, p. 212).

REFLECTION QUESTIONS

1. The ANCC Magnet Model helps reframe the question for an organization from "What do you do?" to "What difference have you made?" (Drenkard, 2010). While understanding that outcomes accomplished are important, what other questions should be asked? Why are these other questions as or more important than identifying the outcome differences you have made?
2. Why is it important for leaders to avoid framing Magnet Status as a destination? If you have worked at a Magnet-recognized organization, how do the leadership and workforce frame this recognition?
3. Does the leadership in your current or most recent work setting recognize the power of organizational culture? If they do, what behaviors or actions do leaders take that make it evident they value the significance of culture? If you perceive that they do not, what makes you think that?

GENERATING AND NURTURING SAFE ENVIRONMENTS WHERE PEOPLE CAN THRIVE

Along the leadership journey to build and sustain a culture of excellence, one of the most important tasks is the creation of a safe environment where all people can thrive—including an organization's providers, staff, patients, and families. While the phrase *safe environment* may conjure images of personal protective equipment, safety programs to avoid back injury or needle sticks, hand hygiene, and clean worksites (which are clearly important), the focus here is on the environmental features that protect against stress, disempowerment, and dissatisfaction among patients and health care workers. Multiple approaches can certainly be used to create such environments, but the four presented here attend to building social relationships and environments that protect, encourage, liberate, and support the health and well-being of all individuals within an organization. Specifically, they include the following: (a) understanding the principles of providing cultural care for patients and families, (b) creating inclusive environments for health care workers, (c) managing power inequities inherent in interprofessional practice, and (d) eliminating incivility and workplace violence to develop a culture of respect and trust.

Providing Cultural Care for Patients and Families

Often, when health care providers and leaders discuss *culture*, we refer to the diverse personal, ethnic, and community contexts of patients and not the *cultures* that exist within the workplace. This focus on cultural care for patients and families is one that has received ever-increasing attention over the past several decades. In fact, it is now commonly accepted that two important steps toward the elimination of health disparities among diverse populations are to (a) create a health care workforce that better reflects the general population in terms of gender, race, and ethnicity, and (b) better prepare health care leaders and providers in culturally competent care (Dogra, Reitmanova, & Carter-Pokras, 2010; Institute of Medicine, 2010).

Though these requirements may be recognized, the action steps needed to fully accomplish them are dawdling at best. For example, while White females comprise only 31.7% of the general U.S. population and White males 30.7% (Pew Research Center, 2015), White women constitute approximately 70% of registered nurses (McMenamin, 2015) and White men 47.5% of physicians (Association of American Medical Colleges, 2015). These staggering differences have implications for addressing the goal of educating providers to deliver culturally competent care. Further, it is unclear whether our predominantly White health care faculty is prepared to teach cultural competence and to integrate cultural competence into pedagogies to further increase the diversity of our health care workforce (Beard, 2013, 2014).

Consequently, it is no surprise that the concept of cultural competence has become such a predominant topic of discussion in health care education and practice (Jeffreys, 2010). Unfortunately, its vague and numerous definitions along with an overuse of the phrase have sustained uncertainty about its original meaning. Meanwhile, other terms have been promoted to extend beyond cultural competence, such as *cultural proficiency*, *cultural humility*, and *cultural sensitivity* (Foster, 2009; Kosoko-Lasaki & Cook, 2009; Purnell, 2013). But these concepts also run the risk of eventually losing their meaning. Thus, instead of providing a list of definitions and characteristics related to different terminology, it may be more helpful to present some of the underlying principles basic to cultural care among patients and families.

The goal of cultural care is not simply to learn and appreciate the culture *of others*, it must also include examining *one's own* biases and cultural limitations (Chang, Simon, & Dong, 2012; Dogra, Reitmanova, & Carter-Pokras, 2009; Hawala-Druy & Hill, 2012; Levi, 2009; Sabin & Greenwald, 2012). Although becoming familiar with aspects of other cultures is desirable, one should not limit oneself to basic familiarity or a "mastery of lists of 'different' . . . beliefs and behaviors supposedly pertaining to certain groups" (Hunt, 2001, p. 135). Rather, those who desire to provide the most excellent cultural care should be willing to engage in lifelong self-awareness and self-critique of the limitations of their own cultural perspectives and openness to new ideas and new cultures. Similarly, sensitive leaders and providers recognize the individual heterogeneity inherent in any cultural group and interact with patients as individuals, not as representatives from a group (Nacoste, 2015). Not every individual of a particular racial, ethnic, religious, or linguistic group possesses identical cultural views and values; rather, views and values are learned and held by individuals who see themselves as members of a certain group (Thagard, 2012). Thus, the sensitive leader and provider examine and consider unconscious bias or prejudice to ascribe cultural characteristics to all from a certain group.

Moreover, cultural care is not a static state that one achieves, but rather a process (Beard, Gwanmesia, & Miranda-Diaz, 2015). It is impossible to know everything about another's culture, and providers will constantly be interacting with patients whose various cultures affect the patient–provider relationship in different ways. As a result, effective leaders commit to modeling and supporting care providers in a lifetime of learning and openness to experiences, to lifelong self-reflection and sensitivity to power imbalances in culture within the patient–provider relationship, and to recognizing the value that these cultural differences provide (Kumagai & Lypson, 2009; PricewaterhouseCoopers, 2014; Simon, Chang, & Dong, 2010; Tervalon & Murray-Garcia, 1998).

Creating an Inclusive Environment for Health Care Workers

The principles and approaches to cultural care described for relationships between health care providers and patients certainly can extend to our direct relationships with staff and colleagues. However, creating an organizational culture that is respectful and inclusive of all people requires much more effort, time, and growth than these individual-level principles can provide and is something that few, if any, organizations in the United States have been able to fully accomplish. Dramatic examples of organizational failures in this area are demonstrated by persistent lower retention rates among women and people of color in the workplace (Ross, 2011). For example, among Fortune 500 companies only 24 (4.8%) women (Swanson, 2015) and five (1%) Black Americans (Wallace, 2015) are chief executive officers, and "glass-ceiling" and other effects persist for women and people of color at all senior levels in industry and higher education, including health care (Cook & Glass, 2013; Jackson, O'Callaghan, & Leon, 2014). Although not apparent in the outcomes of these examples, U.S. academic institutions, health care organizations, and other businesses have actually increased the focus on diversity and inclusion efforts over the past generation. Despite these investments of money and time, "organizations continue to struggle to find effective ways to bring people from diverse backgrounds together with a sense of common purpose and commitment to create new possibilities for action" (Ross, 2011, p. 13).

The reasons for this predicament, and the numerous strategies necessary to change it, are too involved for discussion here. As a health care leader, you have only to look at the current state of affairs in your own organization. Likely, it is not much different from most, which have invested significant time and money into incremental approaches to diversity and inclusion programs, to limited effect (Ross, 2011). If so, you have a critical opportunity to recognize these circumstances and commit to changing them by (a) supporting your organization through an ongoing cultural shift to become an inclusive, respectful, antiracist, multicultural institution accepting of neo-diversity, and (b) taking and persevering in the crucial steps to create these changes (see Box 9.1). Simply put:

> the state of diversity in our country and in our organizations is at
> a point of crisis. . . . at an incipient point of history in which we

BOX 9.1. TOOLS TO ASSESS CULTURAL COMPETENCE

Several tools assess various aspects of an individual's cultural competence, as well as the culture that exists within a health care setting. We encourage you to access one of these tools, complete the questionnaire/assessment, and reflect on what this means for you, your organization, or both. Some tools to consider can be found at **http://iengage. multicultural.ufl.edu/resources/campus_resources/cultural_competence_resources/.**
Additional tools to consider include

- Transcultural Self-Efficacy Tool (TSET)
- Cultural Competence Self-Assessment Questionnaire (CCSAQ)
- Cultural Competence Clinical Evaluation Tool (CCCET)
- Clinical Setting Assessment Tool: Diversity and Disparity (CSAT-DD)
- Cultural Competency Assessment Tool for Hospitals (CCATH)

> have the opportunity to either move into a new future in which we effectively deal with the inevitable and irrevocable movement to a more diverse society and an ever-changing world, or one in which we decline into a deeper and deeper sense of tribalism, one that threatens to tear our society apart. (Ross, 2011, p. 18)

Managing the Power Inequities Inherent in Interprofessional Practice

As discussed previously, there is a growing movement that supports interprofessional practice to improve patient care. Yet, a growing body of evidence also provides insight into the complex assortment of issues inherent in this type of collaboration (Nugus, Greenfield, Travaglia, Westbrook, & Braithewaite, 2010; Reeves et al., 2009). For instance, despite ongoing commitment to interprofessional contributions to patient care, physicians continue to dominate patient management decisions in acute hospital settings, leaving other health clinicians to believe that their opportunities for input are at best *ad hoc*. Interprofessional case conferences, where many patient management decisions are discussed, are commonly led by physicians, managed authoritatively, and dominated by a biomedical discourse and physicians' "talk time." Nugus et al. (2010) reported that 67.9% of talking time in acute case conferences was conducted by physicians compared to 6.6% by nurses, 2.7% by physiotherapists, 0.5% by dieticians, and 0.5% by occupational therapists. Similarly, Reeves et al. (2009) found parallel practices during informal and unplanned interprofessional interactions—that those involving a physician and another health professional were typically terse and unidirectional from physician to other professional (e.g., asking for clinical information or requesting a task for patient care be completed). Yet, those interprofessional interactions observed among nurses, therapists, and other health professionals were often richer and consisted of negotiations related to clinical as well as social content (Reeves et al., 2009).

Among the many explanations for current interactions and barriers to full interprofessional practice, unequal power relations certainly are key. As the preceding examples illustrate, the balance of power is situated with the more established medical profession rather than more recently professionalized disciplines, such as nursing (Roberts, DeMarco, & Griffin, 2009). When there is imbalance in power, the ability to work effectively in interprofessional teams is constrained. The reasons for this power imbalance are rooted in our professional histories.

The sociohistorical circumstances leading to these power inequities, particularly between medicine and nursing, originated with the emergence of the craft guilds in the 1500s. Craft guilds were originally developed to restrict trade in goods and protected and promoted guild members' interests through their controlled ownership of knowledge—a characteristic maintained by many of the professions today (Reeves, Macmillan, & Van Soeren, 2010). During the 1800s, medicine moved from a guild to a profession by establishing itself as the recognized owner of specialized *scientific* knowledge and restricting access to those who could become a physician (via licensure, medical examinations, and creating a single standard for medical education grounded in allopathic medicine). Given that only individuals who passed the medical examination could practice medicine (by an act passed in Britain in 1858) and that few women were able to attend or obtain a university medical degree until the 20th century, medicine continued toward becoming a male-dominated profession and the only legal purveyor of care (Hall, 2005; Reeves et al., 2010).

At the same time medicine was professionalizing, patriarchy was thriving. During this time, a woman's role was either in the private sphere of the home or, if in the workforce, in a profession that embraced the virtues of womanhood (piety, purity, submission of self). Nursing was such a profession. Despite social institutional barriers, nursing itself headed toward professionalism through formalizing education and the registration of trained nurses. Professional self-regulation, however, still did not occur until as late as the 1960s for many European and European-colonized nations—nearly a century after medicine had achieved professional status. Yet, even today, the professional development of nursing continues to lag behind the model set by medicine, as achieving a single standard of nursing education remains an elusive goal in many jurisdictions and the role overlap, confusion, and conflict (e.g., among NPs, nurse anesthetists, and nurse midwives) that continues to threaten medical authority has resulted in nursing practice remaining in many locations under the direction, supervision, and permission of medicine (Caldwell & Atwal, 2003; Hall, 2005; Reeves et al., 2010; Roberts et al., 2009).

Through this history, differences in values, learning styles, and beliefs were produced between the health professions—differences often further advanced through our educational systems today. The opportunities for learners from different health disciplines and professions to interact are severely restricted due to an increasing focus on specialization that addressed the complexity of patient care and professional knowledge (Hall 2005; Reeves et al., 2010), as well as specific curricular patterns and accreditation requirements within each discipline.

"In many ways, the university continued as a 'multiversity' . . . multiple silos under one governance" (Hall, 2005, p. 191). Moreover, our professional regulatory bodies control who enters the profession and legitimize scope of practice for members while restricting select activities to others—further perpetuating a focus on professional *separateness* rather than *togetherness* (Reeves et al., 2010).

The barriers and challenges built and maintained among the health professions are great, but they are not insurmountable to visionary, effective leaders of the future. At an organizational level, leaders can help individuals from various professions work collaboratively, which can be accomplished when a common frame of reference is built from our mutually held values for holistic patient and family outcomes rather than our different professional goals and ideologies (Caldwell & Atwal, 2003; Ross, 2011). Further, health care leaders can ensure that the interprofessional team is prepared with the skills (e.g., conflict resolution, cross-professional communication) to navigate not only challenges related to blending different professional cultures (e.g., different vocabularies, different problem-solving approaches, and different views of issues and values), but the individual personalities that impact group dynamics.

Likely, there are exemplary examples of interprofessional teams already fostering a status-equal basis among members (Hall, 2005) to produce improved patient outcomes. In fact, one important place to look may be in community-based settings, as evidence demonstrates that the effectiveness of care in these settings strongly relates to more collaborative power among the different professions (Nugus et al., 2010). While all of these suggestions may help leaders to advance interprofessional collaboration in their organizations, it is important to remember that the structural configuration of the health professions, *based on a more than 500-year-old system,* "will continue to make the role of leadership a difficult one, especially as long as this history remains a largely unacknowledged factor" (Reeves et al., 2010, p. 263). Thus, it is critical that on the road ahead, health care leaders constantly evaluate progress to combat interprofessional *separateness* and shape environments that reinforce our *togetherness.*

Eliminating Incivility and Workplace Violence to Develop a Culture of Respect and Trust

Workplace violence, incivility, and bullying are barriers to developing safe environments for providers and can occur in any work setting (Luparell, 2011). These harmful events range from overt (e.g., verbally intimidating a coworker) to covert (e.g., withholding vital information to safe work) and occur through a number of actions and inactions (ANA, 2015). Too many nurses have been touched by some form of violence, bullying, and incivility, as self-report rates of these experiences consistently range from one-quarter to two-thirds of study samples (Johnson & Rea, 2009; Simons, 2008; Ulrich et al., 2006). While the level of disrespect varies across these different harmful events—from refusing to assist a coworker to hostile remarks and threats to physically and psychologically damaging actions—all produce well-documented negative outcomes for victims. Some of these include physiological or psychological distress, intention to leave the organization and nursing, and decreased personal health (ANA, 2015; Clark, Farnsworth, & Landrum, 2009; Johnson & Rea, 2009; Wilson, Diedrich, Phelps, & Choi, 2011). Subsequently, all of these outcomes can have real impacts on the care provided to patients, increasing risks to patient safety and quality care (ANA, 2015; Roche, Diers, Duffield, & Catling-Paull, 2010).

So what can be done? Leaders must work to develop and sustain a culture of respect (ANA, 2015). Respect is defined as "open-minded willingness to accept, acknowledge, and value the uniqueness of an individual and her or his knowledge, experiences, and perceptions" (Antoniazzi, 2011, p. 752), and this must be fostered in every work environment. The ANA (2015) has created a position statement to articulate the shared roles and responsibilities of nurses and employers (including nursing leaders) to create environments free of incivility, bullying, and workplace violence. Many recommendations provide strategies to prevent and mitigate these harmful events and are divided by the responsibilities of nurses and those of employers. Some recommendations call on the self-reflection of leaders to recognize any of their own vulnerabilities to acts of bullying and incivility (ANA, 2015). Some in leadership positions (e.g., managers, directors, and charge nurses) have been reported as primary sources of workplace bullying (Johnson & Rea, 2009). Thus, as an introductory step, future leaders should review and adopt these recommendations as they provide tactical strategies to creating respectful work environments for health care providers. (See Table 9.1 for selected recommendations.)

While the ANA provides helpful coverage of strategies that may prevent and manage incidences of incivility, future leaders are challenged to go beyond these recommendations to identify the problems in specific workplace environments. Zero-tolerance policies and recommendations are often instituted and may seem to be effective approaches, but in reality their success is limited as they have not addressed the root causes of incivility, bullying, and violence (Croft & Cash, 2012; Farrell, Shafiei, & Salmon, 2010). Effective leaders broadly consider the organizational rules, norms, and power structures that contribute to these events. For instance, would overtime, high staff turnover, improper patient-to-nurse ratios, constant changes in policies and procedures, and disregard from other health professionals burden and potentially exhaust nurses' time, emotional coping resources, and well-being? Might such burdens contribute to incivility? This example is not offered to "condone or excuse dysfunctional or disruptive behaviors in the workplace, but rather to problematize the reasons why 'self—and profession—defeating behavior' exist and flourish" (Croft & Cash, 2012, p. 231). It is the ethical responsibility of leaders to critically examine their organizational practices to not only identify and condemn individuals acting in uncivil and violent ways, but to "seek to eradicate those conditions that support the acts of those individuals" (Rhodes, Pullen, Vickers, Clegg, Pitsis, 2010, p. 110).

The potential eradication of contributors does not mean that conflict and disagreements will never occur in an organization again. Rather, true

TABLE 9.1 Selected Prevention Recommendations from the American Nurses Association Position Statement on Incivility, Bullying, and Workplace Violence

---

- **Primary Prevention Interventions (for Registered Nurses [RNs])**

  - Commit to and accept responsibility for establishing and promoting health interpersonal relationships with all members of the health care team
  - Be cognizant of own interactions, including actions taken and not taken and communication with others
  - Practice using suggested predetermined phrases of responses so one is prepared to deflect incivility and bullying

- **Primary Prevention Interventions (for Employers and Formal Leaders)**

  - Provide a mechanism for RNs to seek support when feeling threatened
  - Orient employees to conflict resolution and respectful communication strategies
  - Make available education sessions that define incivility and bullying, introduce prevention strategies, and review the organization's policy around bullying and incivility

- **Secondary Prevention Interventions (for RNs)**

  - Use preestablished code words or phrases to seek support when feeling threatened
  - If observing incivility or bullying, offer support to the target and let the perpetrator know his or her actions are not consistent with the organization's culture

- **Secondary Prevention Interventions (for Employers and Formal Leaders)**

  - Recognize and evaluate personal vulnerabilities to incivility and bullying and act in accordance with the organization's policy and culture
  - Implement strategies to reduce both fatigue among employees and incivility associated with fatigue
  - Offer trainings that enhance employees' psychological hardiness and resilience, self-care measures, and self-reflection practices

---

Adapted from American Nurses Association (2015).

communities include conflict as the people involved know the environment is safe enough "for conflicts and controversy to be aired, engaged in, and resolved" (Ross, 2011, p. 203). But, "the emphasis on cost containment, downsizing, skill mix changes, and decentralization" (Croft & Cash, 2012, p. 237) at an organizational level has resulted in nurses' and other health providers' lived reality being "increased workload, overtime, absenteeism, and feelings of disenfranchisement" (Croft & Cash, 2012, p. 237). This reality is often incongruent with organizational mission statements and branding, which may convey a caring and supportive milieu. The dissonance and discord between organizational positions and actual practices leaves workers with an inability to believe in the organization, decreases their emotional well-being, and creates feelings of weakness due to a lack of support in resources and in leadership (Croft & Cash, 2012; Gabrielle, Jackson, & Mannix, 2008; Goldman & Tabak, 2010; Rodwell & Gulyas, 2013).

REFLECTION QUESTIONS

Cox (1995) suggested that civil societies (or workplaces) are those in which "trust, reciprocity, mutuality, co-operation, time, social fabric and social capital are important and cultivated elements." (p. 5). Conversely: "Organizations that are authoritarian, top-down, rule bound, and competitive run the risk of creating communities in which . . . [there is] often reward through patronage, where cliques are formed, change is resisted, and those who criticize are excluded" (Croft & Cash, 2012, p. 239).

Take a moment to critically examine your own organization.

1. What are the characteristics of the work culture?
2. Does the workplace reflect the kind of nursing world in which you want to practice? If not, what is constraining the organization from adopting a safe and nurturing culture?
3. Are there particular hegemonies (i.e., social, cultural, ideological, or economic influences exerted by a dominant group) that are taken for granted within the organization?
4. How should you move forward to achieve the kind of institution you would like to see and how should we do this collectively?

Therefore, at the root of much of this discussion on safe environments is *trust*, and it is critical for leaders of health care organizations to work constantly to build a culture of trust among all members of the organization—between leaders and workers, providers and patients, and among colleagues. The growth of mutual trust may finally contribute to create an environment where all people can thrive.

MENTORING LEADERS FOR THE FUTURE

The transformational leader in health care has a constant eye on and heart for the next generation of leaders. To assure that any culture of practice excellence is sustained, leaders must habitually look beyond the present-day items at hand and focus on developing the leaders of tomorrow. The ever-changing health care industry requires that we cultivate the skillset for future leaders to navigate these dynamic and complex environments. Unfortunately, too many disciplines within health care have a kind of professional hazing (as in, "if I did it, so should you"), and too many of us are still involved in these practices, such as long hours with assigned shift work; sink-or-swim approaches; or see-one, teach-one, do-one. Such traditions simply will not work in complex environments that are constantly striving for safe, effective, and quality patient care. In addition, the skillset and competencies that future leaders need is likely different than those previously required. There are new requirements of leadership, such as having a global mindset regarding nursing and health care, an ability to appropriately intervene in policy development and political processes, a highly developed team-building and collaboration skillset, and an aptitude to actively adapt to constant change and to lead their organizations to become just as adaptive (Huston, 2008).

There are a number of approaches that leaders can use to prepare future leaders. One of the most foundational methods is mentoring. Leaders who mentor have an instinctive generativity—a "concern in establishing and guiding the next generation" (Erikson, 1963, p. 267). Yet, the leader who mentors is not only interested in helping others grow. In a way, the leader who mentors today is a leader of tomorrow—as she or he, too, has a vision for a better future and contributes to this by developing the future's leaders.

Mentoring the next generation is a huge task, but immensely beneficial for all involved. It helps to develop leadership skills; to promote empowerment; to advance and expand individual vision past individual success to the future of the nursing profession; to promote greater career mobility and job satisfaction; and to provide valuable feedback, insight, and support (Block, Claffey, Korow, & McCaffrey, 2005; Ensher & Murphy, 2011; Hart, 2010; Hodgson & Scanlan, 2013). For leaders, mentoring allows them to extend a living legacy of their own efforts, enliven their own everyday experiences, develop a renewed sense of commitment to their profession and organization, and contribute to a positive human investment in making the world a better place (Ensher & Murphy, 2011; Hodgson & Scanlan, 2013). For the organization, mentoring relationships can provide positive outcomes (e.g., increased support, increased productivity, increased work environment stability, and improved nursing retention (Block et al., 2005; Gilbert & Broome, 2015). As a future leader, think of mentorship at two levels: (a) the type of mentorship you will engage in directly with future leaders you want to cultivate, and (b) the type of mentoring culture you want to create throughout your entire organization (Bally, 2007; Jakubik, Eliades, Gavriloff, & Weese, 2011; Latham, Hogan, & Ringl, 2008; Race & Skees, 2010).

Some of the key competencies and skills that effective mentors exhibit to develop the leaders of tomorrow follow. As a mentor you will not be required to include these concurrently; rather, your approach will shift based on each mentee's individual needs and goals.

- *Develop a trusting mentoring relationship*: As a mentor it is critical to develop a relationship that facilitates trust. Treat the mentee as your colleague and equal. Assure the person that you are interested in his or her views and feelings and that a relationship has been created in which it is safe and encouraged to ask questions. Periodically checking in on how the relationship is meeting the mentee's goals and needs is a vital strategy to maintain the relationship. Remember that mentoring is always shared, and thus as the mentor, you are not the only one responsible for creating a successful relationship. The mentee will also need to be flexible, honest, and receptive to feedback and insight (Betty Irene Moore School of Nursing at U.C. Davis, n.d.; Drucker, 2000; Hart, 2010).
- *Advocate and provide opportunities*: Opening doors can have a huge impact for the mentee to develop new leadership skills and gain visibility. Involve the person in committees, work groups, or task forces, and attempt to create opportunities

that best place the mentee as a colleague where he or she can make the greatest contribution. Similarly, monitor the social environment. Are colleagues talking or not talking about your mentee? What is or is not being said? This will allow you to identify potential opportunities for your mentee or potential threats that may require you to act as an advocate (Davis, 2015; Drucker, 2000; Hart, 2010).

- *Guide and counsel*: As the relationship develops over time the mentor may begin to serve as a confidant or sounding board. This is an opportune time for mentors to help mentees understand conflict and various ways to deal with it—particularly when holding a leadership role. It also may be necessary to advise the mentee to make a particular decision or choice, but this should be based on the needs of the mentee or your mutually established goals (Hart, 2010).

- *Teach*: Teaching involves not only imparting knowledge but also sharing personal experiences. Personal stories can be effective. Share the passion and drama of your leadership experiences, how you failed and learned from the failure, what your successes were, and how you learned to survive (Hart, 2010).

- *Model*: Shadowing can be a great benefit to future leaders. Your mentee will pick up simply through observation many of your idiosyncrasies—from your values and beliefs to your style and methods. Therefore, be profoundly aware of your own behavior, for you are always teaching by example (Davis, 2015; Hart, 2010).

- *Motivate, inspire, and encourage*: Positive reinforcement, or telling mentees you see them as future leaders, is critically important to developing their confidence to see this in themselves. At times it may be important to validate a mentee's feelings and experiences. Continue to support and encourage them while letting them know you appreciate their experience (Betty Irene Moore School of Nursing, n.d.; Hart, 2010).

- *Challenge*: Challenging a mentee is a critical responsibility of the mentor and one that must be performed only when trusting relationships exist. Challenging can occur by posing thought-provoking questions that may allow mentees to see new solutions or self-reflect on their own professional blind spots. Challenging can also occur by providing experiences for mentees to develop new skills. Encourage them to take charge of a project at your organization. Provide them with the resources they will need; but then trust in them to take it from there. Strong mentoring focuses more on "teaching people *how* to think rather than telling them *what* to think" (Thompson, 2010, "Skill 1: Mentoring Questions," para. 1). However, challenging is only successful in the appropriate context. Mentees should not feel like these are sink-or-swim exercises. Thus, it is critical to know your mentees' strengths and weaknesses and provide challenges that supportively coach them just to their limits—each time allowing them to grow a little bit more (Betty Irene Moore School of Nursing, n.d.; Davis, 2015; Drucker, 2000; Thompson, 2010).

As a leader, consider the opportunities you are building in your organization for mentoring and future leadership development to thrive. In response to issues of horizontal violence and poor retention, some organizations are realizing the importance of mentoring programs, which can stimulate professional growth and improvements in staff morale, and thus produce positive outcomes related to nursing care (Bally, 2007; Block et al., 2005; Chen & Lou, 2014; Latham, et al., 2008; Race & Skees, 2010). In this view, mentoring and leadership are not seen as mutually exclusive roles, but leadership is rather understood as a collective venture and practice among all people who work together to accomplish mutual work (Ford, 2009; Latham et al., 2008; Raelin, 2015).

Critical to the success of mentorship throughout a workplace is a culture that promotes and sustains mentoring (Bally, 2007; Jakubik et al., 2011; Latham et al., 2008; Race & Skees, 2010). If the organizational culture where you work does not fit with the goals of a mentoring program, then such a program cannot be initiated or sustained. Thus, mentoring goals and values must be embedded and aligned with the organization's values, practices, and cultural environment.

There has been an amazing increase in opportunities for mentoring at all levels outside the individual organization. See Table 9.2 for examples of national mentorship programs and their specific features. Some additional tactics to contemplate when implementing mentorship programs include:

- Collaborating with and empowering staff to develop a mission statement for the work environment that incorporates and guides mentoring activities (Bally, 2007; Race & Skees, 2010)
- Providing an infrastructure that supports mentoring, including administrative support, financial resources, rewards and recognition, staff and scheduling flexibility, and protected time to mentor (Bally, 2007; Chen & Lou, 2014; Jakubik et al., 2011; Latham et al., 2008; Ramani, Gruppen, & Kachur, 2006)
- Establishing committees or a dedicated coordinator/liaison that can consistently support mentorship relationships and mentoring skill development and training (Bally, 2007; Block et al., 2005; Chen & Lou, 2014; Grindel & Hagerstrom, 2009; Latham et al., 2008; Ramani et al., 2006; Race & Skees, 2010)
- Assuring that a firm commitment exists across all levels of an organization's leadership to support the mentoring program (Grindel & Hagerstrom, 2009; Race & Skees, 2010)

This entire book is about becoming a transformational leader. If, as a leader, you want to change the culture of your organization to one of practice excellence, to develop safe environments in which all people thrive, and to help develop the emerging leaders of tomorrow—then the underlying assumption through all of this work is that the people are more important than the task and that authentically serving the people will get the task done.

TABLE 9.2 Selected Mentorship Programs to Develop Leadership Skills

LEADERSHIP PROGRAM/ ORGANIZATION	DESCRIPTION	TARGET AUDIENCE
Leader2Leader Mentorship Program/ AONE (2015)	• Six-month online mentorship program with specific milestones, tasks, and deadlines to develop nursing leadership skills via mentoring and personal relationships • Provides opportunities for long-time leaders to share experiences and emerging leaders to obtain professional guidance • Matching of mentors and mentees based on questions and interests an individual identifies • Communication occurs through online message boards and private messaging system	Experienced nurse leaders and new and emerging nurse leaders
Leadership Academies/ STTI (2015)	• Eighteen-month programs (in Gerontology, Maternal–Child Health, or Nurse Faculty) via workshops, team projects, and presentations to prepare and position nurses in various settings (health care and academy) to lead initiatives in their specific work settings (i.e., improvement of health care quality for their select population; cultivate high-performing, supportive work environments in academia) • Ongoing mentorship from a selected Leadership Mentor is a critical program component • Attendance to workshops is expected of both fellow and Leadership Mentor	Varies; fellows should be working in the area of interest; Leadership Mentors are identified by fellow prior to applying
NONPF Leadership Mentoring Program/ NONPF (2015)	• One-year program via in-person education meetings, virtual-based programs, and periodic check-ins to prepare and empower new and emerging leaders in nurse practitioner education • Mentorship occurs from mentors experienced in nursing education, personal development, program administration, etc. • Mentees meet with mentors in-person at second meeting and monthly via conference call	Nurse practitioner faculty members with 2–5 years of teaching experience
Fellows of the AANP Mentorship Program/ AANP (2016a)	• One-year program connecting motivated nurse practitioner novices with AANP Fellows who are leaders in their field and eager to share their expertise for the development of others • Involves a formalized commitment between mentor and mentee, attendance at the AANP National Conference for both parties, and development of a formalized and focused goal with objectives	Members of AANP possessing personal and professional qualities in relationship building

AANP, American Academy of Nurse Practitioners; AONE, American Organization of Nurse Executives; NONPF, National Organization of Nurse Practitioner Faculties; STTI, Sigma Theta Tau International.

REFERENCES

Aiken, L. H., Cimiotti, J. P., Sloane, D. M., Smith, H. L., Flynn, L., & Neff, D. F. (2011a). Effects of nurse staffing and nurse education on patient deaths in hospitals with different work environments. *Medical Care, 49*(12), 1047–1053.

Aiken, L. H., Sloane, D. M., Clarke, S., Poghosyan, L., Cho, E., You, L., . . . Aungsuroch, Y. (2011b). Importance of work environments on hospital outcomes in nine countries. *International Journal for Quality in Health Care, 23*(4), 357–364.

Alter, A. (2013, June 14). Where we are shapes who we are. *New York Times.* Retrieved from http://www.nytimes.com/2013/06/16/opinion/sunday/a-self-defined-by-place.html?_r=2

American Academy of Family Physicians. (2012). Patient perceptions regarding health care providers. Retrieved from http://www.aafp.org/dam/AAFP/documents/about_us/initiatives/PatientPerceptions.pdf

American Academy of Nurse Practitioners. (2016a). FAANP mentorship program. Retrieved from https://www.aanp.org/fellows-program/faanp-mentorship-program

American Academy of Nurse Practitioners. (2016b). Fact sheet: The medical home: What is it? How do nurse practitioners fit in? Retrieved from https://www.aanp.org/legislation-regulation/federal-legislation/medicare/68-articles/349-the-medical-home.

American Association of Colleges of Nursing. (2015). Nursing fact sheet. Retrieved from http://www.aacn.nche.edu/media-relations/fact-sheets/nursing-fact-sheet

American Association of Retired Persons Public Policy Institute. (2009). Beyond 50.09 chronic care: A call to action for health reform. Retrieved from http://www.aarp.org/health/medicare-insurance/info-03-2009/beyond_50_hcr.html

American Hospital Association. (2011). *TrendWatch: The opportunities and challenges for rural hospitals in an era of health reform.* Washington, DC: Author. Retrieved from http://www.aha.org/research/reports/tw/11apr-tw-rural.pdf

American Nurses Association. (2010). Solving the crisis in primary care: The role of nurse practitioners, certified nurse-midwives, and certified midwives. *ANA Issue Brief.* Retrieved from http://www.nursingworld.org/MainMenuCategories/Policy-Advocacy/Positions-and-Resolutions/Issue-Briefs/APRNs-as-PCPs.pdf

American Nurses Association. (2015). Incivility, bullying, and workplace violence. Retrieved from http://www.nursingworld.org/MainMenuCategories/Workplace Safety/Healthy-Nurse/bullyingworkplaceviolence/Incivility-Bullying-and-Workplace-Violence.html

American Nurses Credentialing Center. (2016). Magnet recognition program new model. Retrieved from http://www.nursecredentialing.org/documents/magnet/newmodelbrochure.aspx

American Organization of Nurse Executives. (2016). AONE leader2leader member community. Retrieved from http://www.aone.org/resources/community.shtml

Antoniazzi, C. D. (2011). Respect as experienced by registered nurses. *Western Journal of Nursing Research, 33*(6), 745–766.

Association of American Medical Colleges. (2015). Section IV: Additional diversity data from the U.S. Census Bureau and the Henry J. Kaiser Family Foundation. In Diversity in the physician workforce: Facts & figures, 2014. Retrieved from http://aamcdiversityfactsandfigures.org/section-iv-additional-diversity-data/#tab2

Baernholdt, M., & Mark, B. A. (2009). The nurse work environment, job satisfaction and turnover rates in rural and urban nursing units. *Journal of Nursing Management, 17*(8), 994–1001.

Bahadori, A., & Fitzpatrick, J. J. (2009). Level of autonomy of primary care nurse practitioners. *Journal of the American Academy of Nurse Practitioners, 21*(9), 513–519.

Bally, J. M. G. (2007). The role of nursing leadership in creating a mentoring culture in acute care environments. *Nursing Economics, 25*(3), 143–148.

Beard, K. (2013). Macy faculty scholar Kenya Beard on multicultural education. Retrieved from http://macyfoundation.org/news/entry/beard-on-multicultural-education

Beard, K. (2014). *The impact of multicultural education training session on the multicultural attitudes and awareness of nurse educations: The METs project.* Poster session presented at the 26th meeting of Eastern Nursing Research Society, Philadelphia, PA. Retrieved from http://www.enrs-go.org/docs/ENRS2014Proceedings.pdf

Beard, K. V., Gwanmesia, E., & Miranda-Diaz, G. (2015). Culturally competent care: Using the ESDT model in nursing. *American Journal of Nursing, 115*(6), 58–62.

Betty Irene Moore School of Nursing at UC Davis. (n.d.). Mentoring future leaders to reach their potential. Portraits of health and nursing leadership. Retrieved from https://www.ucdmc.ucdavis.edu/nursing/Leadership/portraits_of_health/images/health_leadership_hass.pdf

Block, L. M., Claffey, C., Korow, M. K., & McCaffrey, R. (2005). The value of mentorship within nursing organizations. *Nursing Forum, 40*(4), 134–140.

Bodenheimer, T., Grumbach, K., & Berenson, R. A. (2009). A lifeline for primary care. *New England Journal of Medicine, 360*(26), 2693–2696.

Boughton, M., & Halliday, L. (2009). Home alone: Patient and carer uncertainty surrounding discharge with continuing clinical care needs. *Contemporary Nurse, 33*(1), 30–40.

Budzi, D., Lurie, S., Singh, K., & Hooker, R. (2010). Veterans' perceptions of care by nurse practitioners, physician assistants, and physicians: A comparison from satisfaction surveys. *Journal of the American Academy of Nurse Practitioners, 22*, 170–176.

Buerhaus, P. I., DesRoches, C. M., Dittus, R., & Donelan, K. (2015). Practice characteristics of primary care nurse practitioners and physicians. *Nursing Outlook, 63*(2), 144–153.

Caldwell, K., & Atwal, A. (2003). The problems of interprofessional health care practice in hospitals. *British Journal of Nursing, 12*(20), 1212–1218.

Campaign for Action. (2015). Champions of nursing: Aetna and Cigna. Retrieved from http://campaignforaction.org/news/champions-nursing-aetna-and-cigna

Carver, M. C., & Jessie, A. T. (2011, May 31). Patient-centered care in a medical home. *Online Journal of Issues in Nursing, 16*(2), Manuscript 4. Retrieved from http://www.nursingworld.org/MainMenuCategories/ANAMarketplace/ANAPeriodicals/OJIN/TableofContents/Vol-16-2011/No2-May-2011/Patient-Centered-Care-in-a-Medical-Home.html

Chang, E., Simon, M., & Dong, X. (2012). Integrating cultural humility into health care professional education and training. *Advances in Health Science Education, 17*, 269–278.

Chen, C., & Lou, M. (2014). The effectiveness and application of mentorship programmes for recently registered nurses: A systematic review. *Journal of Nursing Management, 22*(4), 433–442.

Clark, C. M., Farnsworth, J., Landrum, R. E. (2009). Development and description of the Incivility in Nursing Education (INE) survey. *Journal of Theory Construction & Testing, 13*(1), 7–15.

Cook, A., & Glass, C. (2013). Above the glass ceiling: When are women and racial/ethnic minorities promoted to CEO? *Strategic Management Journal, 35*(7), 1080–1089.

Cox, E. (1995). A truly civil society. 1995 Boyer lectures. Retrieved from http://www .crcresearch.org/files-crcresearch/File/cox_95.pdf

Croft, R. K., & Cash, P. A. (2012). Deconstructing contributing factors to bullying and lateral violence in nursing using a postcolonial feminist lens. *Contemporary Nurse, 42*(2), 226–242.

Cummins, S., Curtis, S., Diez-Roux, A. V., & Macintyre, S. (2007). Understanding and representing "place" in health research: A relational approach. *Social Science & Medicine, 65,* 1825–1838.

Davis, C. (2015). Mentoring our future nurse leaders [editorial]. *Nursing Made Incredibly Easy!, 13*(4), 4.

Data.Medicare.gov. (2015). Home health care—National data. Retrieved from https:// data.medicare.gov/Home-Health-Compare/Home-Health-Care-National-Data/ 97z8-de96

Dixon-Woods, M., McNicol, S., & Martin, G. (2012). Ten challenges in improving quality in health care: Lessons from the Health Foundation's programme evaluations and relevant literature. *BMJ Quality & Safety, 21*(10), 876–884.

Dogra, N., Reitmanova, S., & Carter-Pokras, O. (2009). Twelve tips for teaching diversity and embedding it in the medical curriculum. *Medical Teacher, 31*(11), 990–993.

Dogra, N., Reitmanova, S., & Carter-Pokras, O. (2010). Teaching cultural diversity: Current status in U.K., U.S., and Canadian medical schools. *Journal of General Internal Medicine, 25*(2), 164–168.

Donelan, K., DesRoches, C. M., Dittus, R. S., & Buerhaus, P. (2013). Perspectives of physicians and nurse practitioners on primary care practice. *New England Journal of Medicine, 368,* 1898–1906.

Drenkard, K. (2010). Going for the gold: The value of attaining Magnet® recognition. *American Nurse Today, 5*(3), 50–52.

Drucker, P. (2000). Managing knowledge means managing oneself. *Leader to Leader, 16,* 8–10.

Duffield, C., Diers, D., O'Brien-Pallas, L., Aisbett, C., Roche, M., King, M., & Aisbett, K. (2011). Nursing staffing, nursing workload, the work environment and patient outcomes. *Applied Nursing Research, 24*(4), 244–255.

Dybwik, K., Tollali, T., Nielsen, E. W., & Brinchmann, B. S. (2011). "Fighting the system": Families caring for ventilator-dependent children and adults with complex health care needs at home. *BMC Health Services Research, 11,* 156.

Ensher, E. A., & Murphy, S. E. (2011). The mentoring relationship challenges scale: The impact of mentoring stage, type, and gender. *Journal of Vocational Behavior, 79*(1), 253–266.

Erikson, E. H. (1963). *Childhood and society.* New York, NY: Norton.

Farrell, G. A., Shafiei, T., & Salmon, P. (2010). Facing up to "challenging behavior": A model for training in staff-client interaction. *Journal of Advanced Nursing, 66*(7), 1644–1655.

Ford, R. (2009). Complex leadership competency in health care: Towards framing a theory of practice. *Health Services Management Research, 22*(3), 101–114

Foster, J. (2009). Cultural humility and the importance of long-term relationships in international partnerships. *Journal of Obstetrical, Gynecological, & Neonatal Nursing, 38*(1), 100–107.

Gabrielle, S., Jackson, D., & Mannix, J. (2008). Adjusting to personal and organizational change: Views and experiences of female nurses aged 40–60 years. *Collegian, 15*(3), 85–91

Gilbert, J., & Broome, M. (2015). Developing and sustaining self. In J. Daly, S. Speedy, & D. Jackson (Eds.), *Leadership and nursing: Contemporary perspectives* (2nd ed., chap. 15). Sydney, Australia: Elsevier.

Goldman, A., & Tabak, N. (2010). Perception of ethical climate and its relationship to nurses' demographic characteristics and job satisfaction. *Nursing Ethics, 17*(2), 233–246.

Goode, C. J., Blegen, M. A., Park, S. H., Vaughn, T., & Spetz, J. (2011). Comparison of patient outcomes in Magnet® and non-magnet hospitals. *Journal of Nursing Administration, 41*(12), 517–523.

Grindel, C. G., & Hagerstrom, G. (2009). Nurses nurturing nurses: Outcomes and lessons learned. *MEDSURG Nursing, 18*(3), 183–194.

Gunnarsdottir, S., Clarke, S. P., Rafferty, A. M., & Nutbeam, D. (2009). Front-line management, staffing and nurse–doctor relationships as predictors of nurse and patient outcomes. A survey of Icelandic hospital nurses. *International Journal of Nursing Studies, 46*(7), 920–927.

Hader, R. (2009). Is being a chief nursing officer in your future? *Imprint, 56*(1), 33–35.

Hall, P. (2005). Interprofessional teamwork: Professional cultures as barriers. *Journal of Interprofessional Care, 19*(Suppl. 1), 188–196.

Hall, M. J., & Owings, M. R. (2014). Rural residents who are hospitalized in rural and urban hospitals: United States, 2010. *NCHS Data Brief* (No. 159). Retrieved from http://198.246.102.49/nchs/data/databriefs/db159.pdf

Hall, P., Weaver, L., Handfeld-Jones, R., & Bouvette, M. (2008). Developing leadership in rural interprofessional palliative care teams. *Journal of Interprofessional Care, 22*(Suppl. 1), 73–79.

Hart, E. W. (2010). Seven ways to be an effective mentor. *Forbes.* Retrieved from http://www.forbes.com/2010/06/30/mentor-coach-executive-training-leadership-managing-ccl.html

Hawala-Druy, S., & Hill, M. H. (2012). Interdisciplinary: Cultural competency and culturally congruent education for millennials in health professions. *Nurse Education Today, 32*, 772–778.

Hayes, P. A. (2006). Home is where their health is: Rethinking perspectives of informal and formal care by older rural Appalachian women who live alone. *Qualitative Health Research, 16*(2), 282–297.

Henriksen, K., Joseph, A., & Zayas-Caban, T. (2009). The human factors of home health care: A conceptual model for examining safety and quality concerns. *Journal of Patient Safety, 5*(4), 229–236.

Hing, E., Hooker, R. S., & Ashman, J. J. (2011). Primary health care in community health centers and comparison with office-based practice. *Journal of Community Health, 36*(3), 406–413.

Hodgson, A. K., & Scanlan, J. M. (2013). A concept analysis of mentoring in nursing leadership. *Open Journal of Nursing, 3*, 389–394.

Hunsberger, M., Baumann, A., Blythe, J., & Crea, M. (2009). Sustaining the rural workforce: Nursing perspectives on worklife challenges. *Journal of Rural Health, 25*(1), 17–25.

Hunt, L. J. (2001). Beyond cultural competence. *Part Ridge Center Bulletin, 24.* Retrieved from https://www.med.unc.edu/pedclerk/files/hunthumility.pdf

Huston, C. (2008). Preparing nurse leaders for 2020. *Journal of Nursing Management, 16*, 905–911.

Institute of Medicine. (2010). *The future of nursing: Leading change, advancing health.* Washington, DC: National Academies Press. Retrieved from http://iom.nationalacademies.org/Reports/2010/The-Future-of-Nursing-Leading-Change-Advancing-Health.aspx

Jackson, J. F. L., O'Callaghan, E. M., & Leon, R. A (Eds.). (2014, August). Measuring glass ceiling effects in higher education: Opportunities and challenges. *New Directions for Institutional Research* (No. 159). Retrieved from http://www.wiley.com/WileyCDA/WileyTitle/productCd-111895629X.html

Jakubik, L. D., Eliades, A. B., Gavriloff, C. L., & Weese, M. M. (2011). Nurse mentoring study demonstrates a magnetic work environment: Predictors of mentoring benefits among pediatric nurses. *Journal of Pediatric Nursing, 26*(2), 156–164.

Jeffreys, M. R. (2010). *Teaching cultural competence in nursing and health care: Inquiry, action, and innovation* (2nd ed.). New York, NY: Springer Publishing Company.

Johnson, S. L., & Rea, R. E. (2009). Workplace bullying: Concerns for nurse leaders. *Journal of Nursing Administration, 39*(2), 84–90.

Kane, G. C., Grever, M. R., Kennedy, J. I., Kuzma, M. A., Saltzman, A. R., Wiernik, P. H., & Baptista, N. V. (2009). The anticipated physician shortage: Meeting the nation's need for physician services. *American Journal of Medicine, 122*(12), 1156–1162.

Kelly, L. A., McHugh, M. D., & Aiken, L. H. (2011). Nurse outcomes in Magnet® and non-Magnet hospitals. *Journal of Nursing Administration, 41*(10), 428–433.

Kibort, P. M. (2005). I drank the Kool-Aid—and learned 24 key management lessons. *Physician Executive, 31*(6), 52–55.

Kosoko-Lasaki, S., & Cook, C. T. (2009). Cultural competency instrument: A description of a methodology. Part II. In S. Kosoko-Lasaki, C. T. Cook, & R. L. O'Brien (Eds.), *Cultural proficiency in addressing health disparities* (chap. 9). Sudbury, MA: Jones & Bartlett.

Kramer, M., & Hafner, L. P. (1989). Shared values: Impact on staff nurse job satisfaction and perceived productivity. *Nursing Research, 38*, 58–64.

Kumagai, A. K., & Lypson, M. L. (2009). Beyond cultural competence: Critical consciousness, social justice, and multicultural education. *Academic Medicine, 84*(6), 782–787.

Latham, C. L., Hogan, M., & Ringl, K. (2008). Nurses supporting nurses: Creating a mentoring program for staff nurses to improve the workforce environment. *Nursing Administration Quarterly, 32*(1), 27–39.

Lee, T., & Schiller, J. (2015). The future of Home Health Project: Developing the framework for health care at home. *Home Healthcare Now, 33*(2), 84–87.

Levi, A. (2009). The ethics of nursing student international clinical experiences. *Journal of Obstetric, Gynecologic, & Neonatal Nursing, 38*(1), 94–99.

Lewis, P. S., & Malecha, A. (2011). The impact of workplace incivility on the work environment, manager skill, and productivity. *Journal of Nursing Administration, 41*(1), 41–47.

Luparell, S. (2011). Incivility in nursing: The connection between academia and clinical settings. *Critical Care Nurse, 31*(2), 92–95.

MacDowell, M., Glasser, M., Fitts, M., Nielsen, K., & Hunsaker, M. (2010). A national view of rural health workforce issues in the USA. *Rural and Remote Health, 10*(3), 1531. Retrieved from http://www.ncbi.nlm.nih.gov/pmc/articles/PMC3760483/

Marshall, E. S. (2008). Home as place for healing. *Advances in Nursing Science, 31*(3), 259–267.

McHugh, M. D., Kelly, L. A., Smith, H. L., Wu, E. S., Vanak, J. M., & Aiken, L. H. (2013). Lower mortality in Magnet hospitals. *Medical Care, 51*(5), 382–388.

McInnes, S., Peters, K., Bonney, A., & Halcomb, E. (2015). An integrative review of facilitators and barriers influencing collaboration and teamwork between general practitioners and nurses working in general practice. *Journal of Advanced Nursing, 71*(9), 1973–1985.

McMenamin, P. (2015). Diversity among registered nurses: Slow but steady progress. Retrieved from http://www.ananursespace.org/blogs/peter-mcmenamin/2015/08/21/rn-diversity-note?ssopc=1

Molony, S. L. (2010). The meaning of home: A qualitative metasynthesis. *Research in Gerontological Nursing, 3*(4), 291–307.

Montour, A., Baumann, A., Blythe, J., & Hunsberger, M. (2009). The changing nature of nursing work in rural and small community hospitals. *Rural & Remote Health, 9*(1), 1089.

Nacoste, R. W. (2015). *Taking on diversity: How we can move from anxiety to respect.* Amherst, NY: Prometheus Books.

National Council of State Boards of Nursing. (2016). Implementation status map. Retrieved from https://www.ncsbn.org/5397.htm

National Organization of Nurse Practitioner Faculties. (2015). NONPF leadership mentoring program. Retrieved from http://www.nonpf.org/?page=MentoringProgram

Newhouse, R. P., Stanik-Hutt, J., White, K. M., Johantgen, M., Bass, E. B., Zangaro G., . . . Weiner, J. P. (2011). Advanced practice nurse outcomes 1990–2008: A systematic review. *Nursing Economics, 29*(5), 1–22.

Nugus, P., Greenfield, D., Travaglia, J., Westbrook, J., & Braithewaite, J. (2010). How and where clinicians exercise power: Interprofessional relations in health care. *Social Science & Medicine, 71,* 898–909.

Parmelli, E., Flodgren, G., Beyer, F., Baillie, N., Schaafasma, M. E., & Eccles, M. P. (2011). The effectiveness of strategies to change organizational culture to improve health care performance: A systematic review. *Implementation Science, 6*(33). Retrieved from http://implementationscience.biomedcentral.com/articles/10.1186/1748-5908-6-33

Pearson, L. J. (2009). The Pearson report. *American Journal for Nurse Practitioners, 13*(2), 8–82.

Petterson, S. M., Liaw, W. R., Phillips, R. L., Rabin, D. R., Meyers, D. S., & Bazemore, A. W. (2012). Projecting US primary care physician workforce needs: 2010–2025. *Annals of Family Medicine, 10*(6), 503–509.

Pew Research Center. (2015). Non-Hispanic white population, by sex and age: 1980–2013. Retrieved from http://www.pewhispanic.org/2015/05/12/statistical-portrait-of-hispanics-in-the-united-states-1980-2013-trends/ph_2015-03_statistical-portrait-of-hispanics-in-the-united-states-2013-trend-19/

Phillips, S. J. (2015). 27th annual APRN legislative update: Advancements continue for APRN practice. *Nurse Practitioner, 40*(1), 16–42.

Poghosyan, L., Boyd, D., & Clarke, S. P. (2016). Optimizing full scope of practice for nurse practitioners in primary care: A proposed conceptual model. *Nursing Outlook, 64*(2):146–155.

Porter-O'Grady, T., & Malloch, K. (2015). *Quantum leadership: Building better partnerships for sustainable health* (4th ed.). Burlington, MA: Jones & Bartlett.

PricewaterhouseCoopers. (2014). Leveraging the power of our differences: Diversity and inclusion. Retrieved from http://www.pwc.com/us/en/about-us/diversity/pwc-diversity.html

Purnell, L. D. (2013). *Transcultural health care: A culturally competence approach* (4th ed.). Philadelphia, PA: F. A. Davis.

Race, T. K., & Skees, J. (2010). Changing tides: Improving outcomes through mentorship on all levels of nursing. *Critical Care Nursing Quarterly, 33*(2), 163–174.

Raelin, J. A. (2015). Rethinking leadership: Businesses need a new approach to the practice of leadership—And to leadership development. *MIT Sloan Management Review, 56*(4), 95–96.

Ramani, S., Gruppen, L., & Kachur, E. K. (2006). Twelve tips for developing effective mentors. *Medical Teacher, 28*(5), 404–408.

Reeves, S., MacMillan, K., & Van Soeren, M. (2010). Leadership of interprofessional health and social care teams: A socio-historical analysis. *Journal of Nursing Management, 18,* 258–264.

Reeves, S., Rice, K., Gotlib Conn, L., Miller, K., Kenaszhuk, C., & Zwarenstein, M. (2009). Interprofessional interaction, negotiation and non-negotiation on general internal medicine wards. *Journal of Interprofessional Care, 23*(6), 633–645.

Rhodes, C., Pullen, A., Vickers, M. H., Clegg, S. R., & Pitsis, A. (2010). Violence and workplace bullying: What are an organization's ethical responsibilities? *Administrative Theory & Praxis, 32*(1), 96–115.

Roberts, S. J., DeMarco, R., & Griffin, M. (2009). The effect of oppressed group behaviours on the culture of the nursing workplace: A review of the evidence and interventions for change. *Journal of Nursing Management, 17,* 288–293.

Robertson, R., & Cockley, D. (2004). Competencies for rural health administrators. *Journal of Health Administration Education, 21*(3), 329–341.

Robezneiks, A. (2012, October 6). Nurses react as AAFP report backs doctor-led medical homes. *Modern Healthcare.* Retrieved from http://www.modernhealthcare.com/article/20121006/MAGAZINE/310069966

Roche, M., Diers, D., Duffield, C., & Catling-Paull, C. (2010). Violence towards nurses, the work environment, and patient outcomes. *Journal of Nursing Scholarship, 42*(1), 13–22.

Rodwell, J., & Gulyas, A. (2013). The impact of the psychological contract, justice and individual difference: Nurses take it personally when employers break promises. *Journal of Advanced Nursing, 69*(12), 2774–2785.

Ross, H. J. (2011). *Reinventing diversity: Transforming organizational community to strengthen people, purpose, and performance.* Lanham, MD: Rowman & Littlefield.

Sabin, J. A., & Greenwald, A. G. (2012). The influence of implicit bias on treatment recommendations for 4 common pediatric conditions: Pain, urinary tract infection, attention deficit hyperactivity disorder, and asthma. *American Journal of Public Health, 102,* 988–995.

Sealover, E. (2015, November 23). Merger creates metro Denver's largest group of primary-care doctors. *Denver Business Journal.* Retrieved from http://www.bizjournals.com/denver/news/2015/11/23/merger-creates-largest-group-of-primary-care.html

Schein, E. H. (2012). What is culture?. In M. Godwyn & J. H. Gittell (Eds.), *Sociology of organizations: Structures and relationships* (pp. 311–314). Thousand Oaks, CA: Sage.

Shi, L., & Singh, D. A. (2015). *Delivering health care in America: A systems approach* (6th ed.). Burlington, MA: Jones & Bartlett.

Sigma Theta Tau International. (2015). Learn and grow: Leadership. Retrieved from http://www.nursingsociety.org/learn-grow/leadership-institute

Simon, M. A., Chang, E., & Dong, S. (2010). Partnership, reflection and patient focus: Advancing cultural competency training relevance. *Medical Education, 44*(6), 540–542.

Simons, S. (2008). Workplace bullying experienced by Massachusetts registered nurses and the relationship to intention to leave the organization. *Advances in Nursing Science, 31*(2), E48–E59.

Smith, K. B., Humphreys, J. S., & Wilson, M. G. (2008). Addressing the health disadvantage of rural populations: How does epidemiological evidence inform rural health policies and research? *Australian Journal of Rural Health, 16*(2), 56–66.

Stanik-Hutt, J., Newhouse, R. P., White, K. M., Johantgen, M., Bass, E. B., Zangaro G., . . . Weiner, J. P. (2013). The quality and effectiveness of care provided by nurse practitioners. *Journal for Nurse Practitioners, 9*(8), 492–500.

Summers, S. (2012). Magnet status: What it is, what it is not, and what it could be. *The Truth About Nursing.* Retrieved from http://www.truthaboutnursing.org/faq/magnet.html

Summers, S., & Summers, H. J. (2015). Magnet status. This nursing process should be a floor, not a ceiling. *Advance for Nurses.* Retrieved from http://nursing.advanceweb.com/Features/Articles/Magnet-Status.aspx

Swanson, A. (2015, June 4) The number of Fortune 500 companies led by women is at an all-time high: 5 percent. *Washington Post.* Retrieved from https://www.washingtonpost.com/news/wonk/wp/2015/06/04/the-number-of-fortune-500-companies-led-by-women-is-at-an-all-time-high-5-percent/

Tervalon, M., & Murray-Garcia, J. (1998). Cultural humility versus cultural competence: A critical distinction in defining physician training outcomes in multicultural education. *Journal of Health Care for the Poor & Underserved, 9*(2), 117–125.

Thagard, P. (2012). Mapping minds across cultures. In R. Sun (Ed.), *Grounding social science in cognitive sciences.* Cambridge, MA: MIT Press.

Thomas, R., Sargent, L. D., & Hardy, C. (2011). Managing organizational change: Negotiating meaning and power-resistance relations. *Organizational Science, 22*(1), 22–41.

Thompson, E. (2010). How to be a better mentor. *Journal of Accountancy.* Retrieved from http://www.journalofaccountancy.com/issues/2010/nov/20091446.html

Torkington, K. (2012). Place and lifestyle migration: The discursive construction of "local" place-identity. *Mobilities, 7*(1), 71–92.

Ulrich, B. T., Lavandero, R., Hart, K. A., Woods, D., Leggett, J., & Taylor, D. (2006). Critical care nurses' work environments: A baseline status report. *Critical Care Nurse, 26*(5), 46–57.

U.S. Agency for Health Care Research & Quality. (2014). Primary care workforce facts and stats (No. 3). Retrieved from http://www.ahrq.gov/research/findings/factsheets/primary/pcwork3/index.html

U.S. Health Resources and Services Administration. (2013). The U.S. nursing workforce: Trends in supply and education. Retrieved from http://bhpr.hrsa.gov/healthworkforce/reports/nursingworkforce/nursingworkforcefullreport.pdf

Wallace, G. (2015, January 29). Only 5 black CEOs at 500 biggest companies. *CNN Money.* Retrieved from http://money.cnn.com/2015/01/29/news/economy/mcdonalds-ceo-diversity/

Wallace, A. E., Lee, R., MacKenzie, T. A., West, A. N., Wright, S., Booth, B. M., . . . Weeks, W. B. (2010). A longitudinal analysis of rural and urban veterans' health-related quality of life. *Journal of Rural Health, 26*(2), 156–163.

Warshawsky, N. E., & Sullivan Havens, D. (2011). Global use of the practice environment scale of the Nursing Work Index. *Nursing Research, 60*(1), 17–31.

Weaver, K. E., Geiger, A. M., Lu, L., & Case, L. D. (2013). Rural-urban disparities in health status among US cancer survivors. *Cancer, 119*(5), 1050–1057.

Wesley, M. (2014, December 1). Culture does indeed eat structure for breakfast [Web blog post]. Retrieved from http://www.thewesleygroup.com/blog/?p=609

Williams, A. M. (2004). Shaping the practice of home care: Critical case studies of the significance of the meaning of home. *International Journal of Palliative Nursing, 10*(7), 333–342.

Wilson, B. L., Diedrich, A., Phelps, C. L., & Choi, M. (2011). Bullies at work: The impact of horizontal hostility in the hospital setting and intent to leave. *Journal of Nursing Administration, 41*(11), 453–458.

Wong, C. A., Cummings, G. G., & Ducharme, L. (2013). The relationship between nursing leadership and patient outcomes: A systematic review update. *Journal of Nursing Management, 21*(5), 709–724.

CHAPTER 10

Building Cohesive and Effective Teams

Marion E. Broome and Elaine Sorensen Marshall

*If your actions inspire others to dream more, learn more, do more and become
more, you are a leader.*
—John Quincy Adams

OBJECTIVES

- *To discuss the centrality of teams and teamwork to the success of any health care
  organization*
- *To discuss the significance of core values in effective networks in organizations*
- *To describe the essential components of followership and how leaders cultivate engaged
  followers*
- *To identify phases of team development, nurturance, and sustenance*
- *To discuss strategies to manage conflict within and across teams*

Leadership by team is the common functional structure and expectation across
business and health care. The power of a leader is magnified by an effective
team, and the leader who empowers team members expands the capacity of the
whole. In the ideal context of complexity science, self-organizing interprofessional teams work on significant issues across systems to accomplish specific
goals of the organization. Such a structure has enormous potential to release
energy, encourage commitment and accountability, and promote creativity. New
interest in interprofessional collaboration, along with technological possibilities
for virtual team membership (Orchard, King, Khalili, & Bezzina, 2012), offer
the promise to expand the concept of teamwork to include consulting experts,
community members, patients, and others. Yet, the full potential of this kind of
teamwork has yet to be realized.

Teams can be found throughout the health care organization. In the broadest sense the concept of team refers to any group of professionals and others working toward a purpose of service in health care. Numerous studies provide rationales for team approaches to governing and decision making in health care (Clark, 2009; Humphrey, Morgeson, & Mannor, 2009; Kearney & Gebert, 2009; Mitchell et al., 2012; Reeves, Perrier, Goldman, Freeth, & Zwarenstein, 2013). Yet, inspiring members of different disciplines to work together naturally and maximize their functioning and effectiveness is not easy.

The Interprofessional Education Collaborative (IPEC), which consists of leaders from six of the national health professions associations, including the American Association of Colleges of Nursing (AACN), outlined four domains of competency for collaborative practice (IPEC, 2011). They are:

1. Values and ethics for interprofessional practice
2. Roles and responsibilities
3. Interprofessional communication
4. Teams and teamwork

Based on a framework developed at the Medical University of South Carolina, a collaborative group of health professionals described four key behaviors required for each team member to transform individual "ways of knowing" regarding how to interact with each other within a team. These behaviors are (a) prepare, (b) think, (c) practice, and (d) act. Successful transformation will rely heavily on a leader who can truly inspire others to move beyond personal professional territories and biases and change personal perspectives of power and influence. The outcome will be improved quality indicators for patients and clients and satisfaction for providers who work on the teams. As a whole, the team must be able to perform as a patient-centered unit whose practice is based on evidence. These teams use information systems in the environment to maximize their efficiency and tailor their interventions to the individual patient to provide the highest quality care (Institute of Medicine, 2003).

BUILDING EFFECTIVE TEAMS: RECRUITING, RETAINING, AND DEVELOPING

In many situations, it is the work of the leader to build the team. In others, the leader must learn to work with existing personnel who are logically, by virtue of their position and scope of responsibility, members of a team. Leadership by team can be inspiring and fulfilling to both the leader and the team members. The leader must balance efforts between building team member satisfaction and pushing for team productivity. It is often tempting to focus on building team processes and dynamics, but the leader who places too great an emphasis on this component risks losing sight of the actual work to be accomplished by the team. Evidence-based practice and current outcomes perspectives require that the team be evaluated primarily in terms of its productivity, patient outcomes, and the success of its work (Körner, Ehrhardt, &

Steger, 2013). Individual commitment, team satisfaction, or impressive team processes cannot substitute for positive effects on clinical and organizational outcomes. Thus, the transformational leader always carries a vision not only for team spirit and activities, but also for the actual accomplishments of the team to improve the lives of the people being served. Leading a successful team is not for the faint hearted.

Among the most important activities for the leader are recruitment, development, coaching, and retention of team members. Indeed, in hospitals, poor management of human resources has actually been linked to patient mortality and exceptional costs in terms of turnover (Needleman et al., 2011). The concept of team in health care is important in the context of acute care hospital environments as well as ambulatory and community care settings. Some of the most effective team models are found in community health and primary care, as well as across settings. In fact, interprofessional collaboration is often stronger and healthier in community environments (Reeves et al., 2011; Thistlethwaite, 2012). The very complexity and pace of health care organizations demand team approaches to problem solving and leaders who understand and promote team achievement. Contemporary and future health care challenges will require changes in the way care is delivered, evaluated, and compensated. As technology evolves, new ways of delivering care will be discussed, and leaders must think through how new care models will be implemented. No single individual can negotiate such complex issues of caring for individuals with complex chronic conditions, nor can even multiple individuals from any single discipline. Varied and diverse perspectives are needed, and it is incumbent upon the leader to not only manage that diversity but embrace it.

Regardless of the setting or task at hand, a recruitment plan for the best team members is critical. The leader's plan for recruitment and assignment of teams should include clear objectives, long-term projections, analysis of potential pools of candidates, and specific strategies to attract and keep the best individuals functioning on the team. Occasionally, as a leader, one is able to hire just the right person to lead an important team-based initiative. But in other cases, one either inherits a team or has limited information to build the right team. These situations will require different approaches.

Recruitment of the best team members is one area where there is a careful dance between immediate needs for effective management and long-term investments in human capital for the future. Every team should have at least one individual who is relatively new to the health care professions or problems being addressed. There are two reasons for this. First, inclusion on the team offers an opportunity for that person to grow and develop team-based skills; and second, the person will likely have a fresh perspective and even suggest solutions for the problem. Unfortunately, when selecting potential team members, we usually default to the person in an administrative position with experience and responsibilities in the specific area. Although an administrative leader who can guide the team is critical, that alone is not sufficient for innovative solutions to challenges. In fact, one needs people close to the process and problem who have

REFLECTION QUESTIONS

Think about a problem or issue where you work. Assume that you need to recruit a team to solve the problem. As you think about how and who to select as the best members of your team, ask yourself the following:

- What is the overall preferred outcome for this team?
- What kinds of skills are needed to achieve that outcome (e.g., process skills to analyze the current problem; financial acumen to examine costs; organizational skills, including time management; consensus-building skills)?
- What individuals in your sphere of influence have each of those skills?
- Whose goals are aligned with learning from a team of diverse individuals to achieve the desired outcome (e.g., someone who has expressed an interest in participating in the leadership of the organization)?
- What would be possible gains or advantages for in it for each individual to join the team?

a vested interest in solving it. This will mean that the leader must build on the strengths of individuals, as well as their ability to work with others to achieve a common goal or reach a common objective.

So how does one assess the strengths of an individual as a potential team member? Further, how does one "sell" that busy person on the need to use those strengths to work with others on a team to achieve an organizational objective? This is where the strategic leader's vision and plan are most useful.

Your responses to the reflection questions are important because they can guide you to recruit members of your team. For instance, you may identify strengths of which a person is unaware, and he or she will be pleased to hear your opinion. That team member most likely will not initially recognize the benefits to be derived from such an experience. Your success at recruiting the best people will be enhanced if you are able to articulate the answers to the reflection questions.

LEADING THE TEAM

Teams Working in Cohesive, Forward-Thinking Cultures

Why is an effective team important to promote a forward-thinking culture? One might ask, "What is a cohesive, forward-thinking culture?" A culture that is forward thinking looks to the future and has clear vision and mission statements about the work it does and the level at which the work is expected to make an impact. These are organizations where individuals think proactively about alternative scenarios that may promote the ability of the organization to seize important opportunities. When problems or challenges arise, the leaders in a forward-thinking culture do not explain away or deny the problem but rather discuss ways the organization should approach the challenge in order to maintain stability and remain effective in meeting its mission. A cohesive culture is transparent about these challenges, and most individuals in the organizations are interested in contributing their efforts to work toward finding solutions for the issue.

This is where teams and their leaders can play a major role. A large part of the job of any leader is to build the team. By building the team, you are building a community that becomes the culture of the organization. Effective, efficient, and caring communities are not convened by magic. Building the effective team requires planning, training, and constant effort (Salas, DiazGranados, Weaver, & King, 2008). Five important functions of the leader in such a setting are (a) environmental monitoring to provide resources and support to the team, (b) organizing activities to enhance team activities, (c) teaching and coaching team members, (d) motivating the team, and (e) intervening appropriately and collaboratively in team activities (Hackman & Wageman, 2005; Klein, Zeigert, Knight, & Xiao, 2006; Morgeson, 2005).

These team-building functions require that the team leader be highly respected and viewed as credible by team members. But leading a team also requires that one selectively and honestly share weaknesses. When a leader demonstrates vulnerability, he or she becomes more approachable and humble. Do not hesitate to rely on intuition (experience and wisdom) to interpret cues in the environment that help team members know when and how to approach problems and make decisions. Manage members of the team with compassion and firmness, a kind of "tough empathy." Team members need to know that the leader is passionate and cares about them and the work they do. Further, do not be afraid to reveal your own differences as a leader, and learn to share what is unique about yourself (Goffee & Jones, 2011).

Effective teams work together over time, sometimes in phases, to create a respectful, shared subculture through the identification of core values. This process allows team members to analyze the evidence that underlies and supports challenges under examination. Team members will come to encourage individual ideas and contributions, mutually think through the unintended consequences of proposed solutions and decisions, and be willing to oversee and champion the implementation of decisions.

Core Values of Organizations and Teams

It is difficult for individuals to work together if they lack shared values and regard for each other. Core values differ from individual to individual and organization to organization and often depend on the vision and mission of the organization. Such values underpin how people work, and how they work *together*. Examples of core values commonly found in organizations are listed in Box 10.1.

The leader of any team must be ready to lead a discussion about core values of the team and how they influence its work in the following ways: (a) to guide the way the team asks questions and addresses challenges, (b) to positively influence how the team holds discussions, (c) to determine and provide information needed by the team, and (d) to guide the team as it makes decisions, especially when there is diversity of perspectives and opinions.

Hence, two different teams, guided by different core values or even different leaders, may reach different solutions about the same problem on a different timetable. This is the scenario presented in Box 10.2.

BOX 10.1. EXAMPLES OF CORE VALUES

Transparency
Accountability
Trust
Openness to new ideas
Flexibility
Caring
Responsibility

BOX 10.2. TEAM-BASED PROCESS IMPROVEMENT

After reading the case example, discuss with a classmate or coworker your responses to the reflection questions that follow.

Team A and Team B are asked to develop a process to improve triage and care in the emergency department in order to decrease wait times and improve satisfaction of patients and families. At an initial meeting, Team A identifies its core values as innovation, transparency, flexibility, and consensus. Team B's core values are teamwork, evidence, inclusiveness, and transparency.

Team A: At the second meeting, Team A's leader encourages the team members to review the data they requested (current wait times, current processes, etc.) and to think about all of the factors that slow the process of placing patients in rooms for care (e.g., the length of time in the room, what they do throughout their visit, etc.). Team members are asked individually to list strategies addressing each factor that leads to increased time and decreased satisfaction. After each person has shared his or her ideas, commonalities across factors are sought and common strategies are identified.

At the third team meeting, the entire group devises pilot tests of changes that could be implemented and evaluated one at a time. At a fourth meeting a week later, the group analyzes the "cost" of time, effort, and disruption each small test of change would require and decides how to evaluate the effectiveness of each change to achieve the goals of increased satisfaction of patients and decreased wait time. They also decide that provider satisfaction is critical, and they incorporate this into their evaluation scheme. Finally, based on these decisions, they prioritize which test of change should be implemented first, second, and so on.

This process took 4 weeks, with one 2-hour meeting each week.

(continued)

BOX 10.2. TEAM-BASED PROCESS IMPROVEMENT (*continued*)

Team B: Team B also asks for data on which to make decisions. Team members spend their time during the second meeting talking about how the data are incomplete and do not capture the entire situation. At the second meeting, the leader asks them to brainstorm about the factors involved and potential strategies. Two members of the group who have worked in the emergency department the longest, and another member who is in the highest position of authority, speak most often and take notes, while others nod their heads in agreement. When the team leader asks if there are any additional ideas, none are offered.

At the third meeting a week later, one-third of the original team does not return due to "time conflicts"; however, both of the experienced individuals return and lead the meeting. One new approach to the problem is identified, and it is decided that this approach will be implemented and evaluated. The formal leader thanks everyone for coming and for thinking about how to work so efficiently "within the constraints we had." This process took 3 weeks.

REFLECTION QUESTIONS

1. How do you think the core values of each team in Box 10.2 influenced the way they approached the challenge they were given?
2. Did any of the core values self-identified by either team as important to them seem less readily apparent to you?
3. One team took less time to devise a solution, and its implementation of the solution appears as if it, too, will take less time. How do you think the members of each team felt about the experience of participating in this effort?
4. Do you think both teams' approaches are equally effective, or would one team's approach produce better results than the other's? Why?

Despite the prevailing discussions about the need for team-based care in health-related organizations, some colleagues remind us of their challenges, particularly in complex health care organizations. Many report that there are relatively few times throughout the day when members of the interdisciplinary team actually function as a team. Most often, they work as individual advocates for the patient through their individual roles, and only in rare instances, such as clinical emergencies, do they step out of the role and truly work together as a synergistic team. Turf battles, differences of knowledge level and experience, and rare opportunities for group conversation can lead to a competitive atmosphere where everyone is struggling to do the right thing (Gerardi, 2010). Among explanations given for this common situation are the following:

• Today's health care professionals did not train together while learning to be a nurse, physician, physical therapist, or other member of the team.

- After individual professionals joined the health care workforce they were not rewarded for their performance as a team member.
- Care delivery and outcomes have not been compensated based on success of team care; rather, care provided by nurses, physicians, and other health providers entails separate costs and charges.
- In many cases, core values of the professions differ and must be shared and discussed if effective and high-performing teams are ever to become hard-wired into health care organizations.

Although much has been said about the preferred characteristics of teams and team members, little evidence has correlated team characteristics with strategies, outcomes, innovations, or decisions in health care environments (Holleman, Poot, Mintjes-de Groot, & van Achterberg, 2009). There is no such thing as the "correct" or "perfect" team member. The very reason we work in teams is that a combination of a several people with individual characteristics and strengths is better than any particular person, no matter how exceptional. Certainly, team members need to have the basic qualities of honesty, respect, and accountability and be willing to participate, but teams do not benefit by selecting dominant personality styles, however, apparently competent.

SUSTAINING HIGH-PERFORMING TEAMS

Leader characteristics are important to the effectiveness of any team. Several studies have confirmed that transformational qualities in the leader contribute to more effective team function. Effective teams require enormous amounts of energy, planning, communication, and investment in others. This is contributed by the identified team leader as well as organizational leaders "at the top." The fine art of team leadership is commonly discussed but uncommonly done with excellence. The work of the team needs to be seamless, with a purpose whose results are greater than the sum of individual efforts. The team leader is critical in setting the tone to ensure that each team member clearly understands his or her role, and that individual members have the resources needed to achieve their goals.

The following are key requisites for any high-performing team:

- Expectations and communications should be clear and open—between leader and all members, and among all members.
- Team consensus must be met about the goal to be achieved, the core values by which dialogue and disagreements will be managed, who will be responsible for bringing what information to the group, and how often and for how long the group will meet before the task is completed.
- Each team member should have full accountability for decision making within his or her team role, and those decisions should be openly shared at each meeting.
- The entire team must be included in the wider strategic decision making.

Teams differ in how they approach a challenge. Some teams make decisions by simple majority vote. This method carries the risk of being less about the team and more about the collection of individuals. In this case, once the vote is taken it is important that all team members support the decision. Other teams are able to work by consensus, which is more challenging but often more effective when the time comes to implement a change. Consensus requires team members to work together until a decision is crafted that reflects the entire team membership without a vote. It has the advantage of engaging team members in coming to mutual decisions. It requires discussion, listening, and compromise. At some point, the entire team must be behind all decisions. A good decision means little without the full support of the team.

A cohesive team becomes like a committed community. Creating a community requires the leader's attention to the details of supporting a sense of belonging. Block (2008) observed that in order to build community on a team, conversations should be structured around questions that do not necessarily evoke answers but rather elicit commitment, accountability, and the possibility for transformation. Block asserted that such questions are of "invitation" rather than mandate or persuasion, "possibilities," "ownership" that guides people to accept responsibility, "dissent" that allows constructive conflict and safe authentic doubt, "commitment" that promotes kept promises and results, and "gifts" that appear when members of the community come together.

Effective teams have a purpose. Members understand their roles and the priorities of their work. They feel appreciated for their contribution. Norms for behavior and conflict management are understood. The decision-making authority of the team is clear, and team members have a vision for what constitutes success. Team members feel free to contribute, recognize, and appreciate differences among members, and they participate. Teams that are high-performing and effective engage in the following behaviors:

- Manage boundaries among their tasks and responsibilities. Effective teams recognize assignments they can assume and others that are not appropriate.
- Challenge the process and be open to change.
- Ask for resources using realistic assessments of what is needed to accomplish their goals.
- Self-manage and support their social climate (Morgeson, DeRue, & Karam, 2010).

Communication and information sharing are probably the most important aspects of team leading and teamwork. It is critical to success that team members individually and collectively use all available sources of information, including members of the team itself. Mesmer-Magnus and DeChurch (2009) performed a meta-analysis of 72 independent studies, totaling 4,795 work teams and a total of 17,279 individuals. The studies explored team information

REFLECTION QUESTIONS

The truth is that from a transformational perspective, we have not even begun to think creatively about teams.

1. Consider an organization with which you are familiar. Why are there so few truly interprofessional teams with clinicians of all kinds, including staff nurses, nurse practitioners, physicians, leaders, community members, patients, and students? What "old" ways of thinking, what values, and what hierarchal structures impede us from thinking inclusively?
2. For areas in which teams do function at a high level, what does that look like to others? How do team members behave? How effective are their outcomes?
3. What current challenge is your organization facing that could be better assessed and managed by an interprofessional team empowered to understand the problem in depth, generate solutions, and oversee implementation of changes?
4. Who would you recruit for that team? How would you evaluate its effectiveness? What role would you play as a transformative leader in its success?

sharing. They found information sharing to be critical to team performance, cohesion, decision satisfaction, and knowledge integration. Information sharing positively predicted team performance across all levels of related factors. Furthermore, in a study among Israeli soldiers, friendship networks (sense of community) within the team (or platoon) were the single mediator of the positive relationship between transformational leadership and climate strength, or agreement among platoon members regarding social climate (Zohar & Tenne-Gazit, 2008).

SHARED LEADERSHIP AND MANAGING TEAM CONFLICT

A new concept has emerged in the literature over the past few years. Called shared leadership, it reflects the complexity of the organizations in which most of us work. In one study (Grille, Schulte, & Kauffield, 2015), the similarity of the leader with members of the team and the individuals' perceptions of their own psychological empowerment and being fairly rewarded were all associated with shared leadership. This would suggest that team leaders must have strong credibility with their team members and engage all in decision-making processes using fair and equitable access to the leader and to information in the organization. In a meta-analysis of studies on shared leadership (D'Innocenzo, Matthieu, & Kukenberger, 2014), scientists found that the degree of complexity of processes and the outcomes expected of a team were not always straightforward. That is, the more complex the task given to a team, the more guidance must be provided from higher in the organization—even with shared leadership on a team.

Despite the strength of shared leadership, when one pulls together or assigns individuals in an organization to achieve goals and engage in regular interaction, conflict results. Diverse teams naturally bring perspectives that vary. One of the challenges of successful team building is the potential discrepancy of perceptions and expectations among team members. Divergent views may exist between team members and the leader (Gibson, Cooper, & Conger, 2009) or among team members—as between physicians and nurses, or among other representatives of distinct different disciplines. In fact, current perspectives suggest that healthy, respectful disagreements among team members ensure open, transparent, and broad-based decision making— sometimes referred to as creative abrasion (Broome, 2015; Leonard-Barton & Swap, 2005). Yet, many team disagreements are anything but open and transparent! Rather, disagreements are often talked about after the meeting—in small groups, in the coffee room, or in hallway conversations—a process that can be disruptive to team functioning and may occasionally become toxic. The leader must bravely face these behaviors and model to the team that it will move forward.

If conflict leaves you frustrated, remember that throughout history, many great leaders were born or made by conflict. Indeed, the first leadership theories were rooted in conflict. Think of the great social and political leaders in world history: Elizabeth I, Abraham Lincoln, Harriet Tubman, Winston Churchill, Indira Gandhi, or Nelson Mandela. They were able leaders when they entered the fray, but they emerged to greatness from the crisis of conflict.

All human dynamics carry the potential for conflict. In any work situation, conflict is inevitable (Greer, Caruso, & Jehn, 2011). Furthermore, to recognize the diversity and fundamental differences in personal experience, viewpoints, and values among human beings is to acknowledge conflict to be a normal characteristic of human interaction. Conflict is a human experience. Especially in complex environments with a highly diverse workforce and laden with high-risk situations, conflict happens.

Nursing and health care organizations can be particularly vulnerable to conflict given the larger number of interactions that occur among individuals with daily varied expectations, roles, and responsibilities. These interactions, when conflictual, may affect safety in the workplace for both patients and professionals (Rosenstein, Dinklin, & Munro, 2014). Conflict cannot be eliminated, particularly in health care organizations, which have a vast range of stressors and diversity of disciplines and professions. A professional mediator observed why the health care environment is particularly fraught with potential for conflict:

> The health care professional's typical day involves a frenetic race to coordinate resources, provide care, perform procedures, gather data, integrate information, respond to emergencies, solve problems, and

interact with diverse groups of people. Regardless of the role of the professional . . . , as a group health care professionals face more conflict and greater complexity than any other profession. Despite the challenges of balancing competing interests, philosophies, training backgrounds, the endless question for adequate resources, and the emotional quality of the work that they do, very few health care professionals have had the opportunity to learn the skills and processes necessary for negotiating their environments. There is little formal training available to them in this area and role models for collaboration and good negotiation are far and few between. As a result, the clinical environment is one of competition, quick fixes, hot tempers, avoidance tactics and at times, hopelessness . . . (Gerardi, 2010)

Other reasons for conflict include (a) disagreements sparked by differences in perspective, competencies, access to information, and strategic focus, (b) lack of clarity about purpose and roles (Rosenstein et al., 2014), and (c) information overload, inaccurate information, and variation in understanding of critical situations (Broome & Gilbert, 2014). The increasing complexity of clinical decision making and range of people making clinical decisions for any particular patient can also create misunderstanding and conflict based on information and practice issues of ambiguity (Sitterding & Broome, 2015).

A positive, healthy professional care environment makes a difference in reducing error, improving safety, alleviating stress, and generally enhancing the patient and caregiver experience (Doucette, 2008). Few individuals have had experience or training in resolving conflict. Thus, fundamental to the role of a leader is the understanding, embrace, and ability to deal effectively with conflict. Conflict is more than a "necessary nuisance" and can be a resource for learning and insight, and most importantly, creative solutions (Broome, 2015). Thus, it is in the leader's best interest for the organization not to eliminate conflict but to embrace it and "institutionalize mechanisms for managing it." Unfortunately,

REFLECTION QUESTIONS

1. How do you *feel* when individuals who hold differing opinions voice them strongly in a meeting?
2. What strategies have you or others used to diffuse a situation in which differing opinions make other team members uncomfortable?
3. As leader of a team, can you envision yourself using the power of negotiation between conflicting perspectives, encouraging those members who are silent to share their ideas, and outlining some potential solutions?
4. If you are not comfortable, or cannot envision yourself using those strategies, are there other leaders you know to be effective from whom you can learn?

neither the clinical nor the leadership training of most health care professionals prepares them for the realities of conflict management and resolution.

Managing conflict well is a fine art. There are a few basic general principles. First, as a leader, it is important to bracket your own emotional responses. Draw upon your highest levels of emotional intelligence, which can help you to frame conflict situations as opportunities for learning. High levels of emotional intelligence in the leader has been associated with staff satisfaction with the leader's method of conflict management (Morrison, 2008).

The effective leader manages conflict with sensitivity, serenity, and wisdom. Useful strategies to employ in conflict situations include the following:

- Stand back, stand firm, reflect the perspectives of both sides, and approach the situation as a compassionate mediator or therapist.
- Remember that you are *the leader*, not the parent or the referee. Examine your own thoughts and feelings about conflict. If it is helpful, share them with a trusted person outside the conflict to assure that your thinking is rational.
- The aim is to support others to work through their disagreements. Plan your response to the people involved in the conflict carefully and fairly.
- Do not respond to ambushes, except to listen. Then listen carefully and responsively, reflecting the viewpoint of the parties in a verbal or written summary.
- As the leader, you set the time, place, and agenda for any official meeting to facilitate resolution. Ask questions, and listen again. Separate fact from opinion, including your own, while considering the perspective of all parties involved.
- Separate people from problems in your own mind. It is rare that a person is simply "being difficult," although frustration may cause you or others to interpret it that way. It is often helpful to think about the context from which the "difficult person" functions to better understand the perspective.
- Finally, hang on to the goal of preserving human respect and working relationships.

Sometimes providing wise interpretation of each other's viewpoints to conflicting parties is enough. If not, take time to plan your response, record it in writing, hold parties accountable, follow up, consult internal or outside experts as appropriate, and be firm but gentle where possible. Promote compromise and collaboration. Help others move out of damaging entrenched positions by constructing graceful ways out of those corners into which acrimony sometimes backs a person. You may need to resort to reassignment or other means to simply separate the parties. Whatever the approach, emphasize the strengths of each person, allow face-saving positive responses, and do not respond to grudges.

You may find it useful to assess your own comfort with conflict before you begin employing any of the tactics described in this section. One most common tools for this purpose is the Thomas-Kilmann Conflict Mode Instrument (Thomas & Kilmann, 1974), also called the Conflict Resolution Scale, which has been used for decades in research and business. It is available online, and there is a small charge for analyzing the results of the tool, but the information gleaned from the assessment may be well worth the cost (http://www.kilmanndiagnostics .com/overview-thomas-kilmann-conflict-mode-instrument-tki).

Occasionally, conflicts may escalate beyond your ability, as the local leader, to resolve them. If the issue is particularly complex or hazardous, it may be helpful to bring in a mediator to avoid full-blown litigation, which is costly to organizational and human resources. Once conflicting parties engage attorneys, the rules change and you are required to work only through your own counsel.

Novice leaders soon learn that part of the mantle of their stewardship as leaders is the burden of carrying confidential knowledge of conflicts, misbehaviors, and mischief of some workers in the organization. Some of that mischief can be directed toward the leader. Hall talk stemming from grudges that may have little to do with you as an individual can generate sentiment directed against you as the leader. Others can talk, but you must carry the burden of confidentiality and simply bear it gracefully.

Intervening in Conflict Situations

Beyond case-by-case real-world conflict resolution, the wise leader provides staff training and education in dealing with conflict. Because the topic is so conspicuously absent or underplayed in the educational programs preparing health professionals, it becomes your responsibility as the leader to raise awareness and educate colleagues. This can be done proactively through grand rounds, continuing education programs, invited experts, staff meetings, retreats, and other programs. It is topically at least as important as any clinical update. Role playing and training across disciplines may be especially helpful.

Health professionals are trained to solve problems. They are experts at assessing problems; developing plans, strategies, and tactics; securing resources; and curing the disease. Engage others in resolving issues that produce conflict:

- Put colleagues to work to identify and address problems related to interpersonal conflicts in their own teams and units using nonthreatening, collaborative goal setting and processes.
- Model openness to alternative solutions to resolve complex problems.
- Encourage creativity beyond a new policy, guideline, or program.
- Provide an environment of trust and support.
- Adding a healthy dose of humor will not hurt and often can help facilitate difficult conversations.

A key aim is to provide a clear process for people to use in resolving issues independently without damage to relationships or organizational morale. Without a dependable structured process, individuals can become mired not only in the end result, but also in how to approach a solution. Furthermore, a systematic approach may promote goodwill and prevent less optimal outcomes in which parties "split-the-difference" or remain deadlocked.

Providing workable mechanisms and fostering openness, support, good-will, and encouragement of thoughtful refection to solve problems across the entire interpersonal environment and across all hierarchical levels of leader-ship are challenging tasks but worth the effort. Successful conflict resolution can result in improved therapeutic environments, strengthened human relation-ships, innovation in processes, shared meaning, and new stories (Rahim, 2011).

Is There Such a Thing as Positive Conflict?

In healthy work environments, sparring, disagreeing, and even construc-tive conflict release creative energy, invite consensus, and promote effective decisions. Beware of a "culture of yes," in which people tell you only what they think you want to hear, or people who disagree sit quietly in meetings, saying nothing, and then undermine leadership and decisions in the hallways. Or, they sit quietly, saying nothing, then passively resist progress or change efforts. Those who are the least likely to express disagreement may be the very ones to whom you should be listening!

Think about it. Knowing who disagrees with a decision and why that person disagrees may actually help you to make a different decision, imple-ment a decision in a more effective way, clarify your rationale, or invite change to a better way. On the other hand, a culture of too much "no," in which workers have all power to veto or resist every decision, can stifle prog-ress. Roberto (cited in Lagace, 2005) also described a "culture of maybe," in which leaders and followers become mired in analysis, resist ambiguity, and continue to gather information, striving for the certainty of just the right answer. Such an environment can immobilize the leader and an entire organi-zation. A bit of constructive conflict in such a situation can move the process toward a decision. Remember, if you make a decision that does not work, you can always make another one!

Leonard-Barton and Swap (2005) discussed how well-managed conflict creates a culture in which individuals can state their opinions and feel free to disagree with each other. This allows others to be more creative and innova-tive in their approaches to solving conflicts and problems. Creative abrasion, mentioned earlier, relies on diverse perspectives and provides for "safe spaces," where those with differing perspectives can express their views. It is critical in these conversations that personal attacks on others and their ideas be prohibited.

Remember, however, that it is *constructive* conflict you seek. This is where the art lies: in determining how to make disagreement and sparring construc-tive. Constructive conflict that fosters critical thinking, active engagement, vigorous debate, and commitment can enhance the quality of decisions while building consensus. (See Box 10.3, which describes one framework, termed *Collective Genius*, for achieving creative resolution of conflict.)

Consensus must be goal and activity oriented rather than emotion based. It helps to establish ground rules for civil dialogue, clarify roles, recognize

BOX 10.3. COLLECTIVE GENIUS

The complex problems of contemporary health care across all settings present many challenges that must be solved to achieve the goals of nurses in practice, education, and research. Our highly regulated profession often reflects rigid approaches to achieving quality and consistency that have unintended consequences, which often results in less educational innovation and higher cost for the innovation and training (Broome, 2015). Resolution of these complex issues requires a more flexible, cohesive, and inclusive approach to ensuring greater access to and higher quality of care for patients. Hill, Bandeau, Truelove, and Lineback (2014) proposed a framework that could promote a process by which such resolution could occur. The framework has three main components.

Creative discourse refers to discussion, debate, and discovery-driven learning about the scope of the complex issue at hand. But discourse goes beyond just talking about the problem. It involves honest, open examinations of the various factors that have contributed to the current situation, as well as the desired future state. To achieve this level of conversation, individuals must let go of their territoriality around ideas and solutions. Transformative leaders must call for, encourage, and then engage in these discussions to motivate and provide role models for others.

Creative agility refers to approaches that are created and implemented using "rapid-cycle" pilots—or small tests of change—that are closely monitored and evaluated to assess their effectiveness in achieving objectives for change. This particular aspect of the collective genius framework has never been a strength of the nursing profession. We tend to prolong discussions about the problem and debate proposed solutions for extended periods of time without coming to "action" and implementation. To adopt creative agility, we need leaders who not only allow pilots of projects for change to move forward, but also hold those testing the pilot projects accountable for assessing their impact, and then communicating the process and outcomes to others.

Creative resolution requires engaged leaders and followers who work together with individuals who have different perspectives and agendas but who can identify common goals and outcomes. Resolution of complex problems comes with a cost to individuals in that no one group or faction achieves the entire outcome wanted. Rather, creative resolutions reflect disparate and opposing views that come together in a way that allows for, and even promotes, innovative approaches to these complex issues.

differences in cognitive and communication styles, and build mutual respect. The process must be fair to promote ultimate commitment to decisions. Constructive conflict will not result in everyone achieving the outcomes that they want. To promote fair, open processes of constructive conflict, Roberto (in Lagace, 2005, p. 3) warned leaders to consider the following "rules of engagement." For people to believe that the process is fair, they must:

1. Have ample opportunity to express their views and to discuss how and why they disagree with other group members.
2. Feel that the decision-making process has been transparent; that is, that deliberations have been relatively free of secretive, behind-the-scenes maneuvering.

3. Believe that the leader listened carefully to them and considered their views thoughtfully and seriously before making a decision.
4. Perceive that they had a genuine opportunity to influence the leader's final decision.
5. Have a clear understanding of the rationale for the final decision (Lagace, 2005, p. 3).

LEADERS STRIVE FOR CONSENUS

It is reassuring for both leaders and followers to know that they are working together. Consensus is not blind. It is achieved through social convergence (Stephen, Zubasek, & Goldenberg, 2015). Consensus is a process that occurs after individuals are able to offer their initial ideas in small groups of two to three, explaining why they think the ideas are useful in addressing the problem at hand. The ideas of these small groups are then fielded within a larger group, and a convergence occurs in which consensus can be reached.

Consensus is generally more effective than a majority vote that automatically elicits the dissenting opinion after the decision is made. Consensus represents a generally high level of commitment to the course of action, a buy-in to the process, and shared understanding of the direction of the work. It is through consensus that teams can move the vision and mission of the organization forward.

Building and sustaining effective teams may be among the most challenging of tasks for the leader. But the rewards of achieving consensus on thorny problems among a variety of minds and hearts go far beyond any unique creative approach offered by an individual. Teamwork is the norm and requirement of decision making and progress in health care. Make it a practice to observe healthy, effective teams and examine the characteristics of their leaders and how they function. Your contribution to a better future in health care may be the work of your own team.

REFERENCES

Block, P. (2008). *Community: The structure of belonging*. San Francisco, CA: Berrett-Koehler.

Broome, M. (2015). Collective genius. *Nursing Outlook, 63*(2), 105–107.

Broome, M. E., & Gilbert, J. (2014). Developing and sustaining self. In J. Daly, S. Speedy, & D. Jackson (Eds.), *Leadership and nursing: Contemporary perspectives* (2nd ed., pp. 199–212). Sydney, Australia: Elsevier.

Clark, P. R. (2009). Teamwork: Building healthier workplaces and providing safer patient care. *Critical Care Nursing Quarterly, 32*(3), 221–231.

D'Innocenzo, L., Mathieu, J. E., & Kukenberger, M. R. (2014). A meta-analysis of different forms of shared leadership–team performance relations. *Journal of Management, 20*(10), 1–28.

Doucette, J. N. (2008). Conflict management for nurse leaders. In H. R. Feldman, M. Jaffe-Ruiz, M. L. McClure, M. J., Greenberg, & T. D. Smith (Eds.), *Nursing leadership: A concise encyclopedia* (pp. 125–128). New York, NY: Springer Publishing Company.

Gerardi, D. (2010). *Conflict management training for health care professionals.* Retrieved from http://www.mediate.com/articles/gerardi4.cfm

Gibson, C. B., Cooper, C. D., & Conger, J. A. (2009). Do you see what we see? The complex effects of perceptual distance between leaders and teams. *Journal of Applied Psychology, 94*(1), 62.

Gilbert, J. H., & Broome. M. E. (2015). Leadership in a complex world. In M. C. Sitterding & M. E. Broome (Eds.), *Information overload: Framework, tips, and tools to manage in complex healthcare environments.* Silver Spring, MD: American Nurses Association Publications.

Goffee, R., & Jones, G. (2011). Why should anyone be led by you? In *Harvard business review, on leadership* (pp. 79–95). Boston, MA: Harvard Business Review Press.

Greer, L. L., Caruso, H. M., & Jehn, K. A. (2011). The bigger they are, the harder they fall: Linking team power, team conflict, and performance. *Organizational Behavior & Human Decision Processes, 116*(1), 116–128.

Grille, A., Schulte, E. M., & Kauffeld, S. (2015). Promoting shared leadership: A multi-level analysis investigating the role of prototypical team leader behavior, psychological empowerment, and fair rewards. *Journal of Leadership & Organizational Studies,* online before print. doi:1548051815570039. Retrieved from http://jlo.sagepub.com/content/early/2015/02/03/1548051815570039

Hackman, J. R., & Wageman, R. (2005). A theory of team coaching. *Academy of Management Review, 30*(2), 269–287.

Hill, L., Bandeau, G., Truelove, E., & Lineback, K. (2014). *Collective genius: The art and practice of leading innovation.* Boston, MA: Harvard Business Review Press.

Holleman, G., Poot, E., Mintjes-de Groot, J., & van Achterberg, T. (2009). The relevance of team characteristics and team directed strategies in the implementation of nursing innovations: A literature review. *International Journal of Nursing Studies, 46*(9), 1256–1264.

Humphrey, S. E., Morgeson, F. P., & Mannor, M. J. (2009). Developing a theory of the strategic core of teams: A role of composition model of team performance. *Journal of Applied Psychology, 94*(1), 48–61.

Institute of Medicine. (2003). *Crossing the quality chasm: A new health system for the 21st century.* Washington, DC: National Academies Press.

Interprofessional Education Collaborative Expert Panel. (2011). *Core competencies for interprofessional collaborative practice: Report of an expert panel.* Washington, DC: Interprofessional Education Collaborative.

Kearney, E., & Gebert, D. (2009). Managing diversity and enhancing team outcomes: The promise of transformational leadership. *Journal of Applied Psychology, 94*(1), 77.

Klein, K., Zeigert, J., Knight, A., & Xiao, Y. (2006). Dynamic delegation: Shared hierarchical and de-individualized leadership in extreme action teams. *Administrative Science Quarterly, 51*, 590–621.

Körner, M., Ehrhardt, H., & Steger, A. K. (2013). Designing an interprofessional training program for shared decision-making. *Journal of Interprofessional Care, 27*(2), 146–154.

Lagace, M. (2005, June 6). Don't listen to "Yes." In *Harvard Business School, working knowledge: The thinking that leads.* Retrieved from http://hbswk.hbs.edu/item/dont-listen-to-yes

Leonard-Barton, D., & Swap, W. (2005). Deep smarts. *Harvard Business Review, 30*(2), 157–169.

Mesmer-Magnus, J. R., & DeChurch, L. A. (2009). Information sharing and team performance: A meta-analysis. *Journal of Applied Psychology, 94*(2), 535.

Mitchell, P., Wynia, M., Golden, R., McNelis, B., Okun, S., Webb, C., . . . Von Kohorn, I. (2012). *Core principles and values of effective team-based health care.* Discussion paper. Washington, DC: Institute of Medicine.

Morgeson, F. P. (2005). The external leadership of self-managing teams: Intervening in the context of novel and disruptive events. *Journal of Applied Psychology, 90*(3), 497–508.

Morgeson, F. P., DeRue, D., & Karam, E. (2010). Leadership in teams: A functional approach to understanding leadership structures and processes. *Journal of Management, 36*(2), 579–587.

Morrison, J. (2008). The relationship between emotional intelligence competencies and preferred conflict-handling styles. *Journal of Nursing Management, 16*(8), 974–983.

Needleman, J., Buerhaus, P., Pankratz, V. S., Leibson, C. L., Stevens, S. R., & Harris, M. (2011). Nurse staffing and inpatient hospital mortality. *New England Journal of Medicine, 364*(11), 1037–1045.

Orchard, C. A., King, G. A., Khalili, H., & Bezzina, M. B. (2012). Assessment of interprofessional team collaboration scale (AITCS): Development and testing of the instrument. *Journal of Continuing Education in the Health Professions, 32*(1), 58–67.

Rahim, M. (2011). *Managing conflict in organizations* (4th ed.). Piscataway, NJ: Transaction Publishers.

Reeves, S., Perrier, L., Goldman, J., Freeth, D., & Zwarenstein, M. (2013). Interprofessional education: Effects on professional practice and healthcare outcomes (update). *Cochrane Database of Systematic Reviews, 3*(3), CD002213.

Reeves, S; Lewin, S; Espin S; Zwarenstein, M. (2011). *Interprofessional care for health and social care.* Oxford, UK: Wiley-Blackwell.

Rosenstein, A., Dinklin, S., & Munro, J. (2014). Conflict resolution: Unlocking the key to success. *Nursing Management, 45*(10), 34–39.

Salas, E., DiazGranados, D., Weaver, S. J., & King, H. (2008). Does team training work? Principles for health care. *Academic Emergency Medicine, 15*(11), 1002–1009.

Sitterding, M., & Broome, M. E. (2015). *Information overload: Framework, tips, and tools to manage in complex healthcare environments.* Washington, DC: American Nurses Association.

Stephen, A., Zubasek, P., & Goldenberg, J. (2015, July 24). People offer better ideas when they can't see what others suggest. *Harvard Business Review.* Retrieved from https://hbr.org/2015/07/people-offer-better-ideas-when-they-cant-see-what-others-suggest

Thistlethwaite, J. (2012). Interprofessional education: A review of context, learning and the research agenda. *Medical Education, 46*(1), 58–70.

Thomas, K. W., & Kilmann, R. H. (1974). *The Thomas-Kilmann conflict mode instrument.* Mountain View, CA: Xicom.

Zohar, D., & Tenne-Gazit, O. (2008). Transformational leadership and group interaction as climate antecedents: A social network analysis. *Journal of Applied Psychology, 93*(4), 744.

CHAPTER 11

Leadership in the Larger Context: Leading Among Leaders

Elaine Sorensen Marshall and Marion E. Broome

Never assume that you see the whole picture.
There is always more. Keep looking.

—*Frank Rivers*

OBJECTIVES

- *To understand the importance of one's ability to take the perspective of other leaders when working on common goals and organizational initiatives*
- *To describe how education and training influence one's perspective and collaborative behaviors*
- *To identify how differences in generational cohorts influence a leader's approach to planning and execution of ideas*
- *To identify the various regulatory and political arenas in which leaders of nursing operate and to recognize strategies to improve the viability of nursing expertise*
- *To describe actions one takes to widen a sphere of influence in the larger community that interacts with health care*

Current health care environments are complex, uncertain, and changing in ways we never imagined. O'Neil (2009) listed four key changes in American demographics that will ensure change in health care: (a) sheer growth in population, (b) increasing racial and ethnic diversity, (c) dramatic aging of the population, and (d) the epidemiology of illness and care moving from acute to chronic, and from hospital to community. We claim to forecast the future (Hegarty, Walsh, Condon, & Sweeney, 2009; Robinson & Reinhard, 2009; Thomas & Hynes, 2009), but no one really knows what is next in practice or leadership.

Even more surprises will happen in health care. Health care institutions are confronting the need to consider business decisions they have rarely faced before. For example, how many primary care practices can one system support in order to provide a "customer base" from which to refer patients to specialists within the system? Must a system maintain all patient care services within its network (e.g., rehabilitation) or is it possible to partner with other independent specialty units more cost effectively? Hundreds of other such questions challenge health care systems at all levels. As accountable care models change the emphasis to one of securing cost-effective, high-quality outcomes within a fully integrated system, leaders of all professions and disciplines will be asked to think in new ways, to work together to generate solutions to system problems, and to support their workforce to enact shared decisions. Such bold, creative moves will surely change how we think about health care financing, coverage, services, and systems. In the past decade, this situation has been called "a perfect storm" (Yoder-Wise, 2007), because a constellation of factors has come together in a figuratively explosive manner. How we predict and prepare for a better future will depend on how we as leaders understand each other and how we all work together.

Never has the need been greater for an army of visionary leaders to join in the transformation of health care to meet the challenges of the next generation. Supreme among the challenges is the requirement to work together and to understand each other. Leaders are serving in a time of challenge when simply understanding the language, practice, and culture of other disciplines is not enough. We must come to the table, speak each other's languages, and communicate with fluency.

KNOWING THE OTHER LEADERS AND TAKING THEIR PERSPECTIVE

The enterprise of health care comprises dozens of different highly trained clinical and management experts representing a broad range of preparation, theoretical perspectives, disciplinary bodies of knowledge, practice experience, and viewpoints. For the most part, we each go on our merry ways inside the silos of our disciplines. Although we interact cordially with professionals from other disciplines, we often approach our work in parallel play without meaningful attention to the perspective of our colleagues. Meanwhile, patients and families rightfully expect that we truly understand each other as we work together.

Throughout the history of health care, members of various disciplines have been educated, trained, and set out to engage in practice almost solely from within the narrow perspective and traditions of a single discipline. On occasion, once we enter the real world of practice, we run into each other in areas where the disparities in power and influence erupt. This sometimes happens when we notice that "someone else" is doing the tasks to which we have become accustomed as our territory. Physicians can become distressed when nurse practitioners write prescriptions; nurses resist registered care technicians at the bedside; radiological technicians are upset when dental assistants take x-rays. Even within disciplines, registered nurses complained when licensed practical nurses first inserted intravenous needles, and radiologists complained when the first obstetricians used the ultrasound machine. We have fought disciplinary battles over obstetrical forceps, venipuncture, ownership of the button on the x-ray machine, and, most recently, who can be addressed as "doctor." We assert authority over the skills and tools we were taught to use. For example, policy statements from medicine continue to set barriers for advanced practice nursing (Hain & Fleck, 2014). Such actions are unbecoming to professions that profess healing and altruism at their core. This cannot continue. Patients, families, and the communities we serve deserve better. The next generation of leaders must respond with authentic interprofessional understanding and collaboration. Excellence in health care demands our ability to understand and work together at the most basic levels.

It is important to understand the context out of which the present situation evolved. Disciplinary boundaries for preparation, expertise, and scope of practice are important to confirm order, develop expertise, and provide clear public information about which professional can be accountable for providing which services. But the public needs to be informed by wisdom and not by squabbles over tools, procedures, and titles. We must work together for the good of our communities, and we must begin to do that by cultivating the basic skill of professional perspective taking.

Perspective taking is the empathetic understanding of another's viewpoint, way of thinking, motivation, or feelings (Dugan, Bohle, Woelker, & Cooney, 2014). It goes beyond simple understanding of the "other" to include the ability to interpret back the other's viewpoint from his or her frame of reference as well as to convey empathy. It requires that we reflect on our own viewpoint, and practice seeing the world through the prism of the other. From an interprofessional viewpoint, we can begin to build authentic working relationships by learning each other's history and traditions; by reflecting on our similarities, differences, and mutual priorities; by reading each other's literature and policies; and by basic respect for and recognition of our need for each other as we work together.

It is simplistic to point to "the other" discipline as the problem, yet too often that is what one hears. First, the unbecoming behaviors of physicians and nurses who continue to point to each other as uncivil and to be blamed for lapses in care delivery have become old, tired and, in many cases, can place patients at risk when communication patterns are broken. Second, we need to move beyond attempts to highlight the virtues of our own discipline over how we work together. For example, often, nurse leaders emphasize the contribution of nursing or herald the "voice of nursing." Although this may be laudable within the discipline and explained reasonably by history and legitimate needs to secure autonomy of practice (Stewart, Stansfeld, & Tapp, 2004), it is often not helpful. Often, what is needed is to take the perspective of other health care disciplines to move the agenda forward for improved health care. Taking the broader perspective enhances understanding of the "whys" of intention and behavior, while not requiring that one agree with that line of reasoning or behavior. Of course, nursing and medicine are not the only disciplines that confront these kinds of tensions; a kind of egocentrism is present to some degree in all professions. The wise leader is at least aware of this tendency and is willing to look at the horizon through a different frame of reference.

Another common problem in professional disciplines is to focus on the time-valued activities within the profession without considering resources or the bottom line for the whole. The worn phrase "Follow the money" is a truism (Steinbrook, 2009). We need another phrase, such as "Follow the care to the patient." (Cassell & Guest, 2012). Disciplines need to come together on quality, patient experiences, and cost, better known as the triple aim. These mandates cross all professional boundaries.

We cannot adequately take the perspective of the other if we do not know about the other. We need to understand the basic philosophies that underpin the knowledge and practices of each discipline, how and why we prepare our clinicians in the way we do, and what are our values are. We need to understand each other's fears, hopes, and aspirations.

Working Across Disciplines, Styles, and Models

There is hope on the horizon. Across the world, health care disciplines are responding to the call to work together. Here we discuss the system's response to calls for collaboration. Burnett (2005) described a phenomenon in Scotland called the *managed clinical network*, which is an interdisciplinary model to provide high-quality, evidence-based, knowledge-based care. It is based on an organizational system of knowledge and information sharing, valuing, acquiring, networking, and using knowledge to improve quality of care. In Canada, authors also described successful collaborations between research and practice in health services (Brazil, MacLeod, & Guest, 2002). Other examples could be reported in all aspects of care. In the United States, we are beginning to foster collaborative ventures between medicine and nursing—especially in professional education—in learning clinical skills (Dillon, Noble, & Kaplan, 2009; Margalit et al., 2009; Reese, Jeffries, & Engum, 2010). Globally, new nurse-led models of care are becoming more prevalent, and the evidence supports their effectiveness in reducing readmissions (Lambrinou, Kalogirou, Lamnisos, & Sourtzi, 2012) as well as improved health outcomes and cost reductions in all settings (Oliver, Pennington, Revelle, & Rantz, 2014).

"Working across styles" refers not only to different characteristics among disciplines or personalities but also to actual styles of practice or practice model designs. Leaders who are multilingual across disciplines are needed to develop and implement such organizing principles. Systems that integrate across disciplines are better able to meet population health care needs, link information systems between providers and patients, and coordinate care across settings. Models that build "integrated practice units" will not only treat disease but engage individuals in care, encourage adherence, provide health education, and support needed behavioral change. However, these processes will demand a "village" approach to care delivery. Teams will have one primary goal: improve outcomes through review of data on performance, develop and test new protocols, collect data to personalize care, and assess changes in both patient and provider performance (Porter & Lee, 2013). Disciplinary squabbles about who does what will detract from optimal performance and affect access, quality, and cost of care.

Primary care is an important example in current health care debates. To meet the needs for primary care, it will be especially important for physicians, physician assistants, and advanced practice nurses (APNs) to work together to understand the perspective of the other in order to best serve the public. This will affect practice, business affairs, educational preparation of practitioners, and licensing regulations. For example, a growing trend in primary care is the retail clinic. Clinics inside drugstores or shopping malls have attracted controversy and debate, largely because they are "different," although their potential has been recognized as valuable for screening, prevention, and as a "safety-net provider for the poor and underserved" (Rudavsky & Mehrotra, 2010, p. 42). The nearly 3,000 such clinics across the United States (a threefold increase since 2010) provide an opportunity for transformational leaders to collaborate not only across disciplines but also across new approaches to care. But the cost-effectiveness of these clinics is influenced by state regulations about scope of practice, which are slow to change (Robert Wood Johnson Foundation [RWJF], 2016).

Another interprofessional model is the "medical home," a concept advocated in 2007 by a consortium representing the American Academy of Family Physicians, the American Academy of Pediatrics, the American College of Physicians, and the American Osteopathic Association. It is officially named the *patient-centered medical home* (Kellerman & Kirk, 2007). Early principles of the medical home included the provision of a personal physician for each patient, a focus on primary care, a physician-directed medical practice, whole person orientation, coordinated or integrated care, quality and safety, enhanced access to care, and payment structures that "recognize the added value provided" (Kellerman & Kirk, 2007, pp. 774–775). The current iteration reflects the team-based model (physician, APNs, physician assistants, and medical assistants) that has expanded to provide chronic illness management in ambulatory care (Bodenheimer, 2011).

Although the basic principle of the medical home is needed and laudable, the initial focus in this model on direct care of all patients by physicians, to the exclusion of other disciplines such as APNs, was unfortunate. There is some evidence that one purpose of the medical home may be to secure interests of physicians (Baron & Cassel, 2008; Dimick, 2008; Fisher, 2008; Rogers, 2008; Rubinstein, 2008; Scherger, 2009). Yet, changes in reimbursement and new care management compensation have mandated change in order to obtain the increased access, decreased cost, and increased quality that drove the initial concept. Struggles in care delivery required redefinition of provider roles, which has created angst for certain providers and remains a challenge (Nutting et al., 2010)

Nevertheless, despite its initial flaws, a model that values a health care "home" for primary care and care coordination for patients and families is highly needed. Our challenge now is to secure the broadest perspective of patients, communities, and health care disciplines in the construction of care models that enhance the patient experience and provider satisfaction. This will be one of the first tasks of doctors of nursing practice working with medicine and other disciplines. As accountable care models evolve, it will be interesting to watch whether and how the concept of medical home is sustained.

Working Across Generations

As the health care workforce becomes more diverse, leaders will have opportunities to work with people not only from a greater variety of disciplinary backgrounds but also across the range of generations. Howe and Strauss (2000, 2007) reminded that as a society, we move across time among different groups born at different times, faced with different generational cultural issues, and shaped by different life experiences as a group or generation. They further asserted that there may be cycles of these generational phenomena. We now recognize some general common characteristics in various generational groups. Of course, those commonalities do not represent specific individuals, but they do provide a general guide to understand generational perspectives.

Current popular concepts recognize traditionalists, born from 1925 to 1945, who have been socialized to stay in a specific workplace, or even the same position, over an entire career and thus may be resistant to change. Baby boomers, born from 1946 to 1964, are also generally loyal to their work and to their employer. On the other hand, Generation X, born between 1965 and 1980, shows no such loyalty but rather may seek immediate rewards, advances, recognitions, and benefits. Generation Xers are individualists who search for career meaning and purpose. They are not impressed by authority or traditional hierarchical organizations. If they do not get what they seek, they will go somewhere else. We are now also working with Generation Y, also known as "millennials," who were born prewired for electronic technology. They seek the immediate and customized service that technology has always provided them, and they are less willing to see the value of personal sacrifice for an employer (Malleo, 2010). Only recently have we recognized generational characteristics in popular culture, although for some time, sociologists have examined social and generational cycles of philosophical and lifetime viewpoints and their associated cultural implications (Howe & Strauss, 2007; Strauss & Howe, 1991, 1997).

Nurses who have been surveyed follow some of the same patterns of beliefs and work-life behaviors. Keepnews, Brewer, Kovener, and Shin (2010) studied 2,369 newly licensed nurses and found significant differences on 12 different dimensions of work life, including job satisfaction, supervisory support, work-to-family conflict, and organizational commitment. The informed leader will cultivate a background in such sociological and cultural information. Keepnews and colleagues reminded us that these differences must be recognized in all aspects of the professional nurse's work climate, from orientation through evaluation. To develop and support the next generation of leaders, doctorally prepared nurse leaders must recognize how younger nurse professionals view their work as well as sources of satisfaction, and then leverage various opportunities to maximize productivity. For instance, work-life balance is clearly more important to younger professionals, which lends another dimension to shaping care delivery.

SUCCEEDING WITH REGULATORY ORGANIZATIONS

Within the culture of professional health care is the ever-present heavy hand of regulation. Indeed, health care has become one of the most regulated industries in modern society. Field (2007, p. 2) claimed that health care regulation in the United States is broad and disjointed:

> At the federal level there is the Department of Health and Human Services and its many components, including the Centers for Medicare and Medicaid Services (CMS), the Centers for Disease Control and Prevention (CDC), and the Food and Drug Administration (FDA), in addition to the Environmental Protection Agency (EPA), the Occupational Safety and Health Administration (OSHA), and numerous other agencies. In each state there are departments of health, welfare, and insurance. In cities and counties there are municipal health departments. Turning to the private side, there is the Joint Commission on Accreditation of Healthcare Organizations (JCAHO), the National Committee on Quality Assurance, and numerous professional boards and societies…. New ones are often added with little consideration for those already in place, sometimes resulting in redundancy and conflict.

In addition, there are other specific compliance requirements, such as privacy protections from the Health Insurance Portability and Accountability Act (HIPAA), protection of human subjects in research, health information technology standards, nondiscrimination regulations, and numerous others. Employees in most health care organizations and schools of nursing are required to complete training (sometimes online, sometimes in person) in as many as five to seven of these various compliance policies and regulations. To the leader at any level, enforcing the vast array of external regulations can be daunting, but they cannot be ignored. Most importantly, it is crucial that the leader set the pace in this area through his or her on-time completion of requirements (many annually) as well as by providing for the success of others.

Although these responsibilities may appear overwhelming, most accredited health care institutions have processes and personnel in place to help the organization sustain compliance with myriad regulations. Your job as leader is to assure that such offices and people perform to their fullest, to support their work, to champion compliance, and to integrate compliance with your own vision as well as quality and performance within your organization.

Beyond the employer, the first-level regulatory body for professional nursing practice in the United States is the state board of nursing, which takes its authority from the state legislature. Each U.S. state has its own practice act that governs the scope of nursing practice and its own regulatory body, usually called the board of nursing. Practice acts outline the authority, scope, and criteria for licensure. State regulatory boards differ considerably, especially in their requirements related to advanced practice nursing and the scope of practice for nurses in each state.

As a leader, it is important to know and understand your local and state regulations. Critical issues related to autonomy and practice authority, particularly for APNs, remain to be resolved. For example, there remains a vast range of state regulations regarding prescriptive authority. Advanced nursing practice has evolved in response to consumer demand and financial issues, yet the role remains constrained in some areas due to public policy challenges at the state level, although some areas of the federal government have changed reimbursement patterns in substantial ways and these are expected to change even more (Iglehart, 2013).

As a leader, you must be visible and build relationships with the regulators, including members of boards of nursing, legislators, and other civic leaders who have influence in health care. Regarding scope of practice, legislators are often heavily influenced by professional organizations, such as the state medical association. Be an active part of your state nurses association and be available to provide testimony to support expansion of APN roles so that patient access can be improved and costs of health care reduced. It is critical as a transformational leader to be an integral member of the professional community at large. Personal relationships have been instrumental in legislative changes more often than well-written, well-reasoned proposals.

Although unions may not be considered regulatory organizations, they can exert considerable influence on regulations and practices within your organization. In 2014, unions represented 11.2% of all workers in the United States and 17% of all registered nurses (Hirsch & Macpherson, 2016). The best known union is probably the United American Nurses, formed in 1999 as an independent affiliate of the American Nurses Association (ANA). Laws related to labor relations in public health care facilities vary across states. Generally, employees have the right to organize and bargain collectively, strike, grieve, and arbitrate issues. Employees have the right to advance notice of union activities and intentions, and regulations usually preclude supervisors or managers from joining union activities (Ballard, 2008).

Regardless of the regulation load, keep your perspective as the leader. Remember that such regulations and programs are designed to make your work better. Do not allow yourself to become either buried in overwhelming "stuff" or beguiled by illusions that compliance guarantees human caring. Remember your vision and your purpose to help others to promote health and care for the sick and suffering. You are the guardian of the human processes and the humanity in your organization.

WORKING WITH THE GOVERNING BOARD

Working with the board of trustees of your organization can be one of the most unique and rewarding aspects of your life as a leader. Boards usually include selected members of the community, representing a broad range of experience in health care from none to considerable. Since boards have a fiduciary responsibility to represent the community, there is increasing expectation of responsibility in financial oversight. This requires considerable orientation, training, and preparation for effective service (Evans, 2009; Walton, Lake, Mullinix, Allen, & Mooney, 2015). That is usually the job of the leader of the organization, working with the director or president of the board.

During your career as a leader, you may be responsible for recruiting or working directly with a board, collaborating with a board, or actually serving on a board (Jumaa, 2008). If you work for a hospital or nonprofit organization, you may work directly with your board of trustees. In 2014 the American Academy of Nursing joined 21 other organizations, including the AARP, ANA, Sigma Theta Tau International (STTI), and the American Organization of Nurse Executives (AONE), to promote the appointment of 10,000 nurses to boards by 2020. This national coalition will implement a strategy designed to bring nurses with their expertise to governing boards in health-related sectors (Campaign for Action, 2014). Regarding the purpose, composition, and actions of a governing board, Nadler (2004, p. 104) asserted that the high-performance board "is competent, coordinated, collegial, and focused on an unambiguous goal. Such entities do not simply evolve; they must be constructed to an exacting blueprint." These boards need the right work, the right people, the right agenda, the right information, and the right culture. Nagler also outlined the agenda, norms, beliefs, and values for effective boards.

Each board, and each situation, is unique. If you have the opportunity to recruit members to your own advisory or governing board, think strategically. Consider special skills, insights, background, community connections, and personality types (Mycek, 2000). Consider needs for the makeup of the board itself, but especially for your organization. All members of the board must care deeply about your organization; loyalty is the prime qualification. If you need fundraising, identify people who will either make significant donations or have connections with those who may. Be prepared to accommodate a range of types of participation. Mycek (2000) described a board member of a children's hospital who was a major contributor to the board, never attended a board meeting, but was essential to community networking. I (Marshall) served on a board where one member seldom engaged directly in board activities but had a key legislative connection. Be creative in including such board members in activities outside the board meetings, in committee subcommittees, and as well-informed advocates or representatives of your organization to the community at large. Make sure that all board members understand the mission of the organization and tell the same story—your story!

As a leader with stature, you will likely be invited to serve on the board of another agency in your community. Some board members are compensated; others are expected to provide voluntary service. If you serve on a board, you can benefit from positive personal relationships with other board members to influence decision making, resource allocation, and the strategic direction of the organization (DiMattio, 2015; Thorman, 2004). This raises a broader concern. Especially in board service, the possibility of conflicts of interest must be considered.

A conflict of interest occurs when personal or private interests exist that may interfere with professional or public responsibilities or interests. As a leader, at some point, you will be confronted with a potential conflict of interest. It may be the offer of an inappropriate personal gift or the opportunity to gain personally from a professional or public endeavor. Conflicts of interest involve the use of position, power, or influence to gain advantage for self or others, and seldom occur because of actual malicious intent. Such advantages may be large or small; personal, political, or financial. A conflict of interest may be actual, perceived, or potential (Greenfeld, 2008).

When you are in the thick of things, it may not always be easy to recognize a conflict of interest. It helps to ask the question, "If I worked for me, would I think this was appropriate?" Or, "If this appeared in the newspaper, would it be something I would be proud of?" Then trust your inner voice. Confer with a wise mentor or leader. Sometimes, it is enough to simply disclose the potential conflict of interest publicly so that everyone involved is aware that you have some personal involvement in the issue. Other times, you must remove yourself from the situation, refuse the offer, or decline the opportunity. It may be helpful to consult with legal counsel within your organization if the potential conflict is significant or even just ambiguous. If the conflict precludes your service on one board, be assured that other opportunities will come. Whatever your action, the ethical response always offers personal peace and potential future opportunities.

Finally, be aware that on occasion decisions you make, or support as a board member will not be popular with other nurses (DiMattio, 2015). This may place you in a difficult position, but if you supported the decision for the right reasons you will sleep better at night. People notice and respect the ethical leader.

WORKING WITH LAWYERS, LEGISLATORS, AND POLICY MAKERS

The practice and leadership of nursing are integrally related to decisions of law, government, public and private payment organizations, and a variety of other legal entities. Such groups affect standards, practices, and payment for care.

If you serve any time as a leader, you may at some point be involved directly or indirectly in litigation. Most often lawsuits involving nurse executives are related to patient safety or breaches in such performed by subordinates who report directly or indirectly to the executive. The leader facing litigation for the first time quickly realizes that he or she did not learn about this in school. And, since no one talks about it at work, he or she may feel totally unprepared and alone. In this situation, it is easy to think, "I must be the only one this has ever happened to." That is not true. Because of the discrete, confidential, and often distressing nature of most issues of litigation, few people talk about them. Usually, these issues have little or nothing to do with the nurse executive personally; rather, he or she is named because of the specific leadership position held. Regardless of the situation, the adversarial nature of such events can be overwhelming and sometimes devastating.

If you find yourself in this situation, seek legal help immediately. Begin by contacting legal counsel within your organization, if such exists. In a position of leadership, you should have already cultivated a positive relationship with your institutional general counsel. If you have a personal issue in the case, seek your own counsel. Remember that the organizational counsel's priority is to protect the corporation, not you personally. If you are called to give a deposition or to testify in a case not related to you, still seek counsel. You need a lawyer to help you prepare. Usually the institution's counsel will help prepare you for any testimony—whether in a deposition or in court. Do not forget the following three simple rules when you are deposed or testifying under oath in court:

1. Listen to the question.
2. Answer the question (and *only* the question).
3. Then stop talking.

Also remember that most legal cases go on for what seems like forever. You must find a way to live your life alongside the case. Let it unfold, attend to it when required, and continue your best performance as the leader you are.

Most activities in the public arena will not have direct legal implications but rather will be related to influencing public policy. Public policy refers specifically to sources of such rules, actions, and decisions specifically from government agencies. Simply stated, policy comprises the official plan, rules, and decisions regarding how resources are allocated to a specific purpose. Health policy includes the "rules, actions, and decisions by government and private bodies—which affect the delivery of health care and the processes by which health care takes place" (Keepnews, 2008, p. 270).

The transformational leader in health care must be fluent in current issues and activities related to health policy. Resources, regulations, and decision making in health care are increasingly influenced by legislative and professional policy. Policy fluency affords the leader the opportunity to provide input and be proactive rather than reactive to measures that affect health care organizations. A significant number of doctor of nursing practice programs include offerings on health policy to improve understanding and skills in negotiating policy issues, such as scope of practice, health care compensation, the impact of care delivery models, and related issues. To improve policy literacy, nurse leaders may participate in policy training programs, graduate courses, or studies of information, which are provided by nearly every major health care organization.

In 2016 there were five nurses serving as legislators in the United States Congress (all in the House of Representatives) and many more in the state legislatures (ANA, 2016). Many of them have shared that their nursing background provided them with interpersonal, analytical, and advocacy skills to represent their constituencies. The Congressional Nursing Caucus is a group of members from both parties whose backgrounds help them provide a voice in Congress for the health care needs and professional values of nursing. These members can be especially helpful to the profession in addressing nursing issues.

In an interview in 2014, two nurse congresswomen, Lois Capps (D-CA) and Diane Black (R-TN), emphasized the critical importance of nurse leaders who can lend voice and skill to the national health care policy agenda (RWJF, 2014). The American Association for Colleges of Nursing (AACN) prepares valuable toolkits each year outlining the issues and talking points for those visiting with their legislators (AACN, 2015).

Key points for interacting with your legislator include the following: (a) be prepared for a 15-minute maximum visit; (b) prepare your elevator speech, which should include only a few powerful salient points; (c) include short data points that support your premise; and (d) use stories or examples of nurses who make a difference. These stories are especially helpful to legislative aides who prepare briefs for the legislators.

To convert your practice, research, or project to policy, observe what kinds of evidence are best accepted by legislators and policy makers and what kinds of projects are funded. Identify networks within your community and become part of them. Lewis (2009, p. 125) called these "networks of influence." Practice-based evidence (Horn & Gassaway, 2007) is a systematic method to provide data directly from what works in practice—this approach is especially useful to influence policy makers. It uses knowledge and practices from frontline care-givers on interdisciplinary teams, and contributes real stories to policy makers, with images that make policy needs real.

Always have your 30-second elevator conversation ready. Practice it to yourself, emphasizing no more than three major points of your issue. Prepare an internal script that you can recite, with passion, in any situation. Keep it short, clear, and compelling. Then watch and wait for the perfect opportunity. I [Marshall] knew of an influential leader who was prepared. She needed support for a major change initiative from the highest level—the president of the corporation. Without regular access or optimal timing, she simply prepared and waited. She practiced her 30-second approach. She watched and waited. Finally, she coincidentally met the president in an airport security line. When he asked the generic innocuous question, "How is it going?" She was ready. She knew she had only about 30 seconds. She did not hesitate; she did not force, mumble, fumble, or whine. She simply repeated the main points she had rehearsed for weeks. She took advantage of the "luck" of the circumstance through supreme preparation. The president responded with interest and intrigue. Soon, she was *invited* to the president's office to share her idea, which eventually culminated in full support for her plan and her inclusion as a trusted professional colleague at the highest level of the institution.

HAVING INFLUENCE IN THE POLITICAL ARENA

Influence is power. It is the capacity to compel change in ideas, action, and results. Having influence is one of the most important and fulfilling gifts of being a leader. It is also one of the gifts one must be careful to use judiciously. It is easy to forget that position alone can influence others to agree with one verbally even when their behavior does not appear aligned with what they say.

Just as policy is ultimately a decision about how resources are allocated, politics is largely the distribution of power. Power involves making decisions to use the resources where one thinks the most benefits will be accrued for the organization's mission, and political power resides in who gets to make the decision (Gebbie, 2010). Resources can be time, people, or money. Leadership includes elements of policy and politics. In the larger arena, health care leadership may include effective *response* to policy and politics but must also include effective *influence on* policy and politics. Lewis (2006) analyzed the history of the influence and power of medicine on policy. All health care disciplines can learn from medicine's example to use ties of association and effective use of positional and personal influence. To be effective as a leader, you will engage in the policy arena and network with other people of influence. A report on the future of nursing from the Institute of Medicine (2010) reminded us that nursing has not maximized its political power and to create long-lasting change we must learn to do so. Education alone will not be sufficient unless we use our political power and influence.

It is well recognized that influence on policy requires collaboration and networking across a variety of interests. "Strategic alliances" are described as a way to promote collaboration across organizations working toward policy-related solutions to common problems. One contemporary example of a constructive alliance is between nursing and the AARP. As leaders in health care increase such alliances, we may expect greater applications of models from business, such as "disruptive innovations" (Huang & Christensen, 2008) and others.

So how does all of this relate to you now? You are likely leading, planning, or even contemplating some extraordinary or innovative project that might be expanded beyond your organization to make a difference in the larger community. At the outset, think larger. Include policy makers on your team. Invite your local government official, state legislator, or even your congressional representative. Become active in understanding and participating in regulatory initiatives. Regulations are most often developed from bad care rather than good works (Mason, 2010). The only way to influence a change is to become involved and to involve policy makers directly in your good work.

Mason (2010) outlined barriers related to policy that restrain the advancement of innovative models of care. They include national position statements and state regulations that limit the scope of practice of nonphysician providers (Pearson, 2009). Other barriers include limitations on reimbursement by insurers and payers to nonphysician providers. These barriers are further extended to definitions and credentialing of the medical or health home. In many cases, such restrictions are not necessary for quality and actually interfere with access. Mason (2010) also pointed to a list of nurse-related barriers to policy that supports innovative programs. The list includes "lack of clinical and financial outcome data," limiting reports to descriptions of programs and recipients served, and "failure to recognize the mandate to translate research into practice and policy." Another key barrier is the inability to translate or "scale up" creative interventions beyond a local use to larger applications (Mason, 2010).

The United States continues to be embroiled in debate regarding national health care policy. The issues are highly entangled regarding health insurance reform, mandated health insurance coverage, health care structures and paradigms such as the medical or health home, education for health professionals, scope of practice and roles of various health professionals, and ongoing issues of cost, access, and quality of health care. Among the most difficult questions are how to support health promotion and disease prevention initiatives in the face of overwhelming emphasis on acute care and large hospital systems, how to promote innovation, how to manage chronic conditions, and how to reach rural and underserved populations. These areas are crying most for creative leadership.

Too many nurses opt out of policy discussions. Coming from educational preparation that provided little or no training in policy, and heavily involved in patient care inside the clinical setting, nurses often do not see policy involvement as a priority. Demands of health care now require that nurse leaders join other professional leaders to influence and implement policy. As an expert clinician moving to the role of transformational leader, you have the preparation and tools to lead, and you have the social responsibility to influence policy. Mason (2010) reminded, "Society, and nurses themselves, should have higher expectations for what nurses can achieve, and . . . nurses should be held accountable for not only providing quality direct patient care, but also for health care leadership [in policy]."

Opportunities to become involved in making a difference in policy and politics abound. Speak up and speak out on institutional and public policy. In your role as expert, communicate on specific issues with policy makers; communicate in public forums through both traditional media and emerging social media; connect and partner with other health care leaders. Think creatively about influencing policy from a new perspective. For example, every state land-grant institution has an agricultural extension service that provides valuable public information. What would happen if we had a health information extension service? Just a thought—what would be the policy implications? Finally, seek and take opportunities to serve on corporate boards, hospital boards, boards of health, and nonprofit organizational boards at the local, state, and national levels. If your professional association is part of the Nurses on Boards Coalition (2016), work through their offices and let them know who you are, what your experience is, and your interest in serving on boards. Think about running for office in your local area, including boards of health, city council, or state legislature. Who knows where it will lead you, and where you will lead? Get your message to the public.

Throughout these experiences take the opportunity to learn from others, read widely, and study the biographies of great public leaders. Join and participate actively in national professional organizations. Collaborate broadly at every opportunity. Mentor, sponsor, and empower others to expand the influence of your own leadership. Think of yourself operating in different spheres: locally, nationally, and globally. Transformational leaders support others to "transcend their own self-interest" and to grow. They generate intellectual stimulation and emotional commitment (Weston, 2008). They recognize and promote the talent of others. They transcend the bureaucracy of their environments to raise all workers to higher levels.

TRANSFORMING PRACTICE AND POLICY IN THE LARGER COMMUNITY

Regardless of your practice or leadership role, your work environment includes the community beyond your institution. Just as individuals must lead from a collaborative interprofessional perspective, organizations within communities are interdependent and function best within the larger community perspective. There are various stimulating ways to serve.

As you continue your journey as a transformational leader, you will have opportunities to work with a variety of community agencies, including nonprofit organizations. In these times of cross-setting collaborations, partnerships, and mergers, the skill of showing authentic interest in working with others for the benefit of all is an art in and of itself. Your leadership and skill in doing this, if genuine, will be recognized. Indeed, as a respected community leader, you may be invited to serve on the board of directors of a nonprofit organization. It is important to understand the general characteristics of nonprofit organizations. Although hospitals are usually considered nonprofit—especially those associated with academic health centers—here we are talking about nonprofit community agencies.

Most nonprofit organizations function with a specific mission. "They rally under the banner of a particular cause" (Rangan, 2004, p. 112) such as homelessness or other underserved populations. Nonprofit organizations are particularly mission driven. Rangan (2004, p. 114) explained, "After all, the mission is what inspires founders to create the organization, and it draws board members, staff, donors, and volunteers to become involved, What's more, the founders often deliberately try to assure that their original vision is embraced by the next generation of leaders." Nonprofit organizations usually depend heavily on a financial base laid by private donations and grants. Thus, nonprofit organizations are closely tied to the community in which they reside, and the contribution of board members usually focuses on helping to secure donors.

Your experience with strategic planning and outcomes evaluation can be especially helpful if you serve with a nonprofit organization or any other community agency. Rangan (2004) asserted that although most nonprofit organizations are strong on mission, they are less able in translating the mission statement to an operational mission and strategy process. Because they are usually single-mission focused, there is little need to identify integration of specific programs. An operational mission can bring quantitative measurement and evaluation to the "lofty" inspiring mission. Then, specific objectives and strategies can be implemented. As a leader in health care this is certainly an area in which you could put your skills to use.

Preparing to Influence

The messages of this book have been directed to expert clinicians who are launching their careers as leaders. As you think about your own preparation to influence, consider advanced leadership preparation beyond the terminal degree. Recall from Chapter 9 that many professional associations, such as STTI and AONE, offer leadership training experiences ranging from short-term conferences to 18-month leadership academies. Take advantage of the opportunity to engage in larger arenas where you might interact with leaders from all disciplines. Make a commitment to never stop learning or growing.

Several formal leadership development programs are designed to help you build on your current preparation and experience to enhance your influence. Some of these were mentioned in Chapter 7. A few others are described briefly here as examples. The Wharton Nursing Leaders Program is directed toward high-level nursing leaders preparing for the role of chief nursing officer of a health care organization or a deanship. The program addresses the complexity of leadership in health care, strategic planning, resource management, decision making, and team building (Wharton Executive Education, 2016). The Harvard Business School (2015) offers several short- and long-term programs in leadership development, including programs in managing health care delivery and higher education.

If you aspire to leadership in higher education, many programs and fellowships are offered by the AACN (2015) and the American Council on Education (ACE, 2016). The Higher Education Resource Services (HERS, 2016) provides short-term residence programs specifically for women aspiring for higher education leadership. The Center for Creative Leadership (2015) also offers a range of programs for women and members of racial minorities in management positions. Specific to health care and nursing leadership, among the best known programs was the Robert Wood Johnson (2016) Executive Nurse Fellows program, which admitted its last class in 2014 and will likely develop new human talent programs in the future. Several creative endeavors to promote leadership development in specific areas offer programs, consulting, or information. For example, the RWJF combined with the Kellogg Foundation to support the National Center for Healthcare Leadership (NCHL), which has created Leadership Excellence Networks as a platform for health care systems to share best practices in leadership development (NCHL, 2016). Many highly reputable university business schools offer executive development programs. Seek out and participate in programs that may be offered at your own institution. A simple search and talking with other leaders will produce a large variety of programs and opportunities. The cost of such programs varies widely, from $1,000 to $10,000. Choose the best and make the case at your organization for the return on their investment in your preparation and networking as a leader. Negotiation for your preparation is instructive in itself to refine skills to negotiate ideas, projects, and changes related to your larger stewardship as a leader.

By the same token, generativity is an important part of your stewardship as a leader. "Paying it forward" includes the development of others and the creation of a learning organization for those within your institution. Supporting people in formal leadership development programs is not only helpful to the individual, but also powerful in the message of support for advancement and excellence in your organization, and it attracts useful networks to your work. Your influence is also critical to the next generation of leaders. Wise influence from a perspective of generativity includes succession planning at all levels. Health care has been behind other industries in succession planning in leadership (Carriere, Muise, Cummings, & Newburn-Cook, 2009; Titzer, Phillips, Tooley, Hall, & Shirey, 2013). Succession planning for positions throughout the nursing organization will require that time be spent identifying potential leaders and providing them with development opportunities outside the organization, feedback on their performance, and regular assessments of their learning.

Leading to Transform

It is important to understand various levels of influence in leadership. Within your health care organization, the primary goal is to support those who deliver direct care for the people or populations served by the agency. At this level nurse managers, directors, and executives now have budgets they must monitor and stay within. They make decisions about resource allocation and management. At higher levels of state, regional, or national service, you have the power to influence regulations, policy, and resources. You and your nurse colleagues at this level will be asked to make decisions regarding how money is allocated and for what services. At the international level, you have the influence to make recommendations for health care policy across nations.

Cook (2001) developed a model for leadership reflecting four elements or levels of the leadership style of the clinician leader: (a) experience, (b) understanding, (c) internal environment (personal values and beliefs), and (d) external environment. She further proposed an ascending order of style that ultimately moves from transformational to what she calls "renaissance leadership," which operates in the realm of holistic care and is characterized by empowering relationships among providers and patients. As a clinical leader, you are prepared to transform practice. You also have the professional responsibility to transform policy in the larger community to reflect the best of practice.

Opportunities to advance your influence abound throughout the world. Do not limit yourself. At the international level, you can influence policy for improved health care across the world. Global issues call for leadership to solve issues of worldwide shortages of health care professionals, especially nurses (Oulton, 2006), and other important issues of international disaster and humanitarian services (Negus, Brown, & Konoske, 2010). Become acquainted with and involved in international efforts. The International Council of Nurses (ICN) is a federation of national nursing organizations from 130 countries, representing over 13 million nurses throughout the world. ICN's current initiatives include championing the contribution and image of nurses worldwide, advocating for all nurses, advancing the nursing profession, and influencing health, social, educational, and economic policy (ICN, 2016). Think global: How might you become involved? What knowledge, skills, and insights as an American nurse might you bring to that arena? What could you learn from international colleagues about health care leadership?

International or global influence may take the form of involvement at the global level, as with the ICN or the World Health Organization, or a more local foreign partnership perspective by collaborating on specific issues with international partners, such as capacity building of nurses in direct care in developing countries, or participating in one of many international nursing mission opportunities. It is challenging, and well worth it, to work with partners in another country. It opens your vision and your view to new perspectives on old problems. You gain insights into cultural influences. You learn new perspectives of time. You discover different priorities. When the needs of your partner in a developing country may be as basic as water sanitation, you learn about different resources. And you share work across different technologies (Riner & Broome, 2014).

When something great is happening in one part of your own organization, it is sometimes difficult to spread the word and even more challenging to spread the positive action. Massoud, Nielsen, Nolan, Schall, and Sevin (2006) called this a "framework for spread," identifying the need for a system to accelerate or elevate improvement simply by getting changes to move across the organization. Others call it diffusion of innovation (Chaudoir, Dugan, & Barr, 2013; Rogers, 2003). It sometimes requires an entire change of culture to accept innovation as a way of living, working, and serving. When you are frustrated with the slow rate of change, remember the following guidelines to promote diffusion of innovation:

- Promote the idea: The innovation must be perceived as better than what people are already doing, so you have some selling to do.
- Provide a reliable source or channel of communication to spread the news that the new idea is better.
- Give people a little time to learn about the innovation, to participate in the decision, and to implement change.
- Make your institution a place of learning (Newhouse & Melnyk, 2009).
- Pay attention to the general culture and other leaders of your community to be sure you have their support (Weston, 2008).

To be able to encourage others to be innovative, you must provide a culture that encourages others to think big and take small risks—not an easy culture to promote in health care. Innovators respond to transformative leaders who support their diverse (and sometimes divergent) perspectives on things (Broome, 2016). To facilitate the diffusion of innovations the leader must be visible in adoption and support of new innovations.

You have prepared and cultivated the characteristics and habits of a transformational leader. You are able to function as a leader in a broad range of contexts, and you understand the power of culture. You embrace challenge. You know when to sustain tradition and when to be bold with innovation. You build and nurture your team. You understand economics and finance. You have prepared to become the leader the world needs.

You will have the greatest positive influence as a transformational leader if you are authentic and speak the truth. Authenticity means that you know and understand yourself. You are aware of your influence and effects on others. You are able to take the perspective of another. You are aware of your own values and strengths, and you are able to recognize the values and strengths of others. You are sensitive to the context in which you work, and you are "confident, hopeful, optimistic, resilient, and of high moral character" (Avolio, Gardner, Walumbwa, Luthans, & May, 2004, p. 804). People can believe you and count on you, and they want to work with you and for you. You live your values.

If you feel like you are not this person described, you can be. You can practice every day. Reflect on your progress at the end of the day, identifying what was the best part of each day. You bring the credibility of experience in expert clinical practice to the joyful places you create as environments for healing. Consider these words, commonly attributed to the poet Carl Sandburg:

> … For what you are … yet more for what you are going to be … not so much for your realities as for your ideals. I pray for your desires that they may be great, rather than for your satisfactions, which may be so hazardously little…. Not always shall you be what you are now. You are going forward toward something great. And I am on the way with you.

REFERENCES

American Association of Colleges of Nursing. (2015). From patient advocacy to political activism: AACN's guide to understanding policy and politics. Washington DC: Author. Retrieved from http://www.aacn.nche.edu/government-affairs/AACNPolicyHandbook_2010.pdf

American Council on Education. (2016). Retrieved from www.acenet.edu.

American Nurses Association (2016). Nurses currently serving in Congress. Retrieved from http://www.nursingworld.org/MainMenuCategories/Policy-Advocacy/Federal/Nurses-in-Congress

Avolio, B. J., Gardner, W. L., Walumbwa, F. O., Luthans, F., & May, D. R. (2004). Unlocking the mask: A look at the process by which authentic leaders impact follower attitudes and behaviors. *Leadership Quarterly, 15*, 801–823.

Ballard, K. A. (2008). Collective bargaining and unions. In H. R. Feldman, M. Jaffe-Ruiz, M. L. McClure, M. J. Greenberg, & T. D. Smith (Eds.), *Nursing leadership: A concise encyclopedia* (pp. 116–117). New York, NY: Springer Publishing Company.

Baron, R. J., & Cassel, C. K. (2008). 21st-century primary care: New physician roles need new payment models. *Journal of the American Medical Association, 299*(13), 1595–1597.

Bodenheimer, T. (2011). Lessons from the trenches: A high-functioning primary care clinic. *New England Journal of Medicine, 365,* 5–8. Retrieved from http://www.nejm.org/doi/full/10.1056/NEJMp1104942#t=article

Brazil, K., MacLeod, S., & Guest, B. (2002). Collaborative practice: A strategy to improve the relevance of health services research. *Healthcare Management Forum, 15*(3), 18–24.

Broome, M. (2016). The innovator. *Nursing Outlook, 64*(1), 1–2.

Burnett, S. (2005). Knowledge support for interdisciplinary models of healthcare delivery: A study of knowledge needs and roles in managed clinical networks. *Health Informatics Journal, 11*(2), 146–160.

Campaign for Action (2014). *Leveraging nursing leadership.* Retrieved from http://campaignforaction.org/campaign-progress/leveraging-nursing-leadership

Carriere, B. K., Muise, M., Cummings, G., & Newburn-Cook, C. (2009). Healthcare succession planning: An integrative review. *Journal of Nursing Administration, 39*(12), 548–555.

Cassell, C. K., & Guest, J. A. (2012). Choosing wisely: Helping physicians and patients make smart decisions about their care. *JAMA, 307*(17), 1801–1802.

Center for Creative Leadership. (2015). *Achieve what matters most.* Retrieved from http://www.ccl.org/leadership/about/

Chaudoir, S. R., Dugan, A. G., & Barr, C. H. (2013). Measuring factors affecting implementation of health innovations: A systematic review of structural, organizational, provider, patient, and innovation level measures. *Implementation Science, 8,* 22.

Cook, M. J. (2001). The renaissance of clinical leadership. *International Nursing Review, 48,* 38–46.

Dillon, P. M., Noble, K. A., & Kaplan, L. (2009). Simulation as a means to foster collaborative interdisciplinary education. *Nursing Education Perspectives, 30*(2), 87–90.

Dimattio, M. K. (2015). A view from the hospital boardroom. *Nursing Outlook, 63,* 533–536.

Dimick, C. (2008). Home sweet medical home: Can a new care model save family medicine? *Journal of the American Health Information Management Association, 79*(8), 24–28.

Dugan, J. P., Bohle, C. W., Woelker, L. R., & Cooney, M. A. (2014). The role of social perspective-taking in developing students' leadership capacities. *Journal of Student Affairs Research & Practice, 51*(1), 1–15. Retrieved from http://leadershipstudy.net/wp-content/uploads/2014/02/dugan-et-al-2014.pdf

Evans, M. (2009). Raising the bar for boards. *Modern Health Care, 39*(9), 1, 6–7, 16.

Field, R. I. (2007). *Health care regulation in America: Complexity, confrontation, and compromise.* Oxford, England: Oxford University Press.

Fisher, E. S. (2008). Building a medical neighborhood for the medical home. *New England Journal of Medicine, 359*(12), 1202–1205.

Gebbie, K. M. (2010, January). *Preparing doctoral students for health policy leadership.* Paper presented at the meetings of the American Association of Colleges of Nursing, Captiva Island, FL.

Greenfeld, D. (2008). Conflict of interest. In H. R. Feldman, M. Jaffe-Ruiz, M. L. McClure, M. J. Greenberg, & T. D. Smith (Eds.), *Nursing leadership: A concise encyclopedia* (pp. 125–128). New York, NY: Springer Publishing Company.

Hain, D., & Fleck, L. M. (2014). Barriers to NP practice that impact healthcare redesign. *Online Journal of Issues in Nursing, 19*(2). Retrieved from http://www.nursingworld.

org/MainMenuCategories/ANAMarketplace/ANAPeriodicals/OJIN/TableofContents/Vol-19-2014/No2-May-2014/Barriers-to-NP-Practice.html

Harvard Business School. (2015). E*xecutive education: Managing healthcare delivery.* Retrieved from http://www.exed.hbs.edu/programs/mhcd/

Hegarty, J., Walsh, E., Condon, C., & Sweeney, J. (2009). The undergraduate education of nurses: Looking to the future. *International Journal of Nursing Education Scholarship, 6*(1), 17.

HERS. (2016). What are the institutes? Retrieved from www.hersnet.org/institutes

Hirsch, B., & MacPherson, D. (2016). Union membership and coverage database from the CPS. Retrieved from www.unionstats.com

Horn, S. D., & Gassaway, J. (2007). Practice-based evidence study design for comparative effectiveness research. *Medical Care, 45*(10), S50–S57.

Howe, N., & Strauss, W. (2000). *Millennial rising: The next generation.* New York, NY: Random House.

Howe, N., & Strauss, W. (2007, July–August). The next 20 years: How customer and workforce attitudes will evolve. *Harvard Business Review.* Retrieved from http://download.2164.net/PDF-newsletters/next20years.pdf

Huang, J., & Christensen, C. M. (2008). Disruptive innovation in health care delivery: A framework for business-model innovation. *Health Affairs, 27*(5), 1329–1335.

Inglehart, J. K. (2013). Expanding the role of advanced nurse practitioners: Risks and rewards. *New England Journal of Medicine, 368,* 1935–1941.

Institute of Medicine. (2010). *The future of nursing.* Washington, DC: National Academies Press.

International Council of Nurses. (2016). *ICN's vision, mission, and strategic plan.* Retrieved from http://www.icn.ch/who-we-are/icns-vision-mission-and-strategic-plan/

Jumaa, M. O. (2008). The F.E.E.L. good factors in nursing leadership at board level through work-based learning. *Journal of Nursing Management, 16,* 992–999.

Keepnews, D. M. (2008). Health policy. In H. R. Feldman, M. Jaffe-Ruiz, M. L. McClure, M. J. Greenberg, & T. D. Smith (Eds.), *Nursing leadership: A concise encyclopedia* (pp. 269–273). New York, NY: Springer Publishing Company.

Keepnews, D. M., Brewer, C. S., Kovner, C. T., & Shin, J. H. (2010). Generational differences among newly licensed registered nurses. *Nursing Outlook, 58*(3), 155–163.

Kellerman, R., & Kirk, L. (2007, September 15). Principles of the patient-centered medical home. *American Family Physician, 76*(6), 774–776.

Lambrinou, E., Kalogirou, F., Lamnisos, D., & Sourtzi, P. (2012). Effectiveness of heart failure management programmes with nurse-led discharge planning in reducing re-admission: A systematic review and meta-analysis. *International Journal of Nursing Studies, 49*(5), 610–624.

Lewis, J. M. (2006). Being around and knowing the players: Networks of influence in health policy. *Social Science & Medicine, 62*(9), 2125–2136.

Lewis, J. M. (2009). Understanding policy influence and the public health agenda. *New South Wales Public Health Bulletin, 20*(7/8), 125–129.

Malleo, C. (2010, February 13). Each generation brings strengths, knowledge to nursing field: A nurse's journal. *Everything Cleveland.* Retrieved from http://www.cleveland.com/healthfit/index.ssf/2010/02/each_generation_brings_strengt.html

Margalit, R., Thompson, S., Visovsky, C., Geske, J., Collier, D., Birk, T., & Paulman, P. (2009). From professional silos to interprofessional education: Campus wide focus on quality of care. *Quality Management & Health Care, 18*(3), 165–173.

Mason, D. (2010, January 28). *Nursing's visibility in the national health care reform agenda*. Paper presented at the meetings of the American Association of Colleges of Nursing Doctoral Education Conference, Captiva Island, FL.

Massoud, M. R., Nielsen, G. A., Nolan, K., Schall, M. W., & Sevin, C. (2006). *From local improvements to system-wide change. IHI Innovation Series white paper*. Cambridge, MA: Institute for Healthcare Improvement.

Mycek, S. (2000). The right fit: Recruiting for your board. *Trustee, 53*(8), 1, 12–15.

Nadler, D. A. (2004, May). Building better boards. *Harvard Business Review, 82*(5), 102–111.

National Center for Healthcare Leadership. (2016). *Leadership excellence networks*. Retrieved from http://www.nchl.org/static.asp?path=2854

Negus, T. L., Brown, C. J., & Konoske, P. (2010). Determining medical staff requirements for humanitarian assistance missions. *Military Medicine, 175*(1), 1–6.

Newhouse, R. P., & Melnyk, B. M. (2009). Nursing's role in engineering a learning health-care system. *Journal of Nursing Administration, 39*(6), 260–262.

Nutting, P. A., Crabtree, B. F., Miller, W. L., Stewart, E. E., Stange, K. C., & Jaen, C. R. (2010). Journey to the patient-centered medical home: A qualitative analysis of the experiences of practices in the National Demonstration Project. *Annals of Family Medicine, 8 Suppl 1*, S45–S56, S92.

Oliver, G. M., Pennington, L., Revelle, S., & Rantz, M. (2014). Impact of nurse practitioners on health outcomes of Medicare and Medicaid patients. *Nursing Outlook, 62*(6), 440–447.

O'Neil, E. (2009). Four factors that guarantee health care change. *Journal of Professional Nursing, 25*(6), 317–321.

Oulton, J. A. (2006). The global nursing shortage: An overview of issues and actions. *Policy & Politics in Nursing Practice, 7*(3 Suppl.), 34S–39S.

Pearson, L. J. (2009). The Pearson report. *American Journal for Nurse Practitioners, 13*(2), 8–82.

Porter, M. E., & Lee, T. H. (2013, October). The strategy that will fix health care. *Harvard Business Review*. Retrieved from https://hbr.org/2013/10/the-strategy-that-will-fix-health-care

Rangan, V. K. (2004, March). Lofty missions, down-to-earth plans. *Harvard Business Review, 82*(3), 112–119.

Reese, C. E., Jeffries, P. R., & Engum, S. A. (2010) Learning together: Using simulations to develop nursing and medical student collaboration. *Nursing Education Perspectives, 31*(1), 33–37.

Riner, M. E., & Broome, M.E. (2014). Sustainability of international nursing programs. In M. Upvall & J. Leffers (Eds.), *Global health nursing: Building and sustaining partnerships* (pp. 285–300). New York, NY: Springer Publishing.

Robert Wood Johnson Foundation. (2014). Two nurses serving in Congress discuss nurse leadership. Retrieved from http://www.rwjf.org/en/culture-of-health/2014/05/two_nurses_servingi.html

Robert Wood Johnson Foundation. (2016). *Robert Wood Johnson executive nurse fellows program*. Retrieved from http://www.executivenursefellows.org/

Robinson, K. M., & Reinhard, S. C. (2009). Looking ahead in long-term care: The next 50 years. *Nursing Clinics of North America, 44*(2), 253–262.

Rogers, E. M. (2003). *Diffusion of innovations* (5th ed.). New York, NY: Free Press.

Rogers, J. C. (2008). The patient-centered medical home movement: Promise and peril for family medicine. *Journal of the American Board of Family Medicine, 21*(5), 370–374.

Rubinstein, H. G. (2008). Medical homes: The prescription to save primary care? *America's Health Insurance Plans Coverage, 49*(1), 44–47.

Rudavsky, R., & Mehrotra, A. (2010). Sociodemographic characteristics of communities served by retail clinics. *Journal of the American Board of Family Medicine, 23*(1), 42–48.

Scherger, J. E. (2009). Future vision: Is family medicine ready for patient-directed care? *Family Medicine, 41*(4), 285–288.

Steinbrook, R. (2009). Easing the shortage in adult primary care: Is it all about money? *New England Journal of Medicine, 360*(26), 2696–2699.

Stewart, J., Stansfeld, K., & Tapp, D. (2004). Clinical nurses' understanding of autonomy: Accomplishing patient goals through interdependent practice. *Journal of Nursing Administration, 34*(10), 443–450.

Strauss, W., & Howe, N. (1991). *Generations: The history of America's future, 1584–2069.* New York, NY: William Morrow.

Strauss, W., & Howe, N. (1997). *The fourth turning: What the cycles of history tell us about America's next rendezvous with destiny.* New York, NY: Broadway.

Thomas, M., & Hynes, C. (2009). The times they are a changin'. *Journal of Nursing Management, 17*(5), 523–531.

Thorman, K. E. (2004). Nursing leadership in the boardroom. *Journal of Obstetrical, Gynecological, & Neonatal Nursing, 33*(3), 381–387.

Titzer, J., Phillips, T., Tooley, S., Hall, N., Shirey, M. (2013). Nurse manager succession planning: Synthesis of the evidence. *Journal of Nursing Management, 21*(7), 971–979.

Walton, A., Lake, D., Mullinex, C., Allen, D., & Mooney, K. (2015). Enabling nurses to lead change: The orientation expenses of nurses to boards. *Nursing Outlook, 63*(2), 110–116.

Weston, M. J. (2008, August). Transformational leadership at a national perspective. *Nurse Leader, 6*(4), 38–40, 45.

Wharton Executive Education. (2016). *Wharton nursing leaders program.* Retrieved from http://executiveeducation.wharton.upenn.edu/for-individuals/all-programs/wharton-nursing-leaders-program

Yoder-Wise, P. S. (2007). Key forecasts shaping nursing's perfect storm. *Nursing Administration Quarterly, 31*(2), 115–119.

INDEX

46227523R00197

Made in the USA
Middletown, DE
25 July 2017